Nanostructures
in Biological Systems

Nanostructures in Biological Systems

THEORY AND APPLICATIONS

Aleš Iglič
Veronika Kralj-Iglič
Damjana Drobne

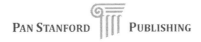

PAN STANFORD PUBLISHING

Published by

Pan Stanford Publishing Pte. Ltd.
Penthouse Level, Suntec Tower 3
8 Temasek Boulevard
Singapore 038988

Email: editorial@panstanford.com
Web: www.panstanford.com

British Library Cataloguing-in-Publication Data
A catalogue record for this book is available from the British Library.

Nanostructures in Biological Systems: Theory and Applications

Copyright © 2015 Pan Stanford Publishing Pte. Ltd.

All rights reserved. This book, or parts thereof, may not be reproduced in any form or by any means, electronic or mechanical, including photocopying, recording or any information storage and retrieval system now known or to be invented, without written permission from the publisher.

For photocopying of material in this volume, please pay a copying fee through the Copyright Clearance Center, Inc., 222 Rosewood Drive, Danvers, MA 01923, USA. In this case permission to photocopy is not required from the publisher.

ISBN 978-981-4267-20-5 (Hardcover)
ISBN 978-981-4303-43-9 (eBook)

Printed in the USA

Contents

Preface   xi

1 **Description of Systems Composed of a Large Number of Constituents**   1
    1.1 Short Survey of the Relevant Physics   1
       1.1.1 Field and Potential   1
       1.1.2 Description of Events   3
          1.1.2.1 Classical mechanics and electrodynamics   4
          1.1.2.2 Quantum mechanics   7
    1.2 Systems Composed of a Large Number of Constituents   11
       1.2.1 Classical Thermodynamics   11
       1.2.2 Statistical Thermodynamics   16
          1.2.2.1 Canonical ensemble   17
          1.2.2.2 Correspondence between statistical and classical thermodynamics   21
          1.2.2.3 System composed of independent constituents   25
          1.2.2.4 Predictability and permutability   26
          1.2.2.5 Configurational free energy and entropy of indistinguishable particles in the lattice model   28
          1.2.2.6 A simple example: equation of state of an ideal gas   30
    1.3 Thermodynamic Description of Living Systems   31
       1.3.1 Thermodynamic Potentials   32
       1.3.2 Chemical Potential   34
          1.3.2.1 Chemical potential of one-component system   35

| | | 1.3.2.2 | Chemical potential of a multicomponent system | 36 |
| | | 1.3.2.3 | Equality of chemical potential as a condition for thermodynamic equilibrium: a simple example | 38 |

2 From Lipid Bilayers to Biological Membranes — 41
- 2.1 Lipid Bilayers — 41
- 2.2 Lipid Vesicles — 41
- 2.3 Biological Membranes and their Composition — 45
- 2.4 Intracellular Membranous Structures — 48
- 2.5 Transmembrane Transport — 49
- 2.6 Cell Shape — 51
- 2.7 Differences in the Membranes of Eukaryotes and Prokaryotes — 53
- 2.8 Consequences of Membrane Damage — 55
- 2.9 Cell Membrane Repair — 58

3 Lipid Vesicles as Experimental Tools — 59
- 3.1 Types of Lipid Vesicles and Their Applications — 60
- 3.2 Vesicles as Cell Membrane Models — 61
- 3.3 Computational Modelling of Lipid Membranes — 62
- 3.4 Preparation of Lipid Vesicles to Serve as Experimental Tools — 63
- 3.5 Examples of Nanoparticle–Membrane Interactions Studies — 64
  - 3.5.1 Morphological Dynamics of Lipid Vesicles — 64
  - 3.5.2 Examples of Nanoparticle–Membrane Interactions: Studies with Artificial Lipid Membranes — 65
  - 3.5.3 Cell Membrane–Nanoparticle Interactions and Internalization — 66
- 3.6 Conclusions — 68

4 Some Experimental Techniques for Studying the Structure and Properties of Lipid Vesicles and Other Lipid Self-Assembled Structures — 71
- 4.1 Light Microscopy — 72

4.2	Atomic Force Microscopy	74
4.3	Small-Angle X-Ray Scattering	75

5 Mathematical Description of the Curvature of Biological Nanostructures — 77

6 Lipid Nanostructures — 83
- 6.1 Polymorphism of Lipid Nanostructures and Intrinsic Shapes of Lipid Molecules — 83
- 6.2 Relevance of Some Non-Lamellar Phases in Biological Systems — 88
- 6.3 Inverted Hexagonal Phase — 89
- 6.4 Phospholipid Nanotubes — 90
  - 6.4.1 Nanotubes of Giant Phospholipid Vesicles — 92
  - 6.4.2 Shape Transformation of the Vesicle with Tubular Protrusion — 97

7 Physics of Lipid Micro- and Nanostructures — 99
- 7.1 Single-Lipid Molecule Energy — 99
- 7.2 Bending Energy of the Anisotropic Lipid Monolayer — 104
- 7.3 Comparison between Planar, Inverted Spherical and Inverted Cylindrical Monolayer Nanostructures — 107
- 7.4 A Detailed Study of the Stability of the Inverted Hexagonal Phase — 112
- 7.5 Nucleation in the Lamellar (L_α) to Inverted Hexagonal (H_{II}) Phase Transition — 126
- 7.6 Bending Energy of the Anisotropic Lipid Bilayer — 135
- 7.7 Stability of Phospholipid Nanotubes Determined by the Anisotropic Properties of Lipid Molecules — 137
- 7.8 Shape Equation and Budding Transition of Phospholipid Vesicles — 146

8 Membrane Nanodomains — 155
- 8.1 Phenomenological Expression for the Energy of a Flexible Membrane Nanodomain — 156
- 8.2 Membrane Nanodomains Induced by Rigid Proteins — 161
  - 8.2.1 Perturbation of Lipid Molecules around Rigid Membrane Embedded Proteins — 161

		8.2.2 Energy of a Membrane Nanodomain Induced by a Single Rigid Membrane Protein	165
	8.3	Estimation of Model Parameters	169
		8.3.1 Basic Model	169
		8.3.2 Advanced model	171
9	**Tubular Budding of Biological Membranes**		**181**
	9.1	Bilayer Membrane with Nanodomains	182
	9.2	Accumulation of Anisotropic Nanodomains and the Stability of Tubular Membrane Protrusions	187
	9.3	Tubular Budding of the Erythrocyte Membrane	195
	9.4	Possible Limiting Shapes of Released Vesicles	200
	9.5	Theoretical Description of Self-Assembly of Anisotropic Nanodomains into Tubular Membrane Protrusions	204
10	**Spherical Budding of Biological Membranes**		**209**
11	**Fusion of Vesicles with a Target Plasma Membrane**		**219**
12	**Exogenous Membrane-Attached Nanoparticles**		**231**
	12.1	Rod-Like Attached Nanoparticles	231
	12.2	Plate-Like Attached Nanoparticles	240
13	**Electric Double Layer Theory**		**245**
	13.1	Charged Biological Systems	245
	13.2	Electrostatic Energy	249
	13.3	Entropy	250
		13.3.1 Solution of Counterions	250
		13.3.2 Solution of Counterions and Coions	253
	13.4	Functional Density Theory of Electric Double Layer for Constant Dielectric Permittivity	256
		13.4.1 Solution of Counterions Only	258
		13.4.1.1 Single double layer	258
		13.4.2 Solution of Counterions and Coions: The Bikerman Equation	261
	13.5	Gouy–Chapman Model: Poisson–Boltzmann Equation	265

13.6	Langevin Poisson-Boltzmann Model	268
13.7	Generalized Langevin–Bikerman Model	275
13.8	Differential Capacitance	285

14 Attraction between Like-Charged Surfaces — 289

- 14.1 Attraction between Like-Charged Surfaces Mediated by Spherical Macro-Ions — 289
  - 14.1.1 Counterions Only — 293
  - 14.1.2 Counterions and Coions — 309
- 14.2 Attraction between Negatively Charged Membrane Surfaces Mediated by Bound-Charged Proteins — 320
- 14.3 Attraction between a Negatively Charged Nanostructured Implant Surface and Osteoblasts — 325
  - 14.3.1 Adhesion of Proteins to a Charged Surface — 328
  - 14.3.2 Electric Field Strength at Highly Curved Edges of the Implant Surface — 332
  - 14.3.3 Clustering of Integrin Molecules in Nanorough Surface Regions with Highly Curved Edges — 335

15 Encapsulation of Charged Nanoparticles (Macro-Ions) — 341

16 Electrostatics and Mechanics of Hydrophilic Pores — 347

17 Membranous Nanostructures as *in vivo* Cell-to-Cell Transport Mechanisms — 371

18 Biological Impact of Membranous Nanostructures — 385

- 18.1 Nanovesiculation and Nanovesicles — 390
  - 18.1.1 Nanovesicles Isolated from Blood — 392
  - 18.1.2 Nanovesicles Isolated from other Body Fluids — 397
- 18.2 Isolated Nanovesicles: Clinically Relevant Artefacts — 404
  - 18.2.1 The Effect of Temperature on Isolates from Blood — 406
  - 18.2.2 Origin of Micro- and Nanovesicles in Blood Isolates — 411

18.3	Post-Prandial Increase in Concentration of Nanovesicles in Isolates from Blood	417
18.4	Mediated Interaction between Membranes	421
18.5	Mediated Interaction between Membranes as a Vesiculation-Suppression Mechanism	427
18.6	The Role of the Stability of Narrow Necks in Suppression of Membrane Vesiculation	436
18.7	Clinical Validation of the Hypothesis of Nanovesiculation Suppression	444
18.8	Concentration of Nanovesicles in Isolates from Blood of Patients with Gastrointestinal Diseases	446
18.9	Perspectives in the Biophysics of Membranous Nanostructures	448

Bibliography   449
Index   507

Preface

This book offers a survey of the theoretical description of and experimental evidence for micro- and nanostructures in biological systems. The book is novel in the sense that biophysical methods are used to describe and manipulate clinically relevant problems which have hitherto been largely described as purely biochemical phenomena.

In the theoretical description, a unifying approach is used starting from the single-particle energy, deriving the free energy of the system and finally determining the equilibrium state by minimizing the system free energy. This approach is basic, transparent and simple so that different systems and interactions can be considered. The method is then applied in describing different electric and elastic phenomena in biological and lipid nanostructures.

Orientational ordering of anisotropic system constituents is found to be an essential mechanism of stabilization of the system configuration in ionic solutions and biological membrane structures. Further, in models based on lattice statistics, a method considering the Boltzmann probability of energy averaged over rotational states is introduced as an improvement over the free energy minimization method.

Experimental evidence for theoretically predicted membranous nanostructures and mediated attractive interactions between these structures is presented. Possible applications in medicine, toxicology and nanotechnology are given, such as the use of the results and methods in the clinically relevant problem of blood clot formation or the fabrication of nanostructured biocompatible implant surfaces.

The book consists of eighteen chapters devoted to the biophysics and biology of biological micro- and nanostructures. Chapter 1 gives a brief review of the basic statistical thermodynamic principles and equations which are then used throughout the book in theoretical description of biological micro- and nanostructures, which are composed of a large number of constituents. The chapter starts with a short survey of the physics involved where some basic definitions of the physical quantities relevant in theoretical consideration of biological systems, like field and potential, are also given. Chapter 2 briefly describes the basic properties of lipid bilayers and biological membranes. Chapter 3 describes lipid vesicles as experimental tools. Different types of lipid vesicles can be used and their preparation and the interpretation of the results is presented. Among the most recent applications of lipid vesicles in scientific studies is their use in the field of nanobiology and nanotoxicology where interactions between nanoparticles and biological systems are investigated. Understanding nanoparticle-induced defects in biological membranes is among the major challenges of bio-nano-related fields of research. In Chapter 4 some basic microscopic techniques for studying the structure and properties of vesicles ranging from direct visualisation (optical or electron microscopy) or scattering techniques (light scattering, LS; small-angle neutron scattering, SANS; small-angle X-ray scattering, SAXS) to polarisation light microscopy; freeze fracture transmission electron microscopy, FF-TEM; and atomic force microscopy. The selection of methods depends on the aim of the study. These methods give information about the morphological features of vesicles and the structural characteristics of lipid bilayers.

In the continuum approach, biological surfaces (e.g., membrane surfaces) may be in the first approximation considered as smooth surfaces that can be theoretically described using the mathematical theory of differential geometry, as shown very briefly in Chapter 5 of the book. Further Chapter 6 describes the polymorphism of lipid nanostructures, including lipid nanotubes, and introduces the concept of anisotropic intrinsic shapes of lipid molecules. Chapter 7 is dedicated to the physics of lipid micro- and nano structures, starting with the concept of the single-lipid molecule energy. Applying the methods of statistical physics, the free energy of a lipid monolayer and bilayer is derived, taking into account the anisotropic shape of lipid molecules. The lipid monolayer and bilayer deviatoric bending energy due to average orientational ordering of lipid molecules is discussed. The influence of lipid anisotropy on the stability of planar, inverted spherical and inverted cylindrical lipid monolayer nanostructures and lipid bilayer nanotubes is presented in detail. At the end of the chapter the shape equation for closed lipid bilayer vesicles is derived and solved in order to describe theoretically the experimentally observed budding transitions of phospholipid vesicles. Chapter 8 gives a derivation of the energy of a single flexible membrane nanodomain. Flexible membrane nanodomains are defined as small complexes composed of proteins and lipids. The so-called membrane raft elements of biological membranes may fall into this category. Membrane nanodomains (inclusions) may also be induced by a single rigid globular membrane protein. Some membrane embedded peptides may induce such nanodomains.

Formation of tubular membrane bilayer structures (nanotubes) is a common phenomenon in both artificial lipid membranes and cellular systems. In Chapter 9 the formation and stability of tubular membrane structures is considered experimentally and theoretically. In Chapter 10 the physical mechanisms of the formation and stabilization of highly curved spherical membrane buds are experimentally and theoretically considered, with special emphasis on the stability of the narrow neck connecting the budding vesicle to the parent membrane. Chapter 11 is dedicated to fusion of a vesicle with the target plasma membrane. Experimental results, along with a theoretical model, are presented to provide a new interpretation of repetitive, transient fusion neck events with narrow neck diameters stabilized by anisotropic membrane components. As the suggested fusion neck stabilization mechanism is nonspecific and as there is no a priori reason why the membrane constituents should be in general isotropic, it could be expected to take place in any cell type. In Chapter 12 we discuss the influence of the intrinsic shape of membrane-attached nanoparticles on the elastic properties of bilayer membranes.

Chapter 13 is devoted to the electrostatic properties of biological systems. It starts with the definition of electrostatic energy and derivation of the configurational entropic part of the free energy of a system composed of finite-sized ions. Then a functional density theory of the electric double layer (EDL) which assumes constant dielectric permittivity is used to derive the standard Poisson–

Boltzmann (PB) equation and the modified PB, i.e., the Bikerman equation. Most models describing the EDL assume constant dielectric permittivity throughout the system. But actually, close to the charged surface, the water dipoles are oriented thus leading to a varying dielectric permittivity. Therefore in this chapter we derive the Langevin Poisson–Boltzmann (LPB) equation for point-like ions, where the orientational ordering of water molecules is taken into account. In order to develop an integrating framework to clarify the factors influencing the relative permittivity, the LPB model within the generalized Langevin–Bikerman model is upgraded to take into account the cavity field as well as the finite size of the molecules.

Subsequently, in Chapter 14 the attraction between like-charged biological surfaces, mediated by spherical macroions are described theoretically and illustrated by different examples observed experimentally, such as the attraction between a negatively charged nanostructured surface and osteoblasts. Chapter 15 briefly describes simulations of the encapsulation of spherical macroions, while in Chapter 16 the electrostatics and mechanics of hydrophilic pores in biological membranes is given. Chapter 17 is dedicated to the role of membranous nanostructures as in cell-to-cell transport mechanisms, where the recently discovered nanotube-mediated mechanism of cell-to-cell communication is described. Chapter 18 presents the liquid crystal mosaic model of the biological membrane as a result of the above generalizations. A pool of membranous nanstructures is biologically important; some clinically relevant mechanisms involving this pool are presented and possible manipulation of these mechanisms in medicine is suggested.

The authors would like to express their gratitude to their colleagues and students, among them especially Aleš Ambrožič, Blaž Babnik, Sebastian Bauer, Apolonija Bedina Zavec, Klemen Bohinc, Goran Bobojevič, Nataliya Bobrovska, Malgorzata Bobrowska-Hägerstrand, Sabina Boljte, Angela Corcelli, Saša Čučnik, Matej Daniel, Gregor Dolinar, Barbara Drašler, Kristina Eleršič, Ana Fortič, Miha Fošnarič, Jan Gimsa, Ulrike Gimsa, Nir Gov, Roman Jerala, Wojciech Góźdź, Volkmar Heinrich, Ines Hribar-Ignaščenko, Roghayeh Imani, Boris Isomaa, Vid Janša, Dalija Jesenek, Jernej Jorgačevski, Ita Junkar, Doron Kabaso, Maša Kandušer, Samo Kralj, Marko Kreft, Mukta Kulkarni, Sunil P.B. Kumar, Maruša Lokar, Mateja

Manček-Keber, Sylvio May, Luczyna Mrówczynska, Sara Novak, Eva Ogorevc, Nataš Poklar Ulrih, Meysam Pazoki, Ulrich Salzer, Patrik Schmuki, Gerhard Schütz, Petra Sušanj, Nejc Tomšič, Ania Wrobel, Jasna Urbanija Zelko, Robert Zorec and Jernej Zupanc. The work presented here is benefitted from their research, writings, conversations, support, and advice over the past years.

We would like to to express our deep gratitude to Ekaterina Gongadze for her support and collaboration in preparation of the electrostatic parts of the book. We highly value the help of Šárka Perutková in preparation of the parts of the book describing the physics of lipid nanostructures and the attraction between like-charged surfaces. Many thanks to Blaž Rozman, Rado Janša and Anita Mrvar-Brečko for pioneering work in clinical biophysics and to Mojca Frank, Vid Šuštar and Roman Štukelj for the many hours spent mastering the method of harvesting membrane nanovesicles from body fluids. We also very much appreciate the continuous support and collaboration of Peter Veranič and Tomaž Slivnik. Special thanks go to Henry Hägerstrand and Michael Rappolt with whom we worked together and had many influential debates over the last years. We also thank Anthony Byrne for linguistic editing of the English and Tatjana Strahija and Jernej Zupanc for technical support with the manuscript.

This work is devoted to our loved ones who define its meaning and provide us with the ultimate dedication.

Aleš Iglič
Veronika Kralj-Iglič
Damjana Drobne
Summer 2015

Chapter 1

Description of Systems Composed of a Large Number of Constituents

1.1 Short Survey of the Relevant Physics

1.1.1 Field and Potential

A scalar field associates a numerical (scalar) value called magnitude to every point of the system (space), while a vector field is a quantity to which at every point of the system, a magnitude and direction are assigned. Examples of scalar fields are temperature, concentration, pressure, and density; examples of vector fields are force and velocity.

A scalar field q may be a source of a vector field $\mathbf{P}$:

$$\nabla \cdot \mathbf{P} = q, \tag{1.1}$$

where nabla (∇) is an operator which in Cartesian coordinates (x, y, z), is written as

$$\nabla = \left(\frac{\partial}{\partial x}, \frac{\partial}{\partial y}, \frac{\partial}{\partial z} \right). \tag{1.2}$$

If we act with the operator ∇ on a field, we are describing changes of this field in space. Symbols $\partial/\partial x$, $\partial/\partial y$ and $\partial/\partial z$ denote partial derivatives with respect to a chosen Cartesian coordinate.

Nanostructures in Biological Systems: Theory and Applications
Aleš Iglič, Veronika Kralj-Iglič, and Damjana Drobne
Copyright © 2015 Pan Stanford Publishing Pte. Ltd.
ISBN 978-981-4267-20-5 (Hardcover), 978-981-4303-43-9 (eBook)
www.panstanford.com

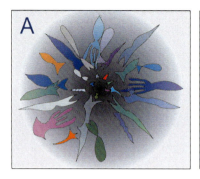 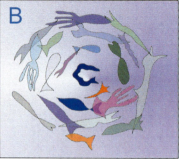

Figure 1.1 Schematic figure of a source of a vector field (a) and a vortex of the vector field (b).

The quantity $\nabla \cdot \mathbf{P}$ is called the divergence of the vector field $\mathbf{P}$, which expresses to what extent an infinitesimal region of space acts as a source or a sink of the vector field. If the divergence of the vector field at some point in space is nonzero, then there is a source of this field (for $q > 0$) or a sink of the field (for $q < 0$).

The vector product of the operator ∇ and the vector field $\mathbf{P}$, which is called a rotor (or curl) of the field ($\nabla \times \mathbf{P}$), describes a vortex of the field. The source and the vortex of the field are schematically represented in Figs. 1.1A and 1.1B, while Fig. 1.2 shows a vector field without sources, sinks and vortices.

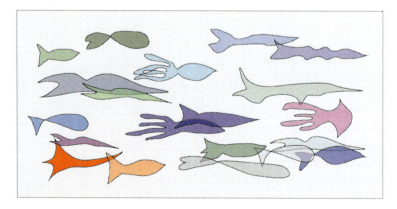

Figure 1.2 Schematic figure of a vector field without sources, sinks and vortices.

If the vector field **P** lacks vortices,

$$\nabla \times \mathbf{P} = 0, \tag{1.3}$$

there exists a scalar function ϕ named scalar potential such that

$$\mathbf{P} = \pm \nabla \phi. \tag{1.4}$$

The expression $\nabla \phi = (\partial \phi/\partial x, \partial \phi/\partial y, \partial \phi/\partial z)$ is called the gradient of the potential. The gradient of the potential is a vector which tells us how the potential (and thus the field) changes in space. The sign is chosen according to the interpretation of the effect of the field.

If there are no static sources or sinks of the vector field, that is, its divergence is equal to 0,

$$\nabla \cdot \mathbf{P} = 0, \tag{1.5}$$

there exists a vector **A** named vector potential such that

$$\mathbf{P} = \nabla \times \mathbf{A}. \tag{1.6}$$

An advantage of introducing potentials is the use of standard mathematical tools and simplification of equations.

1.1.2 Description of Events

Within the framework of a physical description, the same physical laws are valid throughout the entire universe on small- and large scales at low- and high energies. It turns out that under different conditions some effects can prevail so that others can be neglected: we use simplifications and approximations.

In classical mechanics, we introduce a point-like particle to which we ascribe at a given time t, a precisely determined position given by position vector **r** from the origin of the coordinate system to the particular point **r** (Fig. 1.3) and velocity **v**, which is small with respect to the speed of light $c = 3 \cdot 10^8$ m/s. Space is three dimensional, flat and independent of time, while matter and radiation are considered as separate quantities. The laws of classical mechanics are used in description of macroscopic systems.

The microscopic world is described by the laws of quantum mechanics. Within quantum mechanics, we use a dual description: matter and radiation can be described both as particles or as

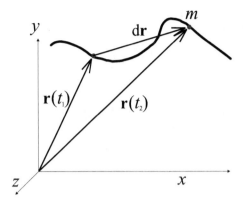

Figure 1.3 Within classical mechanics the motion of a point-like particle with mass m in three dimensional space (x, y, z) is described by time-dependent (t) radius (position) vector $\mathbf{r}(t)$. Here $t_1 < t_2$.

waves. Within quantum mechanics, a system can attain only discrete energies. We say that energy is quantized.

At large velocities, we use the special theory of relativity in which space and time are connected into a four-dimensional vector space-time. An event is given by the four component vector,

$$\mathbf{r} = (x,\ y,\ z,\ c\,t). \tag{1.7}$$

Within classical mechanics and the special theory of relativity, space-time is flat (Fig. 1.4A). The general theory of relativity considers that the presence of mass causes curving of space-time. Greater mass causes stronger curving while the effect is stronger closer to the mass. Figure 1.4B schematically shows curving of two-dimensional space due to the presence of mass.

The string theory is a modern physical theory which connects quantum mechanics and the theory of relativity. The world is described as composed of small strings which oscillate in different ways and thereby, form different constituents of the system.

1.1.2.1 Classical mechanics and electrodynamics

Physical description within classical physics is based on description of the properties of a point-like body, that is, a body with no dimensions. This is a useful approximation for the elements of a

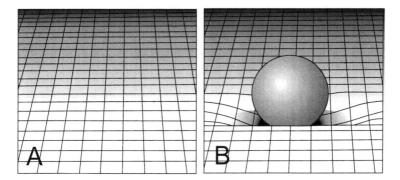

Figure 1.4 A two-dimensional representation of flat space (A). Due to the presence of mass (a sphere), space is curved (B).

system for which the size, shape, and structure are irrelevant in the context considered. The relevant properties of a point-like body are its mass m and electric charge e.

In classical mechanics, the motion of a point-like body is described by a position vector $\mathbf{r}$, velocity $\mathbf{v}$, force $\mathbf{F}$ acting on the point-like body with mass m, momentum $\mathbf{p} = m\mathbf{v}$, angular momentum $\mathbf{\Gamma} = m\mathbf{v} \times \mathbf{r}$, and energy W, which is divided into kinetic energy W_k and potential energy W_p. The kinetic energy of a point-like body with mass m moving with velocity $\mathbf{v}$ is

$$W_k = \frac{1}{2}mv^2, \tag{1.8}$$

where v is the magnitude of the vector $\mathbf{v}$. Kinetic energy is also the stock of work which the body can perform due to its motion, while potential energy is the stock of work which the body can perform due to its position, or due to the mutual positions of its constituents.

Movement of a point-like body with mass m within classical mechanics is described by the three laws of Newton.[a] Newton's first law states that if no net force is acting on a point-like body, the body is at rest or moves with an uniform velocity which defines the inertial frame. The second law gives the relation between the net force acting on the point-like body $\mathbf{F}$ and its momentum $\mathbf{p}$,

$$\mathbf{F} = \frac{d\mathbf{p}}{dt}. \tag{1.9}$$

---

[a] Isaac Newton, 1642–1727.

Newton's third law for two point-like bodies expresses the connection between action and reaction: if body 2 acts on body 1 with force $\mathbf{F}_{1,2}$, then body 1 acts on body 2 with an oppositely directed force of the same magnitude $\mathbf{F}_{2,1}$,

$$\mathbf{F}_{1,2} + \mathbf{F}_{2,1} = 0. \tag{1.10}$$

If the point-like body with mass, m carries an electric charge, e, the force in the electromagnetic field acting on the body is

$$\mathbf{F} = e\left(\mathbf{E} + \mathbf{v} \times \mathbf{B}\right), \tag{1.11}$$

where $\mathbf{E}$ is the electric field strength and $\mathbf{B}$ is the magnetic flux density. The connection between the electric and the magnetic field is given by Maxwell[a] equations. The equation

$$\nabla \cdot \mathbf{D} = \rho_{el}, \tag{1.12}$$

where $\mathbf{D}$ is the electric displacement vector, expresses the fact that charges create an electric field; remember that the divergence of the field describes sources and sinks of the field. The quantity $\rho_{el} = \lim_{\Delta V \to 0} (\Delta e / \Delta V)$ is the volume density of charge where Δe is the charge which is present in a small volume ΔV.

It follows from the equation

$$\nabla \times \mathbf{H} = \mathbf{j}_{el} + \frac{\partial \mathbf{D}}{\partial t}, \tag{1.13}$$

that the magnetic field may be created by electric currents (movement of charges) or an electric field which changes with time. Here, $\mathbf{H}$ is the magnetic field strength and $\mathbf{j}_{el}$, the density of the electric current given by

$$\mathbf{j}_{el} = \frac{dI}{dS}\mathbf{n}, \tag{1.14}$$

where dS is the cross-sectional area carrying an infinitesimal electric current dI and $\mathbf{n}$ is unit vector in the direction of the current.

The equation

$$\nabla \cdot \mathbf{B} = 0, \tag{1.15}$$

where $\mathbf{B}$ is the magnetic flux density, expresses the fact that there are no monopole sources or sinks of the magnetic field. This statement

---

[a] James Clerk Maxwell, 1831–1879.

is based on the experimental fact that isolated magnetic monopoles have never been found.

The equation

$$\nabla \times \mathbf{E} = -\frac{\partial \mathbf{B}}{\partial t}, \qquad (1.16)$$

expresses that in a region with a time-dependent magnetic field an electric field is created.

In free space, $\mathbf{B} = \mu_0 \mathbf{H}$ and $\mathbf{D} = \varepsilon_0 \mathbf{E}$, where, $\mu_0 = 4\pi \cdot 10^{-7}$ Vs/Am is the permeability of free space and $\varepsilon_0 = 8.9 \cdot 10^{-12}$ As/Vm is the permittivity of free space.

Since a magnetic field has no monopole sources or sinks (Eq. 1.15), according to the conditions Eq. 1.5 and Eq. 1.6, we introduce a vector potential $\mathbf{A}$,

$$\mathbf{B} = \nabla \times \mathbf{A}, \qquad (1.17)$$

such that Eq. 1.16 becomes

$$\nabla \times \left(\mathbf{E} + \frac{\partial \mathbf{A}}{\partial t} \right) = 0. \qquad (1.18)$$

The expression in parentheses is a field with no vortices, so we can introduce a scalar potential ϕ as follows:

$$\mathbf{E} + \frac{\partial \mathbf{A}}{\partial t} = -\nabla \phi. \qquad (1.19)$$

From the Maxwell equations follows the wave equations for $\mathbf{E}$ and $\mathbf{B}$—from which it is evident that electromagnetic waves exist and spread in directions perpendicular to the electric field and to the magnetic field, with a constant velocity—the velocity of light c, so that $c = 1/\sqrt{\varepsilon_0 \mu_0}$.

The laws of classical electrodynamics are supplemented by the continuity equation expressing the conservation of charge within a given volume

$$\frac{\partial \rho_{el}}{\partial t} + \nabla \cdot \mathbf{j}_{el} = 0. \qquad (1.20)$$

1.1.2.2 Quantum mechanics

The description of a particle by position, velocity, and energy within classical mechanics is based on simple experiments involving

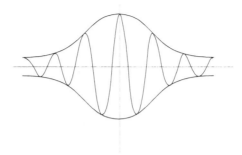

Figure 1.5 A wave packet.

macroscopic bodies from everyday experience. Since microscopic particles (e.g., electrons) in some respects behave similar to macroscopic particles (bodies), attempts have been made to use such a description for microscopic particles as well. However, the similarity between macroscopic and microscopic particles is limited, which is reflected in the fact that the validity of the classical mechanical description of microscopic particles is also limited. It turns out that for microscopic particles the position and velocity can simultaneously be determined only within certain limits given by the Heisenberg[a] uncertainty principle. For a particle moving in the direction of the x-axis with velocity v_x (momentum mv_x), the uncertainty principle gives

$$\Delta x \Delta p_x \geq h, \qquad (1.21)$$

where, Δx is the uncertainty in the particle's position, Δp_x is the uncertainty in the component of momentum and $h = 6.6 \cdot 10^{-34}$ Js is Planck[b] constant, which is characteristic of quantum mechanics.

Since the laws of classical mechanics could not satisfactorily describe the results of some experiments (e.g., interference experiments with electrons, the photo-effect and the characteristic peaks in the spectra of X-rays), a theory has been developed in which two important new concepts were introduced—quantization of energy and the dual nature of the particle-wave. Two equivalent formulations of quantum mechanics were developed almost simultaneously:

---

[a] Werner Heisenberg, 1901–1976.
[b] Max Planck, 1858–1947.

the matrix formulation (Heisenberg, Born,[a] Jordan[b]) and the wave formulation (Schrödinger[c]). Here, we shortly describe some of the basics of the Schrödinger formulation of quantum mechanics, necessary for understanding the principles of statistical mechanics which are used in this book.

To describe material particles within quantum mechanics, we introduce the wave function $\Psi(\mathbf{r}, t)$, so that the probability of a particle existing in the region with infinitesimal volume dV is

$$P(\mathbf{r}, t)\, dV = |\Psi(\mathbf{r}, t)|^2\, dV \qquad (1.22)$$

The quantity $P(\mathbf{r}, t)$ is called the probability density and is an observable quantity.

In quantum mechanics, we use the principle of correspondence, which means that the variables which are used in classical mechanics, the position vector $\mathbf{r}$, momentum $\mathbf{p}$, angular momentum $\mathbf{\Gamma}$, kinetic energy W_k, potential energy W_p, and total energy which is described by the Hamilton[d] function $\mathcal{H}$ (Hamiltonian), are assigned the corresponding operators. The momentum corresponds to the operator $(\hbar/i)\nabla$, kinetic energy corresponds to the operator $-(\hbar^2/2m)\nabla^2$, total energy corresponds to the operator $i\hbar\,\partial/\partial t$, where $\hbar = h/2\pi$. The operators, corresponding to the energy which is used in classical mechanics (sum of the kinetic and potential energies),

$$W_k + W_p(\mathbf{r}) = \mathcal{H}, \qquad (1.23)$$

are applied to the wave function. The equation is rearranged to obtain the Schrödinger equation; that is, the differential equation for the wave function Ψ,

$$-\frac{\hbar^2}{2m}\nabla^2 \Psi(\mathbf{r}) + W_p(\mathbf{r})\Psi(\mathbf{r}) = i\hbar\frac{\partial \Psi(\mathbf{r})}{\partial t}. \qquad (1.24)$$

In the case where the potential energy is independent of time, the solution of Eq. 1.24 can be written as the product of two functions, one of which depends solely on position, while the other on time:

$$\Psi(\mathbf{r}, t) = \psi(\mathbf{r})\exp\left(-\frac{iEt}{\hbar}\right), \qquad (1.25)$$

---

[a] Max Born, 1882–1970.
[b] Pascual Jordan, 1902–1980.
[c] Erwin Schrödinger, 1887–1961.
[d] William Rowan Hamilton, 1805–1865.

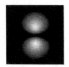 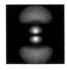

Figure 1.6 Schematic figure of the probability density of an electron in the hydrogen atom. Different probability densities correspond to different eigenstates. Lighter areas mean larger probability densities (image: http://blazelabs.com).

where $\psi(\mathbf{r})$ is the solution of the time-independent Schrödinger equation

$$-\frac{\hbar^2}{2m}\nabla^2\psi(\mathbf{r}) + W_\mathrm{p}(\mathbf{r})\psi(\mathbf{r}) = E\psi(\mathbf{r}). \tag{1.26}$$

The time-independent Schrödinger equation describes the problem of eigenvalues since the operation yields the wave function as a solution. Equation 1.26 can be written by the operator of the total energy $\hat{\mathcal{H}}$,

$$\hat{\mathcal{H}}\psi(\mathbf{r}) = E\psi, \tag{1.27}$$

where

$$\hat{\mathcal{H}} = -\frac{\hbar^2}{2m}\nabla^2 + W_\mathrm{p}(\mathbf{r}). \tag{1.28}$$

Solutions of Eq. 1.27 are eigenfunctions $\psi(\mathrm{r})$, which correspond to particular energies E with discrete values. We call them the eigenenergies of the system. Different eigenfunctions in the atom correspond to different probability densities (Fig. 1.6) and different eigenenergies. We say that the energy of the particles is quantized. Photon emission or absorption can be observed by spectroscopy, in which the spectral wavelengths are a direct measure of the discrete energies of the particle, that is, the differences between them.

An orbital is the region within which the particle exists with high (>95 %) probability. Orbitals determine the shape of more or less stable complexes which are formed from atoms. These complexes are called molecules.

In the description of biological systems composed of a large number of microscopic particles, the methods of statistical physics are used which are based on the energies of particles obtained within a quantum mechanical approach. Therefore in the theoretical description of biological systems, the application of the methods of quantum mechanics cannot be avoided.

1.2 Systems Composed of a Large Number of Constituents

Our everyday experience concerns systems composed of a very large number of constituents (order of magnitude 10^{20} or more). To describe such a system by means of classical mechanics, we would have to write down Newton's laws of motion for every individual constituent. Due to the large number of constituents, this is practically impossible.

If we are describing the macroscopically observable properties of systems containing large numbers of particles by a small set of relevant variables, we say that we are describing the system within *classical thermodynamics*. In order to study the physical properties of the *thermodynamic system*, we should first define the system and the surroundings and describe the relations between their elements. Within classical thermodynamics, it is important that we deduce the facts and the properties which enable us to predict the future behaviour of the system. The properties of the system are given by thermodynamic variables and functions of state of the system, while the facts are expressed by the laws which connect these variables and functions of state. Thermodynamic variables include, for example, temperature, volume, and concentration, while functions of state include, for example, internal energy, enthalpy, entropy, and free energy. The contents of the laws of classical thermodynamics refer to transformations of energy and determination of the equilibrium state of the system. A deeper understanding of the underlying reasons is not possible in such a description. If we want to achieve a deeper understanding, we should consider the features of a system on the microscopic level.

1.2.1 *Classical Thermodynamics*

We first describe some special functions which are used within classical thermodynamics. A system is an entity separated from its surroundings, where everything that is not the system is defined as the surroundings of the system. The state of the system is defined by the set of all the macroscopic properties connected with the system. The equilibrium state of the system is the state in which there are no changes of macroscopic properties with time. The system and the surroundings are separated by a boundary which can isolate the system from the surroundings, or it can allow the exchange of energy and matter between them. If matter can migrate between the system and the surroundings, the system is considered to be open, while it is considered to be closed if such transport is not allowed.

In describing the system within the laws of classical thermodynamics, we are interested in the energy which is connected to the inner state of matter. This energy is called the internal energy W_n. Within quantum mechanics, we say that the internal energy derives from the eigenenergies of the system, while within classical mechanics the internal energy derives from the potential and kinetic energy of the system constituents.

Energy is transported across the boundaries of the system by means of work A and heat Q. Heat is connected to the change of the internal energy of the system due to the temperature difference between the system and the surroundings. Work is connected to the change in the internal energy of the system due to other thermodynamic variables.

The change in the internal energy of the system due to transport of energy across its boundaries is expressed by the first law of thermodynamics:

$$\mathrm{d}W_n = \mathrm{d}A + \mathrm{d}Q, \qquad (1.29)$$

where $\mathrm{d}A$ is a small amount of work which was performed upon the system ($\mathrm{d}A > 0$) or by the system ($\mathrm{d}A < 0$), and $\mathrm{d}Q$ is a small amount of heat which was transported from the surroundings ($\mathrm{d}Q > 0$) or to the surroundings ($\mathrm{d}Q < 0$). The internal energy is changed by $\mathrm{d}W_n$. The first law of thermodynamics also expresses the fact that the total energy of the system and the surroundings is conserved and it is therefore, a conservation law. Further, in the case of an isolated system which performs or receives no work, the internal energy of the system is conserved.

Mechanical work is expressed as

$$\mathrm{d}A = \mathbf{F} \cdot \mathrm{d}\mathbf{r}, \qquad (1.30)$$

where $\mathbf{F}$ is the force and $\mathrm{d}\mathbf{r}$ is the displacement vector (Fig. 1.3). The work which is a consequence of the change of the volume of the system ($\mathrm{d}V$) is given by,

$$\mathrm{d}A = -p\,\mathrm{d}V, \qquad (1.31)$$

where p is the pressure within the system. The volume of the system is diminished if it is squeezed. We say that if the system undergoes a decrease in the volume ($dV < 0$), it accepts work. We can take the standpoint that the work received by the system is positive ($dA > 0$). Work is negative if the system expands ($dA < 0$, if $dV > 0$). We say that, in this case the system performs work. According to such a choice of interpretation, we chose in Eq. 1.31 above a minus sign.

If two thermodynamic systems are connected so that energy can cross the boundary, we say that the systems are in *thermodynamic equilibrium* if there is no transfer of energy across the boundary. We also say that such systems have the same temperature. Once transferred to the system and becoming the internal energy, work and heat cannot be distinguished by the first law of thermodynamics.

Namely, the *internal energy* can be understood as composed of the potential and kinetic energies of its constituents. Nevertheless, work differs from heat. Experience indicates that all work can be transformed into heat, while it is not possible to transform all heat to work without changing the state of the surroundings. Among the processes which are allowed by the first law of thermodynamics, only some of them will actually take place. If two bodies with different temperatures are brought into contact, heat is transferred from the body with higher temperature to the body with lower temperature. Salt dissociates in water, but the reverse process is possible only if the system is acted upon from the outside. The displacement in the oscillations of a pendulum become smaller with time while the mechanical energy of the oscillations is transformed into heat. The above processes are spontaneous and proceed in a definite direction, while the probability of their proceeding in the opposite direction is very small. Such processes are called irreversible processes.

A process is irreversible if the system and the surroundings cannot be returned to the original state. All real processes are irreversible.

A reversible process is an idealization; the process can take place in the reverse direction by passing through the same sequence of equilibrium states. In reversible processes the system and the surroundings can be returned to the original state.

Processes which are so slow that they can be reversed at any time by performing an infinitesimal change in the surroundings can be considered as reversible. The infinitesimal change moves the system from one equilibrium state of the system to another one.

A function called entropy S in introduced and is the subject of the second law of thermodynamics,

$$dS \geq \frac{dQ}{T}. \tag{1.32}$$

The equality in Eq. 1.32 holds for reversible processes, while the inequality holds for irreversible processes. The origin of entropy is

$$S(T = 0) = k \ln \Omega(E_0), \tag{1.33}$$

where $\Omega(E_0)$ is the degeneration of the lowest energy state with energy E_0 expressing how many states of the system correspond to the lowest energy. The origin of entropy is the subject to the third law of thermodynamics: the entropy of a system with a non-degenerate ground state at $T = 0$ is equal to 0.

While seeking for the equilibrium state of a system it is convenient to know some function which describes the system at the given conditions and at equilibrium attains an extreme value. Functions which in the equilibrium state attain an extreme value are called thermodynamic potentials.

Entropy S is a thermodynamic potential of an isolated system. This means that in the equilibrium state of the isolated system entropy attains its maximum. If the system is thermally isolated ($dQ = 0$), it follows from the second law of thermodynamics (Eq. 1.32) that

$$dS \geq 0. \tag{1.34}$$

The entropy of an isolated system increases until the system reaches the equilibrium state where the entropy attains its maximal value.

Therefore, in a reversible process, the change of the entropy of the system is equal to the negative change of entropy of the surroundings, while the total entropy of the system and the surroundings remains unchanged. In an irreversible process, entropy determines the direction of the development of the system. Entropy plays an important role whenever certain processes are not allowed.

In the description of a system which is not thermally isolated, but is kept at constant temperature and at constant volume, an appropriate thermodynamic potential is the free energy F, where

$$F = W_n - T S. \tag{1.35}$$

The infinitesimal change in the free energy is

$$dF = dW_n - T\, dS - S\, dT. \tag{1.36}$$

Considering Eqs. 1.29, 1.32, and 1.36 yields

$$dF \leq dA - S\, dT. \tag{1.37}$$

In this expression equality corresponds to reversible changes.

Let us limit our description to changes in which the work exchanged between the system and the surroundings originates solely from the change of volume of the system,

$$dA = -p\, dV. \tag{1.38}$$

In this case, it follows from Eqs. 1.29 and 1.32 that

$$dW_n \leq -p\, dV + T\, dS, \tag{1.39}$$

while it follows from Eqs. 1.37 and 1.39 that

$$dF \leq -p\, dV - S\, dT. \tag{1.40}$$

If the temperature and the volume are kept constant ($dT = 0$, $dV = 0$), it follows that

$$dF \leq 0. \tag{1.41}$$

At constant temperature and volume, the free energy of the system decreases until the system reaches the equilibrium state. There, the free energy attains its extreme (minimal) value. It can be seen that the free energy is an appropriate thermodynamic potential for systems at constant temperature and volume.

In describing a system which is not thermally isolated, but is kept at constant temperature and pressure, we introduce a function of state called enthalpy, H, where

$$H = W_n + p V. \tag{1.42}$$

The thermodynamic potential, which is appropriate for description of a system at constant temperature and constant pressure, is the free enthalpy G,

$$G = H - T S = W_n + p V - T S. \tag{1.43}$$

Limiting ourselves to systems in which the only type of work exchanged with the surroundings is work due to the change of volume, the infinitesimal change in the free enthalpy is

$$dG = -p\,dV + dQ + p\,dV + V\,dp - T\,dS - S\,dT. \quad (1.44)$$

Considering Eq. 1.32 gives

$$dG \leq V\,dp - S\,dT. \quad (1.45)$$

In this expression equality corresponds to reversible changes. If the change is performed at constant temperature and constant pressure ($dT = 0$ and $dp = 0$), Eq. 1.45 gives

$$dG \leq 0. \quad (1.46)$$

At constant temperature and pressure, the free enthalpy of the system decreases until the system reaches the equilibrium state. There, the free enthalpy attains its extreme (minimal) value. It can be seen that the free enthalpy is an appropriate thermodynamic potential for systems at constant temperature and volume.

1.2.2 Statistical Thermodynamics

Consider a representative system with a large number of constituents (N) and volume V. The system is in contact with a heat reservoir with temperature T. Imagine a set of a large number $\mathcal{M}$ of systems, which are macroscopically equal to the system under consideration, that is, each of the systems has the same values of the thermodynamic variables (N, V, T) and is in contact with the same heat reservoir as the representative system. This imaginary set of systems is called an ensemble.[a] Although all the systems are equal from a macroscopic point of view, they are not necessarily equal from a microscopic point of view. In general, there are a large number of different quantum states which correspond to a given macroscopic state, since three variables, say N, V, and T are insufficient for a detailed microscopic description of a system with 10^{20} constituents. By the expression "quantum states", we mean the eigenstates determined by solutions of the stationary Schrödinger

---

[a] John Willard Gibbs, 1839–1903.

equation with corresponding energy eigenvalues. We now state the two postulates of statistical thermodynamics (Hill, 1986).

The first postulate states that the long-term time average of a mechanical variable X in a given thermodynamic system—representative of the ensemble of $\mathcal{M}$ systems—is in the limit of $\mathcal{M} \to \infty$ equal to the ensemble average of X.

In other words, the average of a mechanical variable of a given system over time can be replaced by the average of the instantaneous values of this variable over a large number of systems which are macroscopically equal to the given system.

The ensemble which describes an isolated system (fixed energy of the system) is called the microcanonical ensemble, the ensemble which describes a closed system (fixed number of particles) at constant temperature is called the canonical ensemble and the ensemble which describes an open system at a constant temperature is called the grand canonical ensemble. The first postulate is valid for all three types of ensembles.

The second postulate (the principle of equal *a priori* probabilities) is valid only for the microcanonical ensemble. The second postulate states that in a microcanonical ensemble with $\mathcal{M} \to \infty$, the systems are distributed evenly over all possible quantum states (the number of possible quantum states is denoted by Ω), which correspond to the macroscopic state (N, V, E) of a given isolated system. In other words, every quantum state of the system is equally probable and is represented by the same number of systems in the ensemble.

Joining both postulates gives the quantum ergodic hypothesis, which states that an isolated system, if observed long enough spends equal time in each of Ω possible quantum states. Such a system is called an ergodic system.

1.2.2.1 Canonical ensemble

The system that we wish to describe has a fixed volume V, a fixed number of constituents N and is immersed in a heat bath at temperature T. Imagine an ensemble composed of a large number of systems which are thermodynamically identical to the chosen system. If we wish the ensemble to describe the chosen system,

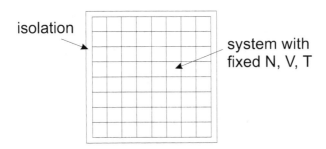

Figure 1.7 Scheme of a canonical ensemble, composed of $\mathcal{M}$ systems. Each system has volume V and N constituents. The temperature in all the systems is T. The ensemble, isolated with respect to the surroundings, is considered as a supersystem with volume $\mathcal{M}V$, number of constituents $\mathcal{M}N$, and energy E_t.

each system in the ensemble must also be in contact with the heat reservoir at temperature T. We compose the ensemble so that $\mathcal{M}$ macroscopic systems, each with N constituents and volume V, are tightly packed together (Fig. 1.7). The boundaries between the systems are such that energy can be transmitted through them while matter cannot. The whole ensemble is then isolated.

All systems in the canonical ensemble have the same V, the same N, and the same set of possible quantum states. Let us denote the possible quantum states by the values of their eigenenergies: E_1, $E_2, \ldots, E_j, \ldots, E_r$. Each state is written separately even if some states are degenerate (have the same energy). Let us denote the number of systems which at a given instant of time are in the state with the energy E_j by M_j. The list $\underline{M} = M_1, M_2, \ldots, M_j, \ldots, M_r$ is called the distribution over quantum states $\underline{M}$.

When the equilibrium state is reached, the outer walls are thermally isolated (Fig. 1.7). The entire canonical ensemble is an isolated system with volume $\mathcal{M}V$, number of constituents $\mathcal{M}N$ and total energy E_t,

$$\sum_j M_j = \mathcal{M}, \tag{1.47}$$

$$\sum_j M_j E_j = E_t. \tag{1.48}$$

Each system in the canonical ensemble is in contact with the heat reservoir at temperature T, where the remaining $\mathcal{M} - 1$ systems serve as a heat reservoir. The entire canonical ensemble, schematically shown in Fig. 1.7, can be considered as a thermodynamic system determined by the given volume $\mathcal{M} V$, number of systems $\mathcal{M} N$ and energy E_t. We name this system a supersystem. The supersystem is a closed system with a fixed number of constituents and constant temperature. Since it is isolated, it has a fixed energy, therefore it can be considered as a microcanonical system and is subject to the second postulate. For the supersystem, all possible quantum states are equally probable.

We would like to determine a quantity $\Omega_t(\underline{M})$ expressing in how many ways at constraints 1.47 and 1.48 we can distribute $\mathcal{M}$ states, of which there are $M_1, M_2, \ldots M_r$ indistinguishable, over $\mathcal{M}$ systems. Using combinatorics, we get

$$\Omega_t(\underline{M}) = \frac{\mathcal{M}!}{M_1! M_2! M_3! \cdots M_r!}. \tag{1.49}$$

The number $\Omega_t(\underline{M})$ depends on the distribution $\underline{M}$.

There are many possible different distributions which are consistent with the constraints (Eqs. 1.47 and 1.48), but as there are many systems in the supersystem we assume that the most probable one prevails. This means that only the distribution which is the most probable and for which the permutability, that is, the number of ways $\mathcal{M}$ states are distributed among the systems, is the largest, actually occurs. In other words, the most probable distribution is the distribution with the largest $\Omega_t(\underline{M})$. For convenience, we state an equivalent problem of seeking the distribution which yields the maximum of the function $\ln(\Omega_t(\underline{M}))$ with constraints (Eqs. 1.47 and 1.48).

As N is very large, the energy levels are very close together while many quantum states correspond to each energy level. So M_j, $j = 1, 2, \ldots r$ are very large numbers and we can use the Stirling approximation stating that for large x, $\ln(x!) = x \ln x - x$, so that

$$\ln \Omega_t(\underline{M}) = \left(\sum_{j=1}^{r} M_j \right) \ln \left(\sum_{j=1}^{r} M_j \right) - \sum_{j=1}^{r} M_j \ln M_j. \tag{1.50}$$

In order to minimize $\ln \Omega_t(\underline{M})$ subject to constraints (Eqs. 1.47 and 1.48), we use the method of undetermined multipliers and construct a functional $\mathcal{L}$,

$$\mathcal{L} = \left(\sum_{j=1}^{r} M_j\right) \ln \left(\sum_{j=1}^{r} M_j\right) - \sum_{j=1}^{r} M_j \ln M_j - \alpha \left(\sum_{j=1}^{r} M_j - \mathcal{M}\right)$$
$$- \beta \left(\sum_{j=1}^{r} M_j E_j - E_t\right), \qquad (1.51)$$

where α and β are the Lagrange multipliers. The conditions for the existence of the extremum of the functional $\mathcal{L}$ are

$$\frac{\partial \mathcal{L}}{\partial M_j} = 0 \qquad j = 1, 2, \ldots, r. \qquad (1.52)$$

Differentiation of the expression in Eq. 1.51 with respect to M_j and using the conditions in Eq. 1.52 gives

$$\ln\left(\sum_{i=1}^{r} M_i^*\right) - \ln M_j^* - \alpha - \beta E_j = 0, \qquad j = 1, 2, \ldots, r, \qquad (1.53)$$

from which it follows that the most probable distribution M_j^* is

$$M_j^* = \mathcal{M} e^{-\alpha} e^{-\beta E_j}, \qquad j = 1, 2, \ldots, r. \qquad (1.54)$$

The Lagrange multiplier α is obtained by substituting the distribution Eq. 1.54 into Eq. 1.47,

$$e^{\alpha} = \sum_{j=1}^{r} e^{-\beta E_j}. \qquad (1.55)$$

The Lagrange multiplier β is associated with temperature T (for the proof, see Hill (1986) and references therein),

$$\beta = \frac{1}{kT}, \qquad (1.56)$$

where, $k = 1.38 \cdot 10^{-23}$ J/K is the Boltzmann[a] constant. Its value is determined by the correspondence of the results of statistical thermodynamics and the results of experiments.

The probability P_j of finding a chosen system of the canonical ensemble in the state with energy E_j is

$$P_j = \frac{M_j^*}{\mathcal{M}}. \qquad (1.57)$$

---

[a] Ludwig Boltzmann, 1844–1906.

Taking into account Eqs. 1.54 and 1.55, we get from Eq. 1.57

$$P_j = \frac{e^{-\beta E_j}}{\sum_{i=1}^{r} e^{-\beta E_i}}. \qquad (1.58)$$

Since β is a positive quantity, the probability that a chosen system in a canonical ensemble is in a state with a given eigenenergy E_j decreases exponentially with eigenenergy. The temperature of the system plays an important role.

The average value of a chosen variable X over the ensemble is

$$\bar{X} = \sum_{j=1}^{r} X_j P_j, \qquad (1.59)$$

where, X_j is the value of the variable X which corresponds to the state with the energy E_j. Taking into account the expression for the probability P_j (Eq. 1.58), we get

$$\bar{X} = \frac{\sum_{j=1}^{r} X_j e^{-\beta E_j}}{\sum_{j=1}^{r} e^{-\beta E_j}}. \qquad (1.60)$$

In the above Eq. 1.60, the values of the Boltzmann factors

$$e^{-\beta E_j}, \qquad (1.61)$$

determine the average value of the chosen thermodynamic variable ($\bar{X}$). In the following chapters of this book Eq. 1.60 will be used in various statistical thermodynamic models to calculate the average value of different thermodynamic variables.

In the language of statistical physics, thermodynamic equilibrium means a state which has the most probable distribution of the systems over the eigenenergies. The most probable distribution means the state with the highest degree of randomness or disorder. If the state is not the most disordered, then it is not the most probable. A state with a high degree of order is called a non-equilibrium state. A system in a non-equilibrium state spontaneously approaches an equilibrium state.

1.2.2.2 Correspondence between statistical and classical thermodynamics

Pressure p in classical thermodynamics corresponds to the average pressure $\bar{p}$ in statistical thermodynamics. Internal energy W_n in classical thermodynamics corresponds to average energy $\bar{E}$. In symbols,

$$p \leftrightarrow \bar{p} \quad \text{in} \quad W_n \leftrightarrow \bar{E}. \tag{1.62}$$

The average energy is

$$\bar{E} = \sum_{j=1}^{r} E_j P_j = \frac{\sum_{j=1}^{r} E_j(N, V) e^{-\beta E_j(N, V)}}{\sum_{j=1}^{r} e^{-\beta E_j(N, V)}}, \tag{1.63}$$

while its differential is

$$d\bar{E} = \sum_{j=1}^{r} P_j dE_j + \sum_{j=1}^{r} E_j dP_j. \tag{1.64}$$

The first term in the above equation corresponds to work and the second corresponds to heat. It can be seen that there is a conceptual difference between work and heat. Work is connected to change of the eigenstates of the system, while heat is connected to change in the distribution of systems within the ensemble over the eigenstates.

In the first term of the expression (Eq. 1.64) we took into account that N is constant so that E_j depends solely on V, $E_j \equiv E_j(V)$, so that

$$dE_j = \left(\frac{\partial E_j}{\partial V}\right)_N dV, \tag{1.65}$$

while E_j expressed from Eq. 1.58,

$$E_j = -\frac{1}{\beta} \ln P_j - \frac{1}{\beta} \ln \sum_{i=1}^{r} e^{-\beta E_i}, \tag{1.66}$$

is substituted in Eq. 1.64 to get

$$d\bar{E} = \sum_{j=1}^{r} P_j \left(\frac{\partial E_j}{\partial V}\right)_N dV - \frac{1}{\beta} \sum_{j=1}^{r} \ln P_j \, dP_j - \frac{1}{\beta} \ln \mathcal{Q} \sum_{j=1}^{r} dP_j, \tag{1.67}$$

where the quantity $\mathcal{Q}$ is defined as a canonical partition function (see Eq. 1.55):

$$\mathcal{Q} = e^{\alpha} = \sum_{j=1}^{r} e^{-\beta E_j}. \tag{1.68}$$

Using the relation

$$d\left(\sum_{j=1}^{r} P_j \ln P_j\right) = \sum_{j=1}^{r} \ln P_j \, dP_j + \sum_{j=1}^{r} dP_j, \tag{1.69}$$

and considering that the probability that a system has any energy is 1,

$$\sum_{j=1}^{r} P_j = 1, \qquad (1.70)$$

so that

$$d\left(\sum_{j=1}^{r} P_j\right) = \left(\sum_{j=1}^{r} dP_j\right) = 0. \qquad (1.71)$$

It follows from Eqs. 1.69 and 1.71

$$\sum_{j=1}^{r} \ln P_j \, dP_j = d\left(\sum_{j=1}^{r} P_j \ln P_j\right). \qquad (1.72)$$

Considering the thermodynamic relation

$$p_j = -\left(\frac{\partial E_j}{\partial V}\right)_N, \qquad (1.73)$$

yields from Eq. 1.67

$$d\bar{E} = -\sum_{j=1}^{r} p_j P_j \, dV - \frac{1}{\beta} d\left(\sum_{j=1}^{r} P_j \ln P_j\right). \qquad (1.74)$$

Taking into account the definition of the average value as described in Eq. 1.59, it follows that the average pressure is

$$\bar{p} = \sum_{j} p_j P_j. \qquad (1.75)$$

Combining Eqs. 1.74 and 1.75 yields

$$d\bar{E} = -\bar{p} \cdot dV - \frac{1}{\beta} d\left(\sum_{j=1}^{r} P_j \ln P_j\right). \qquad (1.76)$$

The above expression for $d\bar{E}$ is compared with the differential of the internal energy (Eq. 1.39),

$$dW_n = -p\,dV + T\,dS. \qquad (1.77)$$

to get the relation

$$T\,dS \leftrightarrow -\frac{1}{\beta} d\left(\sum_{j=1}^{r} P_j \ln P_j\right). \qquad (1.78)$$

Substituting Eq. 1.56 in Eq. 1.78 and integrating yields the expression for the entropy of the system S

$$S \leftrightarrow -k \sum_{j=1}^{r} P_j \ln P_j . \tag{1.79}$$

The definition of the canonical partition function (Eq. 1.68) and the expression for the probability (Eq. 1.58) yields

$$P_j = \frac{e^{-\beta E_j}}{Q} . \tag{1.80}$$

Substituting Eq. 1.80 in the expression for entropy (Eq. 1.79) gives

$$S = -k \sum_{j=1}^{r} P_j \ln \left(\frac{e^{-E_j/kT}}{Q} \right) . \tag{1.81}$$

Further, rearrangement of the above expression gives

$$S = \frac{1}{T} \sum_{j=1}^{r} P_j E_j + k \ln Q \sum_{j=1}^{r} P_j . \tag{1.82}$$

Considering Eqs. 1.63 and 1.70, Eq. 1.82 transforms into

$$-kT \ln Q = \bar{E} - TS . \tag{1.83}$$

By taking into account the correspondence $\bar{E} \leftrightarrow W_n$ and by comparing Eqs. 1.83 and 1.35, we can express the free energy of the system by the canonical partition function as

$$F = -kT \ln Q . \tag{1.84}$$

Equations 1.79 and 1.84 give important and useful connections between classical and statistical thermodynamics. Other thermodynamic functions can be derived from the equations of classical thermodynamics which take into account the free energy $F = -kT \ln Q$. Entropy can thus be expressed as

$$S = -\left(\frac{\partial F}{\partial T} \right)_{V, N} . \tag{1.85}$$

Considering Eq. 1.84 the above equation reads

$$S = kT \left(\frac{\partial \ln Q}{\partial T} \right)_{V, N} + k \ln Q . \tag{1.86}$$

1.2.2.3 System composed of independent constituents

The constituents of a system always interact else the system would not be able to reach the equilibrium state. The simplest problems in statistical mechanics, however, consider constituents (molecules, groups of molecules or degrees of freedom) as effectively independent, while the only interaction is the interaction which allows for the equilibration of the system, for example, collisions between the constituents and the container walls. Within such a description direct interactions between the constituents are not considered. An example of such a system is an ideal gas. The number density of molecules in an ideal gas is so small that the direct interactions between molecules can be neglected, and the system reaches the equilibrium state by means of collisions between molecules and the container walls.

Let $\mathcal{H}$ be the Hamiltonian function which describes the energy of a certain system with a large number of constituents for which the corresponding quantum mechanical time-independent Schrödinger equation is (see Eq. 1.27):

$$\hat{\mathcal{H}} \psi = E \psi, \tag{1.87}$$

where, $\hat{\mathcal{H}}$ is the Hamilton operator, ψ is the eigenfunction of the stationary Schrödinger equation, and E is the eigenenergy of the system.

If the system is composed of independent molecules or subsystems, $\mathcal{H}$ is equal to the sum of the contributions of the constituent parts of the system,

$$\mathcal{H} = \mathcal{H}_a + \mathcal{H}_b + \mathcal{H}_c \ldots, \tag{1.88}$$

where $\mathcal{H}_a, \mathcal{H}_b, \mathcal{H}_c, \ldots$ are contributions of the respective constituent parts of the system. Likewise, it follows for the Hamilton operator

$$\hat{\mathcal{H}} = \hat{\mathcal{H}}_a + \hat{\mathcal{H}}_b + \hat{\mathcal{H}}_c \ldots. \tag{1.89}$$

The eigenvalues of the operators $\hat{\mathcal{H}}_a, \hat{\mathcal{H}}_b, \hat{\mathcal{H}}_c, \ldots$ are denoted by $\mathcal{E}_a, \mathcal{E}_b, \mathcal{E}_c \ldots$, while the corresponding eigenfunctions are denoted by $\psi_a, \psi_b, \psi_c \ldots$. The ansatz for the solution

$$\psi = \psi_a \psi_b \psi_c \ldots \tag{1.90}$$

is substituted in Eq. 1.87,

$$\begin{aligned}
\hat{\mathcal{H}} \psi &= (\hat{\mathcal{H}}_a + \hat{\mathcal{H}}_b + \hat{\mathcal{H}}_c \ldots)\psi_a \psi_b \psi_c \ldots \\
&= \psi_b \psi_c \ldots \hat{\mathcal{H}}_a \psi_a + \psi_a \psi_c \ldots \hat{\mathcal{H}}_b \psi_b + \psi_a \psi_b \ldots \hat{\mathcal{H}}_c \psi_c + \ldots \\
&= \psi_b \psi_c \ldots \mathcal{E}_a \psi_a + \psi_a \psi_c \ldots \mathcal{E}_b \psi_b + \psi_a \psi_b \ldots \mathcal{E}_c \psi_c + \ldots \\
&= (\mathcal{E}_a + \mathcal{E}_b + \mathcal{E}_c + \ldots) \psi = E \psi.
\end{aligned}$$

It follows from the above equation that the possible eigenvalues of the energy of the whole system are equal to the sum of the eigenenergies of the constituent parts of the system,

$$E = \mathcal{E}_a + \mathcal{E}_b + \mathcal{E}_c \ldots . \tag{1.91}$$

If the constituents are independent we can solve the Schrödinger equation with say 10^{20} coordinates by solving a small number of simple equations $\hat{\mathcal{H}}_a \psi = \mathcal{E}_a \psi$. We introduce partition functions (see Eq. 1.68) which correspond to individual constituents of the system,

$$q_a = \sum_j e^{-\mathcal{E}_{aj}/kT}, \quad q_b = \sum_j e^{-\mathcal{E}_{bj}/kT}, \ldots \tag{1.92}$$

where we sum over the eigenenergies of the molecules or subsystems. The product $q_a q_b \ldots$ generates all possible values of the eigenenergies of the system,

$$\mathcal{Q} = q_a q_b \ldots = \left(\sum_j e^{-\mathcal{E}_{aj}/kT}\right) \left(\sum_j e^{-\mathcal{E}_{bj}/kT}\right) = \sum_j e^{-E_j/kT}. \tag{1.93}$$

We conclude that the canonical partition function of the system which is composed of effectively independent constituents is equal to the product of the partition functions of the individual constituents.

1.2.2.4 Predictability and permutability

Let us consider the simple example of the outcome of tossing a coin. We say that tossing a coin is a casual event. For unbiassed coin, the probabilities for heads or tails are both equal to 0.5. The probability for each possible sequence in a series of N tosses are equally probable, that is, equal to $(1/2)^N$. However, each composition (defined by the number of heads (H) in a sequence of N tosses) is not equally probable (Dill and Bromberg, 2003). For example, in a series of four tosses ($N = 4$) the composition with two heads ($H = 2$) and two tails ($T = 2$) is more probable than the composition with four heads ($H = 4$) and no tails ($T = 0$) since only one of the 16 possible sequences has ($H = 4$), while there are six possible sequences corresponding to the composition with $H = 2$ and $T = 2$. In general, the number of possible sequences (defined here as the permutability of the outcome) for the composition with H heads in a series of N tosses is (Dill and Bromberg, 2003)

$$W(N, H) = N!/H!(N-H)!. \qquad (1.94)$$

It can be seen that if we throw the coin four times ($N = 4$) and each time the outcome is heads ($H = 4, T = 0$), then the calculated permutability of the outcome $W(4, 4) = 4!/4!\,0! = 1$. The reader can easily find that the composition which yields the largest permutability is composed of two heads and two tails, where $W(4, 2) = 4!/2!\,2! = 6$. This composition therefore, is six times more abundant (probable) than the composition with four heads. To conclude, if we throw a coin four times, it is most probable that we will obtain one of the sequences with two heads and two tails, since out of 16 possible sequences six sequences correspond to $H = 2$ and $T = 2$. We can see that even at small N compositions with the largest permutability $W(N, H)$ strongly prevail. For a larger number of throws (i.e., larger N) the sequences with the largest permutability $W(N, H)$ strongly prevail (Dill and Bromberg, 2003).

Based on Eq. 1.94 it can be calculated that if we throw the coin 100 times, the permutability of the most probable composition with $H = 50$ and $T = 50$ is equal to $W = 100!/50!\,50! = 10^{29}$, while the permutability of the composition with $H = 25$ and $T = 75$ is equal to $W = 100!/25!\,75! = 2.4 \times 10^{23}$, which is 6 orders of magnitude smaller. The composition with $H = 100$ ($W = 100!/100!\,0! = 1$) is possible, but according to its permutability the probability of such a composition is so small that it is in a human lifetime spent continuously tossing a coin practically unattainable (Dill and Bromberg, 2003).

In conclusion, although tossing a coin is a casual event for which there is an equal probability of heads or tails, the outcome for a

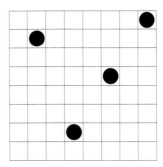

Figure 1.8 Two dimensional representation of a lattice with $M = 64$ sites and $N = 4$ system constituents.

group of such events can be predicted. The predicability of the outcome is better the larger the number of throws is.

1.2.2.5 Configurational free energy and entropy of indistinguishable particles in the lattice model

To describe a system of N constituents, a lattice with M equal sites is constructed. It is assumed that each site is either occupied by one constituent or empty (Fig. 1.8). It is of interest to calculate in how many ways N constituents can be distributed over M sites. The first constituent can chose any of M sites. For the second, there are $M-1$ available sites since one site is already occupied, the third can be placed on any of $M-2$ sites, for the last there are $M-N+1$ available sites. If the constituents are distinguishable, the number of possible configurations of N molecules over M sites (the permutability) is equal to

$$W_\mathrm{d} = M(M-1)(M-2)\ldots(M-N+1). \tag{1.95}$$

In quantum mechanics, constituents of the same species cannot usually be distinguished. In the lattice model, the indistinguishable nature of the constituents is taken into account in determination of the permutability by the factor $N!$ in the denominator of W,

$$W_\mathrm{i} = \frac{M(M-1)(M-2)\ldots(M-N+1)}{N!}. \tag{1.96}$$

Both the numerator and the denominator are supplemented so that we get in the numerator $M!$,

$$W_i = \frac{M(M-1)(M-2)\ldots(M-N+1)(M-N)((M-N)-1)\ldots(3)(2)(1)}{N!(M-N)((M-N)-1)\ldots(3)(2)(1)}, \tag{1.97}$$

which can be written as

$$W_i = \frac{M!}{N!(M-N)!}. \tag{1.98}$$

The canonical partition function of a system composed of N effectively independent, identical, indistinguishable constituents, which are distributed over M sites in the lattice, is

$$Q = W_i q^N = \frac{M!}{N!(M-N)!} q^N, \tag{1.99}$$

where q is the partition function of a single particle.

The configurational free energy which corresponds to the above partition function (Eq. 1.99) is (see also Eq. 1.84)

$$F = -kT \ln W_i - kT N \ln q. \tag{1.100}$$

It follows from Eqs. 1.99 and 1.100 by using the Stirling approximation that

$$F = -kT (M \ln M - M - N \ln N + N$$
$$-(M-N) \ln(M-N) + (M-N)) - kT N \ln q. \tag{1.101}$$

Taking into account that $M = N + (M-N)$,

$$F = -kT ((N + (M-N)) \ln M - M - N \ln N + N$$
$$-(M-N) \ln(M-N) + (M-N)) - kT N \ln q \tag{1.102}$$

and rearranging,

$$F = kT \left[N \ln \frac{N}{M} + (M-N) \ln \frac{(M-N)}{M} \right] - kT N \ln q. \tag{1.103}$$

The first term in the above equation is the configurational free energy

$$F_{config} = kT \left[N \ln \frac{N}{M} + (M-N) \ln \frac{(M-N)}{M} \right], \tag{1.104}$$

while the second term is the contribution of the independent particles' eigenenergies

$$F_0 = -kT N \ln q. \tag{1.105}$$

The configurational entropy S_{config} is obtained if according to Eq. 1.85, F_{config} is differentiated with respect to temperature T,

$$S_{config} = -k \left[N \ln \frac{N}{M} + (M - N) \ln \frac{(M - N)}{M} \right]. \qquad (1.106)$$

If the number of occupied sites is much smaller than the number of sites M (for very dilute systems), ($N \ll M$), we use the approximation $\ln(1 - N/M) \simeq -N/M$. This yields

$$F = kT \left[N \ln \frac{N}{M} - N \right] - kT \, N \ln q \qquad (1.107)$$

and

$$S_{config} = -k \left(N \ln \frac{N}{M} - N \right). \qquad (1.108)$$

The expression in Eq. 1.99 is generalized to the case where there are s species of molecules in the system. The configurational contribution to the partition function is

$$W_i = \frac{M!}{N_1! \, N_2! \, \ldots \, N_s! \, (M - \sum_{j=1}^{s} N_j)!}. \qquad (1.109)$$

while the configurational entropy is

$$S_{config} = k \ln \left(\frac{M!}{N_1! \, N_2! \, \ldots \, N_s!(M - \sum_{j=1}^{s} N_j)!} \right). \qquad (1.110)$$

If all sites in the lattice are occupied, then $M - \sum_{j=1}^{s} N_j = 0$ so that

$$W_i = \frac{M!}{N_1! \, N_2! \, \ldots \, N_s!}, \qquad (1.111)$$

since $0! = 1$. In this case, the configurational entropy is

$$S_{config} = k \ln \left(\frac{M!}{N_1! \, N_2! \, \ldots \, N_s!} \right). \qquad (1.112)$$

1.2.2.6 A simple example: equation of state of an ideal gas

We show below that within the lattice model, the state with the largest permutability corresponds to the equilibrium state of a system of effectively independent particles, expressed by a relation known as the equation of state of an ideal gas.

In very diluted systems we can neglect direct interactions between the particles and treat them as independent. Further, using the lattice model, we can assume that the number of lattice sites occupied by particles N is much smaller than the number of sites M. The free energy can be written by using Eqs. 1.105 and 1.107,

$$F = kT\left(N \ln \frac{N v_0}{V} - N\right) + F_0. \tag{1.113}$$

where the volume of the system V is written as the product of the number of sites M and the volume occupied by a single site (v_0),

$$V = M v_0. \tag{1.114}$$

Recalling that the infinitesimal free energy difference in Eq. 1.40 is,

$$dF = -S dT - p dV, \tag{1.115}$$

it follows that

$$p = -\left(\frac{dF}{dV}\right)_T. \tag{1.116}$$

Differentiation of Eq. 1.113 with respect to volume V and considering Eq. 1.116 yields

$$p = \frac{N kT}{V}, \tag{1.117}$$

that is, the equation of state for an ideal gas,

$$pV = N kT. \tag{1.118}$$

Note that the same result may be obtained by considering a different approach in which the particles in the gas convey momentum to the walls while their velocities are distributed according to the Maxwell–Boltzmann distribution function (see Hill, 1986).

1.3 Thermodynamic Description of Living Systems

The basic unit of a living organism is the cell. In the cell, energy is used for the synthesis of molecules, while the chemical energy of biological molecules is transformed into mechanical energy of muscle contraction and electrical energy of signals conveyed by nerve cells. These transformations can be described by the laws of classical and statistical thermodynamics.

Living organisms are open thermodynamic systems which can exchange matter and energy with their surroundings and

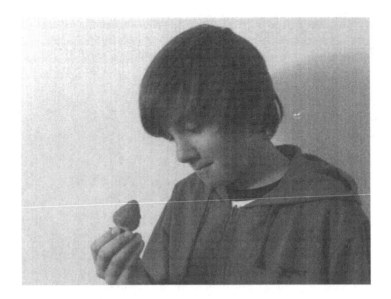

Figure 1.9 A living organism is an open system.

have a characteristic ordered structure. Namely, the condition for thermodynamic equilibrium that the thermodynamic variables are constant with time would mean that the organism is dead. Further, the system is incontinently fluctuating, so living organisms are in a non-equilibrium state. All processes which take place in a non-equilibrium state are irreversible. A non-equilibrium thermodynamic system can be close to equilibrium or far from it. Processes that take place slowly enough in stable biological systems (such as, transmembrane transport) are processes which take place close to equilibrium and can be described as equilibrium processes using the laws of equilibrium classical and statistical thermodynamics, within which the changes of thermodynamic variables between infinitesimally close equilibrium states of the system can be described.

1.3.1 *Thermodynamic Potentials*

Previously, we have described work conveyed to the system by means of a change in its volume (Eq. 1.31). Such a definition of work is not the most important in biological systems where there are more important forms deriving from mechanical, chemical, electrical, and osmotic effects. Therefore, we rewrite the first law of thermodynamics (Eq. 1.29) in the form

$$dW_n = -p\,dV + d\tilde{A} + dQ, \tag{1.119}$$

where $d\tilde{A}$ is the work of all external forces except $-p\,dV$. In general,

$$d\tilde{A} = \mathbf{X} \cdot d\tilde{\mathbf{r}}, \tag{1.120}$$

where $\mathbf{X}$ is the generalized force and $d\tilde{\mathbf{r}}$ is the conjugated generalized infinitesimal displacement. Work $d\tilde{A}$ is done because the force $\mathbf{X}$ causes displacement $d\tilde{\mathbf{r}}$. For example, we have shown above that a physical system in thermodynamic equilibrium attains a configuration which is the most probable under the given circumstances. Since the system is composed of a very large number of constituents, seeking the most probable configuration results in a generalized force that will actually move particles within the system.

The differential of the free energy according to Eq. 1.36 is

$$dF = dW_n - T\,dS - S\,dT. \tag{1.121}$$

If we also consider Eq. 1.119, we get

$$dF = -p\,dV + d\tilde{A} + dQ - T\,dS - S\,dT. \tag{1.122}$$

From the second law of thermodynamics (Eq. 1.32), it follows that $dQ \leq T\,dS$, so that Eq. 1.122 can be written as

$$dF \leq -p\,dV + d\tilde{A} - S\,dT. \tag{1.123}$$

This equality is valid for reversible changes. For isothermal changes ($dT = 0$) which take place at constant volume ($dV = 0$), it follows from Eq. 1.123

$$dF \leq d\tilde{A}. \tag{1.124}$$

The difference between the values of the free energy of the initial and the final equilibrium state of the system at constant temperature and constant volume is the maximal quantity of work other than $-p\,dV$ which the system can perform while approaching the equilibrium state.

In describing a system which is not thermally isolated and has a constant temperature and pressure, the infinitesimal change of the free enthalpy is according to Eq. 1.44 is

$$dG = dW_n + p\,dV + V\,dp - T\,dS - S\,dT. \tag{1.125}$$

Taking into account Eqs. 1.119 and 1.32, we get from Eq. 1.125 for an infinitesimal change the expression

$$dG \leq d\tilde{A} + V\,dp - S\,dT. \tag{1.126}$$

For isothermal changes ($dT = 0$) taking place at constant pressure ($dp = 0$)

$$dG \leq d\tilde{A}. \tag{1.127}$$

When the change takes place at constant temperature ($dT = 0$) and constant pressure ($dp = 0$), the free enthalpy of the system decreases until the system reaches the equilibrium state. In the process the system can perform work $d\tilde{A}$.

1.3.2 Chemical Potential

In systems with s species of particles we can write the infinitesimal change of the free energy as

$$dF \to dF + \sum_{i}^{s} \mu_i\,dN_i, \tag{1.128}$$

and the free enthalpy as

$$dG \to dG + \sum_{i}^{s} \mu_i\,dN_i. \tag{1.129}$$

Here, N_i is the number of particles of the i-th species, $i = 1, 2, \ldots s$, while the conjugated variable μ_i is the chemical potential of the i-th species. It follows from Eq. 1.128 or 1.129 that

$$\mu_i = \left(\frac{\partial F}{\partial N_i}\right)_{T,V,N_{j\neq i}} = \left(\frac{\partial G}{\partial N_i}\right)_{T,p,N_{j\neq i}}. \tag{1.130}$$

Using the connection between classical and statistical thermodynamics (Eq. 1.84), we can rewrite the chemical potential using the partition function $\mathcal{Q}$ as

$$\mu_i = -kT\left(\frac{\partial \ln \mathcal{Q}}{\partial N_i}\right)_{T,V,N_{j\neq i}}. \tag{1.131}$$

1.3.2.1 Chemical potential of one-component system

Consider a system composed of N indistinguishable molecules of the same species, distributed over M lattice sites (Fig. 1.8). We neglect direct interactions between the molecules and consider only interaction collisions of constituents with the container walls to assure the possibility for the system attaining thermodynamic equilibrium. We assume that the volume, pressure, and temperature are constant and use the lattice model in the approximation that the number of occupied sites is much smaller than the number of sites. In this case the free energy is given by Eq. 1.107

$$F = kT \left(N \ln \frac{N}{M} - N \right) - kT\, N \ln q. \qquad (1.132)$$

It follows from the definition of the chemical potential (Eq. 1.130) and Eq. 1.132 that

$$\mu = kT \left(\frac{\partial F}{\partial N} \right)_{T,V} = kT \left(\ln \frac{N}{M} - \ln q \right). \qquad (1.133)$$

Usually, instead of the number density of constituents, we rather use the concentration of the constituents:

$$c = \frac{N}{N_A V}, \qquad (1.134)$$

where V is the volume of the system (solution) and N_A, the Avogadro number. We also introduce the concentration of lattice sites c_M:

$$c_M = \frac{M}{N_A V}. \qquad (1.135)$$

The expression for the chemical potential is therefore:

$$\mu = \mu^0 + kT \ln \left(\frac{c}{c_M} \right), \qquad (1.136)$$

where

$$\mu^0 = -kT \ln q. \qquad (1.137)$$

1.3.2.2 Chemical potential of a multicomponent system

Biological systems are in general composed of many species of molecules or constituents. Molecules of different species are distinguishable while molecules of the same species are indistinguishable. Again, we limit our consideration to systems in which the volume, pressure, and temperature can be considered constant.

Imagine a simple model of solution in which there are two species of molecules which we denote by numbers 1 and 2. In the system, there are N_1 molecules of species 1 and N_2 molecules of species 2. Direct interactions between molecules are again neglected and only indirect interactions through collisions with the container wall are allowed to ensure the possibility of reaching the equilibrium state of the system. Each species of molecules has a distinct set of eigenenergies so that the particle partition function of the molecules 1 is

$$q_1 = \sum_i e^{-\varepsilon_{1,i}/kT} . \tag{1.138}$$

while the particle partition function of the molecules 2 is

$$q_2 = \sum_i e^{-\varepsilon_{2,i}/kT} . \tag{1.139}$$

Index i runs over all eigenstates of each kind of molecules, respectively.

Molecules are distributed over M sites in the lattice. Each lattice site is occupied by one molecule only and there are no empty sites, therefore

$$M = N_1 + N_2 . \tag{1.140}$$

According to Eq. 1.99, the partition function of the system is

$$Q = \frac{M!}{N_1! N_2!} q_1^{N_1} q_2^{N_2} . \tag{1.141}$$

The free energy expression follows from the relation $F = -kT \ln Q$ (Eq. 1.84)

$$F = -kT \, (M \ln M - M - N_1 \ln N_1 + N_1 \tag{1.142}$$
$$- N_2 \ln N_2 + N_2 + N_1 \ln q_1 + N_2 \ln q_2) ,$$

where we applied the Stirling approximation. Taking into account Eq. 1.140, it follows from above equation:

$$F = -kT((N_1 + N_2)\ln M - (N_1 + N_2) - N_1 \ln N_1 + N_1 - N_2 \ln N_2 + N_2 + N_1 \ln q_1 + N_2 \ln q_2)$$

and after rearranging

$$F = kT\left(N_1 \ln \frac{N_1}{M} + N_2 \ln \frac{N_2}{M} - N_1 \ln q_1 - N_2 \ln q_2 + M - N_1 - N_2\right). \quad (1.143)$$

In accordance with the definition of the chemical potential (Eq. 1.130), we calculate the chemical potential of the molecules 1 by partial differentiation of Eq. 1.143 over N_1:

$$\mu_1 = \left(\frac{\partial F}{\partial N_1}\right)_{T, V, N_2} = kT\left(\ln \frac{N_1}{M} - \ln q_1\right). \quad (1.144)$$

Similarly, we get by partial differentiation of Eq. 1.143 the chemical potential of molecules 2

$$\mu_2 = \left(\frac{\partial F}{\partial N_2}\right)_{T, V, N_1} = kT\left(\ln \frac{N_2}{M} - \ln q_2\right). \quad (1.145)$$

In the following, we consider concentrations of molecules and sites rather than their numbers, therefore we introduce

$$c_1 = \frac{N_1}{N_A V}, \quad c_2 = \frac{N_2}{N_A V}, \quad c_M = \frac{M}{N_A V}, \quad (1.146)$$

to get

$$\mu_1 = \mu_1^0 + kT \ln\left(\frac{c_1}{c_M}\right), \quad (1.147)$$

$$\mu_2 = \mu_2^0 + kT \ln\left(\frac{c_2}{c_M}\right), \quad (1.148)$$

where we introduced

$$\mu_1^0 = -kT \ln q_1 \quad (1.149)$$

and

$$\mu_2^0 = -kT \ln q_2. \quad (1.150)$$

Consider a simple example of a solution where molecules 1 represent the solute and molecules 2 the solvent and assume that the solution is everywhere very dilute, ($c_1 \ll c_M$ and $c_2 \simeq c_M$). We introduce the fraction

$$c_1/c_M \simeq \xi, \qquad (1.151)$$

and according to Eq. 1.140

$$c_2/c_M \simeq 1 - \xi, \qquad (1.152)$$

where ξ is small. The chemical potential of the solute is then:

$$\mu_1 = \mu_1^0 + kT \ln \xi, \qquad (1.153)$$

while the chemical potential of the solvent is

$$\mu_2 = \mu_2^0 + kT \ln(1 - \xi). \qquad (1.154)$$

For small ξ, the second term in Eq. 1.154 is very small since $\ln(1-\xi) \simeq -\xi$ and can therefore be neglected so that the expression for the chemical potential of the solvent is

$$\mu_2 \simeq \mu_2^0. \qquad (1.155)$$

The expression for the chemical potential of the solute in Eq. 1.153 can also be used in systems where there are many species of molecules. Considering the assumptions regarding the effective independence and indistinguishability of molecules, the chemical potential of molecules of the i-th species of the solute is

$$\mu_i = \mu_i^0 + kT \ln\left(\frac{c_i}{c_M}\right). \qquad (1.156)$$

1.3.2.3 Equality of chemical potential as a condition for thermodynamic equilibrium: a simple example

Consider a closed system divided by an impermeable wall into two compartments of *equal volume* in which there are very dilute solutions of the same species of particles. In the first compartment of the system there are N_a particles while in the second compartment there are N_b molecules. We use the lattice model where we assume that, in each compartment there are M sites. The wall is now removed and the particles are free to redistribute. It is of interest to find the distribution of molecules when the system reaches thermodynamic equilibrium and to determine the behaviour of the chemical potential in the process.

The free energy is composed of contributions of both compartments

$$F = F_a + F_b, \qquad (1.157)$$

where according to Eq. 1.107,

$$F_a = kT \left(N_a \ln \frac{N_a}{M} - N_a \right) - kT\, N_a \ln q_a, \qquad (1.158)$$

and

$$F_b = kT \left(N_b \ln \frac{N_b}{M} - N_b \right) - kT\, N_a \ln q_b, \qquad (1.159)$$

so that

$$F = kT \left(N_a \ln \frac{N_a}{M} - N_a \right) - kT\, N_a \ln q_a \qquad (1.160)$$
$$+ kT \left(N_b \ln \frac{N_b}{M} - N_b \right) - kT\, N_a \ln q_b.$$

The total number of solute molecules in both compartments N is fixed since the system is closed and cannot exchange matter with the surroundings,

$$N_a + N_b = N. \qquad (1.161)$$

Assume that the set of eigenenergies in both compartments is the same, so that

$$q_a = q_b = q. \qquad (1.162)$$

Using Eq. 1.161, we can express the number of molecules in the first compartment by the number of molecules in the second compartment,

$$N_b = N - N_a \qquad (1.163)$$

and insert it into the expression for the free energy from Eq. 1.160,

$$F = kT \left(N_a \ln \frac{N_a}{M} - N_a \right) \qquad (1.164)$$
$$+ kT \left((N - N_a) \ln \frac{(N - N_a)}{M} - (N - N_a) \right) - kT\, N \ln q.$$

We use the condition that in equilibrium the free energy of the system is minimal, so that

$$\frac{dF}{dN_a} = 0. \qquad (1.165)$$

From Eqs. 1.164 and 1.165 we get:

$$\ln \frac{N_a}{(N - N_a)} = 0. \tag{1.166}$$

so that

$$\frac{N_a}{(N - N_a)} = 1, \tag{1.167}$$

and finally

$$N_a = N/2. \tag{1.168}$$

It follows then from Eq. 1.161 that

$$N_b = N/2. \tag{1.169}$$

It can be seen that in thermodynamic equilibrium the molecules of the solute are evenly distributed over both compartments. Taking into account the expression for the chemical potential from Eq. 1.156 it can also be seen that in equilibrium the chemical potential is equal in both compartments

$$\mu_1 = \mu_2 = \mu^0 + kT \ln \left(\frac{c_{equ}}{c_M} \right), \tag{1.170}$$

where

$$\mu^0 = -kT \ln q \tag{1.171}$$

and

$$c_{equ} = N/2N_A V. \tag{1.172}$$

Equality of chemical potential over a system in the equilibrium state is valid in general and is equivalent to the condition that a system in equilibrium attains the state with minimal total free energy or minimal total free enthalpy.

Chapter 2

From Lipid Bilayers to Biological Membranes

2.1 Lipid Bilayers

A bilayer of lipid molecules (Fig. 2.1) represents the basic building block of the plasma membrane (Cevc and Marsh, 1987; Lasic and Barenholz, 1996; Rappolt et al., 2004; Rappolt and Pabst, 2008; Tien and Ottova, 2003), enclosing the cell interior. The lipid bilayer is composed of two layers of lipid molecules (Fig. 2.2) (Israelachvili, 1997; Rappolt et al., 2004), which have a water-soluble polar headgroup and a hydrophobic non-polar tail(s). The water-soluble headgroup (Fig. 2.2) is usually charged, having a net positive or negative electric charge or dipole–quadrupole moment. The hydrophobic part of the lipid molecule usually has one or more hydrocarbon chains and is not charged.

2.2 Lipid Vesicles

When closed into "bubbles", bilayers provide a barrier between the "inside" and "outside"; that is, they define closed "compartments". Bubbles of some microns in diameter are often called "vesicles".

Nanostructures in Biological Systems: Theory and Applications
Aleš Iglič, Veronika Kralj-Iglič, and Damjana Drobne
Copyright © 2015 Pan Stanford Publishing Pte. Ltd.
ISBN 978-981-4267-20-5 (Hardcover), 978-981-4303-43-9 (eBook)
www.panstanford.com

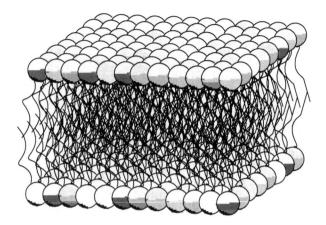

Figure 2.1 Schematic depiction of the lipid double layer; lipids in the lipid bilayer are oriented with their hydrophobic tails towards the centre of the bilayer. Namely, the lipid headgroups have the lowest free energy when in contact with the surrounding polar water molecules, while the hydrocarbon tails have the lowest free energy if they are hidden from the surrounding water (Israelachvili, 1997; Rappolt et al., 2004; Rappolt and Pabst, 2008). The thickness of the lipid bilayer is about 5 nm. The bilayer forms a vesicle, because this is energetically favourable. In this way, contact of hydrocarbon chains with water at the boundaries is avoided (Alberts et al., 2008) (Fig. 2.3). This specific arrangement of the lipid bilayer prevents diffusion of polar solutes like amino acids, nucleic acids, carbohydrates, and proteins across the membrane (see Cevc and Marsh, 1987; Lasic and Barenholz, 1996). Lipids in the bilayer are free to move around on the two-dimensional surface.

Lipid vesicles with only one phospholipid bilayer are called unilamellar vesicles, while those with more bilayers are multi-lamellar vesicles (see Fig. 2.4A,B).

Lipid vesicles have a rich diversity of shapes. They are found to transform sequentially through one of several transformation pathways. Even minute asymmetries in the lipid bilayers can cause deformations of the vesicle from spherical to pear-shaped, cup-shaped, budded and string-of-pearls formations (Leirer et al., 2009; Lipowsky, 1991; Markvoort et al., 2006). The variety of shapes is described elsewhere in this book.

Sakashita et al. (2012) reported that the most prominent feature of the observed shape transformations is their step-like progression.

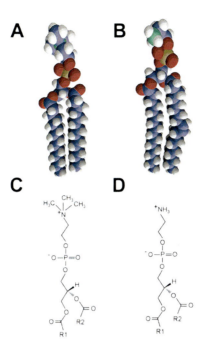

Figure 2.2 Calotte models of the lipids dimyristoyl-phosphatidylcholine (DMPC) (A) and palmitoyl-oleoyl-phosphatidylethanolamine (POPE) (B). PC and PE lipids differ mainly in their headgroup composition (panels C and D, respectively) (Rappolt et al., 2004).

They observed a circular biconcave form as the initial shape in all the pathways and its transformation is reversible up to a certain point in each pathway.

The shape of lipid vesicles is determined mainly by the minimal bending energy for an area to volume ratio (Leirer et al., 2009; Lipowsky, 1991; Mukhopadhyay et al., 2002). The bending energy of lipid membranes and their curvature is frequently studied due to its importance in understanding membrane-related biological processes (Pencer et al., 2001; Umalkar et al., 2011).

The lipid bilayer also undergoes thermal fluctuations (Cevc and Marsh, 1987; Duwe et al., 1990; Faucon et al., 1989; Milner and Safran, 1987; Rappolt and Pabst, 2008). At lower temperatures the lipid bilayer can adopt a solid–gel phase state, while at higher

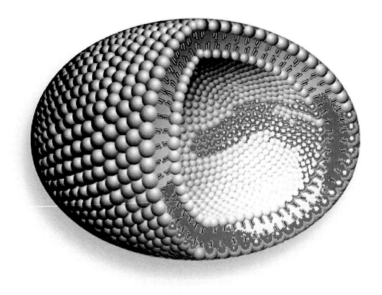

Figure 2.3 Schematical depiction of a unilamellar spherical lipid vesicle.

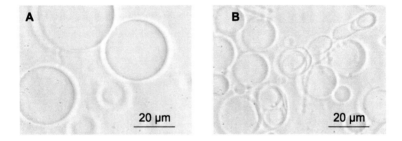

Figure 2.4 Light micrograph showing (A) unilamellar POPC vesicles and (B) a mixture of unilamellar and multilamellar POPC vesicles.

temperatures it undergoes a phase transition to a fluid state (Israelachvili, 1997; Leirer et al., 2009; Rappolt and Pabst, 2008). Unlike the liquid phase, lipids in the gel phase do not exchange positions. In cell membranes, the two phases coexist in spatially separated regions (Israelachvili, 1997). At a given temperature, some of the components of a complex mixture of lipids are liquid, while others are in the gel phase.

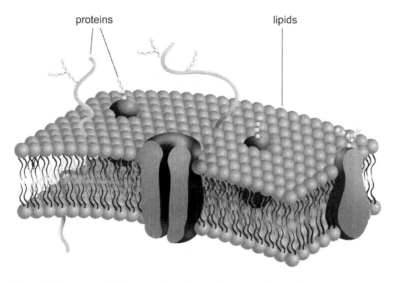

Figure 2.5 Schematic figure of a cell membrane and its major components: lipids, proteins, and carbohydrates.

2.3 Biological Membranes and their Composition

In all cell types, prokaryotic and eukaryotic, the membrane envelops the cell interior and separates it from the environment. The cell membrane is sometimes referred to as the plasmalemma. In addition to an external cell membrane, eukaryotic cells also contain internal membranes that form the boundaries of organelles such as mitochondria, chloroplasts, peroxisomes, and lysosomes. These structures are important for functional specialization of intracellular compartments (Berg et al., 2002).

Biological membranes are two-dimensional constituents of a large number of different components (Israelachvili, 1997). The major constituent of any biological membrane is the phospholipid bilayer (Figs. 2.1 and 2.5) which forms a flat sheet around cells of all living organisms and many viruses. It may have a variety of protrusions, which are fundamental to cell shape change and locomotion. In addition, apical evaginations of some epithelial cells like microvilli (Fig. 2.6) are involved in a wide variety of functions, including absorption, secretion, cellular adhesion, and others.

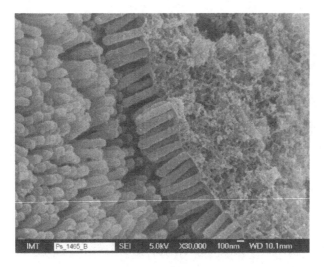

Figure 2.6 Scanning electron micrograph of a mechanically opened digestive gland cell. The mechanical break exposed the cell interior which has a sponge-like appearance. The shape and size of microvilli can be clearly seen. Microvilli cover the apical parts of the digestive gland cells of a terrestrial crustacean. They are formed as cell extensions from the plasma membrane surface (Photo courtesy: Agron Millaku, IMT, Ljubljana).

Apart from lipid molecules (Fig. 2.1), the cell membrane is also composed of proteins and carbohydrates (Fig. 2.5). Proteins may constitute up to 50% of the membrane content. Carbohydrates account for less than 10% of the mass of most membranes and are generally bound either to the lipid or protein components of the membrane.

There are many different types of lipids in cell membranes. The most abundant in biological membranes are phospholipids, which have hydrophlic heads that are soluble in water and hydrophobic tails which are hydrocarbon chains of about 10 carbons (Fig. 2.2). The smaller lipid molecules between the phospholids are cholesterols which strongly influence the mechanical properties of biological membranes. Without cholesterol, cell membranes would be more fluid and more permeable to some molecules. The amount of cholesterol may vary with the type of membrane. Plasma membranes, for example, may have up to one cholesterol molecule per phospholipid, while some other membranes like those around bacteria have no cholesterol at all (Alberts et al., 2008). The main types of lipids in cell membranes are cholesterol, glycolipids, phosphatidylcholine, sphingomyelin, phosphatidylethanolamine, phosphatydilinositol, phosphatidylserine, phosphatidylglycerol, diphosphatidylglycerol (cardiolipin), and phosphatidic acid (Cevc and Marsh, 1987; Israelachvili, 1997; Lasic and Barenholz, 1996; McMahon and Gallop, 2005). Each type of cell or organelle has a differing proportion of each lipid, protein, and carbohydrate.

The regions of the cell membrane which generally contain twice the amount of cholesterol, as found in the surrounding membrane, are called lipid rafts (Lingwood and Simons, 2010). They are small nanodomains ranging from 10–200 nm in size. Membrane rafts are assumed to play an important role in cellular signalling, trafficking, structural, and some other processes.

Membrane proteins, the other large group of membrane constituents, are attached to the inner or outer membrane surface, or embedded in the membrane of the cell or organelle (Fig. 2.5). Proteins float in lipids and act as channel proteins, carrier proteins, receptor proteins, cell recognition proteins, or simply enzymatic proteins (Alberts et al., 2008). Proteins are also involved in cell to cell adhesion and attach the membrane to the cytoskeleton. Membrane proteins are very important in cell to cell communication and may be targets of many drugs and diagnostic agents, but also of many toxins and pesticides (Vachon et al., 2012). For example, many organophosphates, which are potent nerve agents, function by inhibiting the action of acetylcholinesterase (AChE) in nerve cells (Williams et al., 2000).

The third large group of membrane components are sugar molecules, which are attached to proteins and lipids on the outer membrane surface (Fig. 2.5) to form glycoproteins and glycolipids, respectively. Carbohydrates are found on the outer surface of all eukaryotic cell membranes and form the cell coating or glycocalyx outside the cell membrane. When they are attached to proteins the complex is called a glycoprotein, while when they are attached to phospholipids they are called glycolipids. Carbohydrates are composed of a variety of different monosaccharides. The glycocalyx has a versatile function in cell protection and recognition. For example, carbohydrates may help to hold adjoining cells together, or act as sites where viruses, or hormones can be attached (Alberts et al., 2008).

2.4 Intracellular Membranous Structures

In eukaryotes, a variety of membranous structures are found inside cells. Intracellular membrane structures include the endoplasmic reticulum, Golgi apparatus, lysosomes, mitochondria, and chloroplasts. Another intracellular membrane structure is the nuclear membrane which surrounds the cell nucleus. It consists of two lipid bilayers: the inner and outer nuclear membranes. In plants, there is another membranous intracellular structure, the tonoplast which encloses the vacuole of plant cells (Alberts et al., 2008; Cammack et al., 2006). Among the intracellular membranous structures which are less known are lamellar bodies composed of several layers of densely packed membranes (Fig. 2.7).

Multilamellar intracellular structures have been found and described in various vertebrate and invertebrate cell types under normal, stressed, and pathological conditions (see Drobne et al., 2008). Concentric or intracellular lamellar inclusions have a variety of names, for example, lamellar granules, lamellar lysosomes, lamellar bodies, membrane-coating granules, Orland bodies, multilamellar lipids, concentric membranous structures, myelinoid bodies, myelin forms, myelinosomes, cytosomes, multilamellar bodies, osmiophilic lamellar bodies, lamellar structures or lamellar whorls, phospholipid whorls, etc. In the older literature, laminated membranous structures were mainly termed myelinoid bodies or myelinosomes (Drobne et al., 2008). The term "myelin" was primarily used to describe certain fatty substances which, when mixed with water, produce laminated membranous structures. A very detailed morphological description of multilamellar cellular structures was provided for lamellar bodies in lung type II alveolar cells. The lamellar inclusions found in some invertebrate cells are termed lamellar bodies, though their function is not entirely clear yet (Schmitz and Müller, 1991).

Structural investigations of multilamellar cellular inclusions were not possible until the application of lipid-retaining tissue

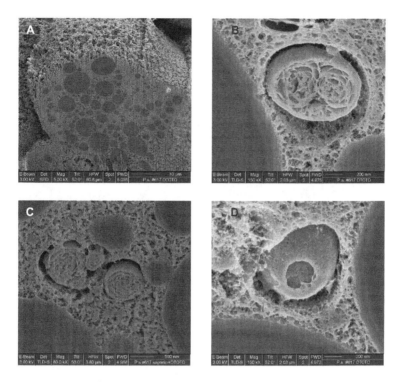

Figure 2.7 Membranous vesicles inside cells (see Drobne et al., 2008). (A) Scanning electron micrograph of focused ion beam (FIB) milled cell; (B–D) different FIB-milled lamellar bodies inside a cell.

preparation procedures in electron microscopy and freeze-fracturing techniques. The application of focused ion beam (FIB)–scanning electron microscopy (SEM) offered new possibilities in structural research on cellular lamellar structures (Fig. 2.7) (Drobne, 2013).

2.5 Transmembrane Transport

The plasma membrane acts as a selectively permeable membrane that defines the boundary and protects the essential intracellular environment of the cell (Verma and Stellacci, 2010). It physically separates the intracellular components from the extracellular environment. Due to its hydrophobic nature the lipid membrane prevents hydrophilic molecules from freely crossing the membrane.

By mediating the transport of ions across the membrane, the membrane maintains the electrochemical gradient across the membrane (Cooper, 2000). The ionic gradient is generated and maintained by energy-dependent processes. Due to this gradient the transmembrane electric potential difference is created. This potential difference may help in the exchange of charged particles across the membrane (Alberts et al., 2008; Heinrich et al., 1982; Iglič et al., 1997; McLaughlin, 1989). In mitochondria and chloroplasts, the proton gradient generates a chemiosmotic potential (Alberts et al., 2008).

Cell membrane permeability can be affected by many external factors. Among them are various chemical pollutants and toxins. Toxins are poisonous substances produced by organisms. They are capable of interacting with biological macromolecules and causing disruption (Baptista, 2013). Some toxins create unregulated pores in the membrane of targeted cells. Some of the best known are produced by the bacteria *Clostridium septicum* and *Staphylococcus aureus* and the sea anemone *Actinia equina* (Baptista, 2013).

Cell membrane destabilization can also be caused by many other chemical pollutants and by nanoparticles (see Fig. 2.8A,B). At present, it is believed that products of nanotechnology on coming unintentionally into contact with biological systems first affect cell membranes and only subsequently provoke other cytotoxic responses.

The regulation of cellular transport may be disrupted by formation of a membrane pore leading to various deleterious effects for cells. One of the consequences is uncontrolled entry of water through the membrane pores causing the cell to swell up uncontrollably (Kaneko and Kamio, 2004).

In addition, a rise in the intracellular Ca^{2+} concentration triggers activation of the Ca^{2+} signal pathway which is accompanied by morphological shape changes in microvilli (Lange et al., 1997; Lange, 2000).

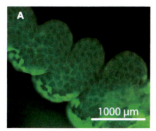 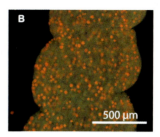

Figure 2.8 The change of membrane permeability of the cells that are affected by nanoparticles may be visualized by diffusion of fluorescent molecules such as ethidium bromide (EB) across the membrane into the cells and subsequently, into the nuclei. The Figure shows light micrographs of the median part of the digestive gland tube of woodlouse, *Porcellio scaber*. (A) In control, untreated animals the nuclei are not stained. (B) In animals treated with TiO_2 nanoparticles, the added EB molecules are taken up by cells of the digestive gland tube after nanoparticles destabilize the cell membranes. After diffusion across the cell membrane, EB molecules are intercalated into nuclear DNA where they emit orange fluorescence light. Reprinted from Valant, J., Drobne, D., Sepcic, K., Jemec, A., Kogej, K., and Kostanjsek, R. Hazardous potential of manufactured nanoparticles identified by in vivo assay. *J. Hazard. Mater.*, 171, 1–3, pp. 160–165. Copyright 2009, with permission from Elsevier.

2.6 Cell Shape

The other very important function of cell membranes is their involvement in maintaining cell shape (Boal, 2002; Canham, 1970; Deuling and Helfrich, 1976; Evans, 1974; Evans and Skalak, 1980; Hägerstrand et al., 2006; Helfrich, 1973; Iglič, 1997; Karlsson et al., 2001; Kralj-Iglič, 2002; Lange, 2000; Lipowsky, 1991; Sackmann, 1994; Zimmerberg and Kozlov, 2006). The actin cytoskeleton has been implicated in altering the membrane shape and form during cell migration, endocytosis, and secretion, and has been postulated to work synergistically with dynamic and coating proteins in several of these important processes (McNiven et al., 2000; Pollard and Cooper, 2009).

The cell membrane is a dynamic structure allowing the cell to grow and change shape as a response to changes in environmental conditions, or as a part of the cell's normal function (Fig. 2.9). Many cells in the body exhibit dramatic changes in their morphology.

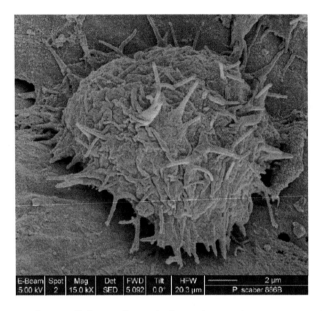

Figure 2.9 Some cells have a dynamic shape. Among them are macrophages with many cell membrane protrusions. The macrophage imaged is attached to the external surface of a digestive gland tube of an invertebrate (terrestrial isopod, *Porcellio scaber*, Isopoda, Crustacea; Photo courtesy: Francesco Tatti, FEI, Italy).

For example, muscle cells change shape due to contraction, nerve axons due to elongation, many epithelial cells form cell-surface protrusions, etc. One of the possible responses of cells to mechanical stress is a change in their shape. Cells may reduce their size or swell during normal activity or as a response to stress. Many cells change size and shape as a result of stress (Figure 2.10A,B). Lange proposed a mechanism of cellular volume regulation based on transport and ion channel regulation via microvillar structures (Lange, 2000). Cell swelling, using membrane portions of the microvilli, results in shortening of the microvilli. The pool of available membrane lipids is then used for cell swelling, which is proportional to the length and number of microvilli per cell (Lange, 2000).

Cell shape alterations were observed many times as a consequence of exposure of organisms to elevated concentrations of metals (Fig. 2.10A,B)

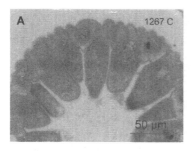 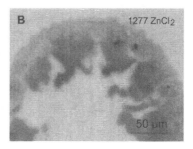

Figure 2.10 Some cells change shape as a result of stress. Digestive gland cells alter their shape from (A) dome shaped to flat with various intermediate shapes, which include the (B) folded-like appearance of an apical cell membrane.

2.7 Differences in the Membranes of Eukaryotes and Prokaryotes

There are two major groups of cells, prokaryotes and eukaryotes. Among the major differences between them are differences in the composition and function of their cell membrane. In eukaryotic cells, the basic building block of the cytoplasmic membrane is a phospholipid bilayer (Fig. 2.1) containing sterols. Prokaryotic cells lack sterols. Due to the ordering properties of sterols the eukaryotic cell membrane is capable of forming liquid-ordered phases. Very recently, Sáenz et al. (2012) provided evidence of bacterial "sterol surrogates" that are hopanoids. They have the ability to assemble saturated lipids to form a liquid-ordered phase in model membranes. These observations suggest that the evolution of an ordered biochemically active liquid membrane could have developed before oxygenation of the Earth's surface and the emergence of sterols.

The two cell types also differ in their cell walls. Among the eukaryotes plant cells have a cell wall. The eukaryotic cell wall is chemically different from the prokaryotic cell wall and never contains muramic acid. Muramic acid is a form of sugar acid, which has many biological functions as a component in many typical bacterial cell walls. The prokaryotic cell wall is composed of proteins or long chain carbohydrates, but not lipids. Another major difference

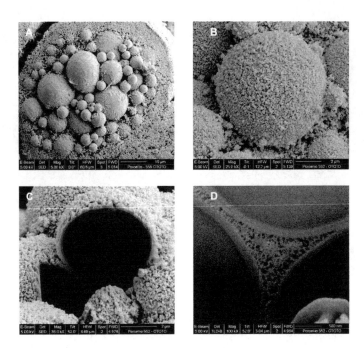

Figure 2.11 SEM micrograph of lipid droplets on the cell surface (A, B). Some lipid droplets were focused ion beam (FIB) milled (C,D). The composition of a lipid droplet is homogenous. (Photo courtesy: Francesco Tatti, FEI, Italy).

regarding membranes between eukaryotes and prokaryotes is related to their internal membranous structures. Eukaryotes have complex internal membranous compartmentalization, containing endoplasmic reticulum, Golgi bodies, lysosomes, mitochondria, etc. (Alberts et al., 2008). These sub-cellular compartments are surrounded by one or more lipid bilayer membranes. They compose the majority of the lipid bilayers in the eukaryotic cell (see Fig. 2.11A,B).

Prokaryotes usually have a simple and often transient internal membranous compartmentalization, if present at all. The intracellular structures which can be seen as primitive organelles in some groups of prokaryotes are in the form of protein-bounded and lipid-bounded organelles. These membranous vacuoles or membrane systems have special metabolic properties (Murat, 2010).

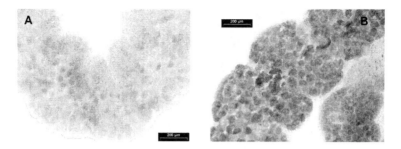

Figure 2.12 Lysosomal membrane permeability assay shows that the control (non-stressed) animals have stable lysosomal membrane (A), whereas the stressed animals have destabilized lysosomal membrane (B).

2.8 Consequences of Membrane Damage

Cellular membranous compartments may be damaged by a variety of factors. A consequence of all types of cell injury is loss of the capacity of the plasma membrane to maintain a proper ionic balance between the intra- and extracellular compartments (Stark, 2005). Under stress, the barrier function of all membranes is affected, not just the plasma membrane. Alterations in mitochondrial outer membrane permeabilization (MOMP) lead to apoptotic and necrotic cell death. Mitochondria serve as the prime source of reactive oxigene species (ROS), as well as being a target for their damaging effects. The earliest consequence of ROS burst is peroxidation which is a critical early event in apoptosis (Ott et al., 2007). As well as MOMP, lysosomal membrane permeabilization (LMP) is also emerging as an important trigger of cell apoptosis (Boya and Kroemer, 2008). Lysosomal membrane permeabilization is a potentially lethal event because it causes the release of cathepsins and other hydrolases from the lysosomal lumen to the cytosol. Lysosomal proteases in the cytosol cause digestion of vital proteins and activate hydrolases, including caspases. The lysosomal membrane is often a target for different contaminants so that membrane permeability is an early indication of the effects caused by chemical pollutants (Fig. 2.12) (Svendsen et al., 2004).

The lysosomal latency (LL) assay and the neutral red retention (NRR) assay are most frequently used for measuring lysosomal membrane stability. The LL assay estimates differences in the permeability of the lysosomal membrane, measuring the optimal reaction time for lysosomal N-acetyl-b-hexosaminidase activity (Nolde et al., 2006). This biomarker has been well established as one of more reliable of the recommended biomarkers in water quality assessment (UNEP, 1997). The NRR assay is another technique applied for monitoring alterations in the permeability of the lysosomal membrane. This test is based on the retention of the cationic probe neutral red within the lysosomal compartment over time (Fig. 2.12).

Cell damage, including cell membrane damage, if severe enough leads to autophagy. Autophagy is a vital catabolic process that degrades cytoplasmic components within the lysosome. Autophagy operating under normal and pathological conditions plays an essential quality-control function in the cell by promoting basal turnover of long-lived proteins and organelles, as well as by selectively degrading damaged cellular components (Murrow and Debnath, 2013). It is manifested by the presence of autophagic vacuoles. These are double-membraned vacuoles containing cytoplasmic material (Pavelka and Roth, 2010). They undergo a stepwise maturation including fusion with both endosomal and lysosomal vesicles and thus, do not have a constant ultrastructural appearance (Fig. 2.13).

Another disturbance related to phospholipids is cellular phospholipid storage disorder, termed phospholipidosis. Phospholipidosis is the excessive accumulation of intracellular phospholipids due to interactions of different substances (cationic amphiphilic structures) with phospholipids or the enzymes that affect their metabolism (Reasor and Kacew, 2001). This accumulation results in a unique structure in the cells noted as electron-dense lamellar whorls in the cytoplasm when observed with transmission electron microscopy. Electron microscopy is the widely accepted standard for classification of the phospholipidosis effect (Monteith et al., 2006).

Almost 500 compounds were described to induce phospholipidosis (Goracci et al., 2013). These compounds share several common physiochemical properties, including a hydrophobic ring structure on the molecule and a hydrophilic side chain with a charged cationic amine group, hence the class term cationic amphiphilic drugs

Consequences of Membrane Damage | 57

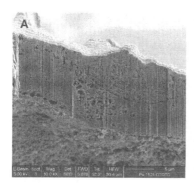 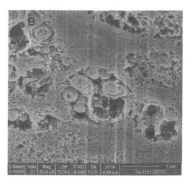

Figure 2.13 An autophagous vacuole as seen by SEM after FIB milling of a digestive gland epithelium. Note that the digestive gland epithelium is flat (A), which is an indication that the organism is under severe stress. (B) Membrane around a targeted region of the cell. (Photo courtesy: Francesco Tatti, FEI, Italy).

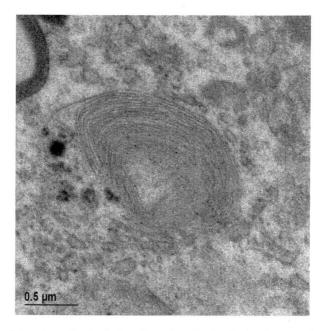

Figure 2.14 Lamellar body in a digestive gland cell of TiO_2 treated model animal, terrestrial isopod *Porcellio scaber* (Unpublished, Photo courtesy: Živa Pipan Tkalec).

(CADs) (Reasor and Kacew, 2001). Phospholipidosis is not directly linked to toxic effects but nevertheless it has to be considered as early as possible during drug discovery. Recently, nanoparticles were also found to provoke phospholipidosis, posing the need for a better understanding and control of this phenomenon (Wang and Petersen, 2013) (Fig. 2.14).

2.9 Cell Membrane Repair

Membrane damage is a reversible process. Rapid plasma membrane repair is essential for cellular survival. Different mechanisms are employed for resealing a membrane lesion, depending on the dimensions of membrane damage (Tam et al., 2010). When cell lesions are below one micron as in electroporation, lipid flow is unimpaired by the tension of the cytoskeleton and membrane repair is independent of calcium and exocytosis. In membrane ruptures near one micron and above, elevation of Ca^{2+} levels triggers fusion of lysosomes with the plasma membrane (Palm-Apergi and Hallbrink, 2011; Steinhardt, 2005). When a much larger area of membrane is damaged, a massive endocytosis is needed to seal the rupture. The motor proteins kinesin and myosin have been proposed to deliver vesicles to the cell periphery where Ca^{2+}-dependent exocytosis repairs the damaged membrane (Steinhardt, 2005).

Chapter 3

Lipid Vesicles as Experimental Tools

Due to the high degree of resemblance to biological membranes, lipid vesicles are attracting a great deal of attention as a model cell membrane system. Since the cellular membrane function is fundamentally related to its essential constituent, the phospholipid bilayer (Fig. 2.1), the lipid vesicle studies could provide many answers related to biological membranes (Fig. 3.1). Vesicles enable studies to be made of biological membrane structure, self-assembly properties, phase behaviour, transport, and elasticity properties, as well as their interactions with ions, macromolecules, or products of nanotehnologies.

Lipid vesicles are closed structures in which one lipid bilayer separates an aqueous inner compartment from the external aqueous medium. Since the same situation occurs in the membranes of biological cells, lipid vesicles have therefore been considered as possible cell precursors during the prebiological era on Earth (Luisi et al., 1999). In addition, the high molecular complexity of the lipid bilayer due to controlled peptide binding may be crucial in allowing early evolution of life on Earth.

The first boundary membranes were most probably formed by spontaneously aggregating amphiphiles, synthesized in prebiotic

---

Nanostructures in Biological Systems: Theory and Applications
Aleš Iglič, Veronika Kralj-Iglič, and Damjana Drobne
Copyright © 2015 Pan Stanford Publishing Pte. Ltd.
ISBN 978-981-4267-20-5 (Hardcover), 978-981-4303-43-9 (eBook)
www.panstanford.com

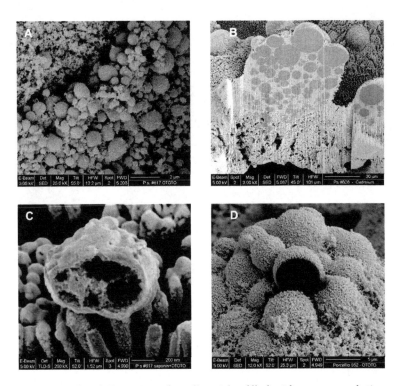

Figure 3.1 (A, B) Extrusion of small vesicles filled with aqueous solution, which was removed during the preparation procedure and thus, the vesicle appears empty. The images (C, D) show vesicles opened by focused ion beams in order to expose the contents. The upper and lower left images show the extrusion of vesicles filled with a lipid non-water soluble content. The sample preparation procedure selected preserved the lipids. The images were taken from the digestive gland cells of an invertebrate (terrestrial isopod, *Porcellio scaber*, Isopoda, Crustacea (Photo courtesy: Francesco Tatti, FEI, Italy).

conditions. Such vesicles can enclose functional polymers, take up precursors, and even grow and divide (Laiterä and Lehto, 2009).

3.1 Types of Lipid Vesicles and Their Applications

Very early knowledge on biological membranes came from experiments on erythrocytes. Already in 1925, Gorter and Grendel (1925) performed a very interesting experiment which demonstrated that a lipid bilayer is an element of the cell membrane structure. They extracted the lipid from human erythrocytes and introduced this lipid to an air–water interface. At this interface, the lipid formed a monolayer. They measured the area of the interface covered by the lipid and found the relationship between the surface area of the monolayer and the surface area of the red blood cell. The surface area of the lipids corresponded to twice the surface area of the erythrocyte (Gorter and Grendel, 1925).

Already in the 1960s, lipid vesicles were studied in many laboratories as model membranes (Miyamoto and Stoecken, 1971) (Fig. 2.4). In the 1970s, several practical applications of lipid vesicles emerged, most notably in drug delivery (see Lasic, 1998). Up to now, thousands of papers on numerous medical applications of lipid vesicles in various pre-clinical models were published (Lasic, 1998). Now we know that lipid vesicles are an indispensable tool in different disciplines, including theoretical physics, biophysics of membranes, membrane chemistry, and membrane biology (Lasic, 1998; Iglič, 2004; Rappolt et al., 2004; Rappolt and Pabst, 2008).

Lipid vesicles vary in size, surface charge, shape, and number of lamellae. According to the number of lamellae, they are classified as unilamellar or multilamellar (Walde et al., 2010). Their surface charges, then classifies vesicles into anionic, cationic, and neutral lipid ones. On the basis of their size, they are categorized into three groups, that is, vesicles with a diameter ranging from (i) 30 to 50 nm are referred to as small vesicles (SUVs); (ii) 100 to 200 nm are referred to as large vesicle (LUVs), and (iii) those reaching a size up to 100 μm are giant vesicles (GUVs). The GUVs are visible under the light microscope and as such, of particular interest as experimental tools.

3.2 Vesicles as Cell Membrane Models

Natural membranes are very complex, therefore many different model systems have been created to simplify the system so that the roles of individual components, their organization and dynamics can be assessed (for a review see Chan and Boxer, 2007).

The model membrane systems are versatile (see Tien and Ottova, 2003). They include vesicles where a lipid bilayer is rolled up into a spherical shell, planar supported bilayers which sit on a solid support, tethered bilayer lipid membranes where the bilayers are tethered to a surface by hydrophilic segments, low molecular weight polymers, bilayer islands wrapped by proteins, fragments from natural cell membranes, etc. Micelles, bicelles, and nanodiscs also form a group of model membrane systems. In micelles, the hydrophilic heads of lipids are exposed to a solvent and their hydrophobic tails are oriented to the centre. Bicelles are made of two lipids, one of which forms a lipid bilayer while the other forms an amphipathic, micelle-like assembly shielding the bilayer centre from surrounding solvent molecules. Nanodiscs consist of a segment of bilayer encapsulated by an amphipathic protein coat (Chan and Boxer, 2007).

Of all these, GUVs are best suited to serve as model cell membrane systems. Therefore, they are considered as abiomimetic cell-sized reactors or model membrane systems (Martinho et al., 2011; Umalkar et al., 2011). The GUVs can be formed from different lipid mixtures and they sustain a wide range of physical conditions such as pH, pressure, or temperature. In comparison to SUVs and LUVs, they have larger diameters and possess a much higher average membrane curvature which is similar to that of cell membranes. In addition, morphological information about SUVs and LUVs is difficult to obtain owing to their invisibility to conventional microscopic approaches. However, the average diameter of the GUVs reaching up to 100 μm could be investigated by means of a fluorescent or confocal microscope. For such purposes an appropriate fluorescent probe is incorporated into the lipid phase during vesicle formation.

3.3 Computational Modelling of Lipid Membranes

Modern investigations of molecular structures are highly dependent on computational modelling. Computer simulations have become a well-established tool in lipid membrane research (Rabinovich and Lyubartsev, 2013). This approach can give essential structural and dynamic information with atomic level resolution.

A characteristic feature of lipids in bilayers, *in vivo* under physiologically relevant conditions is that they exist in a liquid crystalline phase. This state is characterized by a high degree of disorder, making its detailed structure difficult to describe.

Consequently, experimental measurements of the structural and dynamic properties of a disordered system give averages of the behaviour of many lipids over a time interval and not individual ones. In such cases, numerical simulation is often a useful tool for investigating the behaviour of such complex systems (Rabinovich and Lyubartsev, 2013). The first simulation of a lipid monolayer using molecular dynamics was made in the 1980s (Kox et al., 1980). It is now known that computer simulations of various lipid membrane systems allow an understanding of the molecular basis of the relations between chemical structure and physical properties of various lipid molecules and membrane inclusions.

3.4 Preparation of Lipid Vesicles to Serve as Experimental Tools

Lipid vesicles occur naturally or can be prepared artificially from surfactants, phospholipids, or block copolymers. Their common feature is the presence of hydrophilic heads and hydrophobic tails in the molecules and when exposed to water, they avoid exposure of their hydrophobic core to water (Li, 2013). Both lipid vesicles and polymer vesicles are used as experimental tools. They are both composed of a bilayer of amphiphiles enclosing an aqueous compartment. But they differ in the characteristics of their building blocks. Lipid vesicles are composed of phospholipids with a molecular weight well below 1 kDa, whereas polymer vesicle are built of amphiphilic copolymers with a molecular weight up to 100 kDa (Li, 2013). The latter are tougher, less permeable and with a more robust membrane. They are therefore, alternatives to lipid vesicles in, *in vivo* imaging and cellular delivery.

Different preparation methods provide different types of vesicles which vary in size, polydispersity, surface potential, degree of ionisation, thermotropic phase behaviour, permeability, physical stability, etc. (Segota and Tezak, 2006).

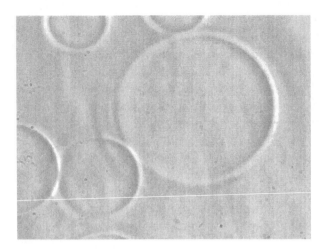

Figure 3.2 Phase-contrast optical microscopy of POPC lipid vesicles.

As unilamellar vesicles are often the preferred ones for different experimental purposes, several methods have been developed for their formation, including sonication, reverse evaporation from organic solvents, detergent dialysis, pressure–mechanical filtration, the swelling of phospholipid bilayers in water in the presence of an AC electric field, etc. (for a review see Segota and Tezak, 2006).

In biochemical and biophysical studies of membranes, vesicles of different sizes are very often prepared in aqueous buffer solutions by electroformation. The preferred diameter of GUVs varies from 10 to 60 μm (Fig. 3.2).

3.5 Examples of Nanoparticle–Membrane Interactions Studies

3.5.1 *Morphological Dynamics of Lipid Vesicles*

Shape transformation is an intrinsic characteristic of vesicles, reflecting changing environmental conditions (Hirst et al., 2013; Yuan et al., 2010). Since GUVs are large enough to allow direct microscopic observation, many investigations have been carried out on their morphological dynamics in response to temperature, chemicals, osmotic stress, detergents, a magnetic field or nanomaterials (Diguet et al., 2012). At a given area to volume ratio, membrane shape transformations are governed by the minimum of the membrane elastic free energy (Boal, 2002; Canham, 1970; Deuling and Helfrich, 1976; Evans, 1974; Evans and Skalak, 1980; Hägerstrand et al., 2006; Helfrich, 1973; Iglič, 1997; Kralj-Iglič et al., 2001b; Leirer et al., 2009; Lipowsky, 1991; McMahon and Gallop, 2005; Sackmann, 1994; Zimmerberg and Kozlov, 2006). Understanding membrane curvature (see Chapter 5) is important for elucidating membrane-related biological processes (Deserno, 2009; Tomita et al., 2011).

Vesicles were found to transform sequentially in a well-defined manner through one of several transformation pathways. A prominent feature of the shape transformations of vesicles is their step-like progression (Sakashita et al., 2012). These authors observed a circular biconcave form as the initial shape in all pathways and its transformation is reversible up to a certain point in each pathway. Consequently, polydispersity of shapes is a characteristic of a population of vesicles and has to be considered before any application or experimental use (Bibi et al., 2011).

3.5.2 Examples of Nanoparticle–Membrane Interactions: Studies with Artificial Lipid Membranes

Among the most recent applications of lipid vesicles in scientific studies are those in the field of NP–biological membrane interactions (Li and Malmstadt, 2013; Zupanc et al., 2012). Nanoparticles (NPs) are particles having at least one dimension below 100 nm. Material of this size has numerous novel properties which distinguish it from bulk material. This is because NPs have a greater surface area per weight than larger particles rendering them more reactive. When used in medicine, pharmacy, or the food industry. They come into direct contact with biological membranes purposely or unintentionally (Karagkiozaki et al., 2012). Understanding the interaction of NPs with biological membranes and their trafficking across the cell membrane is imperative for their successful application (Verma and Stellacci, 2010).

On the basis of research with GUVs, Li and Malmstadt (Li and Malmstadt, 2013) reported that NP interactions with membranes are nonspecific, driven by the electrostatic interaction between the lipid phosphate group and the NP surface. Nanoparticle binding to the membrane could be accompanied by many events. Among them are membrane pore formation (Li and Malmstadt, 2013) which is reported to be a result of both positively or negatively charged particles (Negoda et al., 2013). The results of these authors suggest that NP adhesion imposes surface tension on biomembranes via a steric crowding mechanism, leading to poration. The phenomenon is potentially a physiologically relevant mode of interaction between NPs and biomembranes, and may help in explaining observed plasma membrane permeabilization in the presence of broad classes of NPs (Fig. 2.8) (Valant et al., 2012). Changed membrane permeability could also arise from a reduction in density of the plasma membrane or changes in plasma membrane content (Leroueil et al., 2007).

3.5.3 Cell Membrane–Nanoparticle Interactions and Internalization

The effects of the surface properties of NPs on their interactions with cell membranes were reviewed by Verma and Stellacci (2010). In medical applications, most interest is focused on NP internalization.

For the cellular uptake of materials, both active and passive internalization have been proposed (Iversen et al., 2011). Specific internalization requires the cell to have an active role, while non-specific internalization is a random processes in which the cell has no active involvement. An important example of the specific uptake mechanism is receptor-mediated endocytosis. This includes selected extracellular macromolecules and inter-cellular signalling. This process is regulated by plasma membrane receptors that are only activated by receptor-specific ligands. Non-specific cellular uptake refers to the process of receptor-free material internalization. In almost all eukaryotic cells, non-specific uptake is dominated by pinocytosis (Alberts et al., 2008).

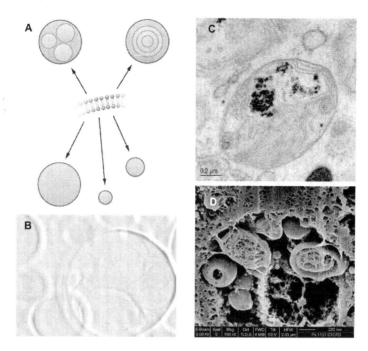

Figure 3.3 (A) Vesicles may undergo dynamic shape transitions in time and as a result of external agents; (B) Micrograph of POPC lipid vesicles; (C,D) Variety of intracellular vesicles investigated by (C) TEM (Photo courtesy: Ž. Pipan Tkalec) and (D) FIB/SEM (Photo courtesy: F. Tatti, FEI Italy, Italy).

To improve particle recognition and specific uptake by cells, efforts have been devoted to the surface modification of materials with ligands that bind specifically to membrane receptors (Ding and Ma, 2012; Kelf et al., 2010). These authors reported that not only the chemical but also the physical parameters of ligands can govern the NP–cell interaction, which may give some significant insights into future NP design for drug delivery.

Nanoparticles were also reported to be taken up following a passive uptake process, consisting of two steps (Ding and Ma, 2012). First, the particles are adsorbed on the plasma membrane, which could be followed by internalization.

In nanotoxicity, all types of interactions between NPs and cells are studied, as well as their consequences. It was reported that neutral functional groups are less active in unwanted NP–biological

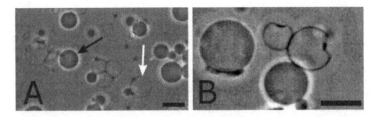

Figure 3.4 Lipid vesicles incubated with buffer solution of plasma apolipoprotein H. After addition of apolipoprotein H adhesion between vesicles took place. Also, the membrane of some vesicles became permeable to sugar so the inside and the outside solutions mixed (A, white arrow). Lateral segregation of membrane material was also observed (B). Bar = 100 μm.

interactions, whereas most charged functional groups actively interact with NPs (Verma and Stellacci, 2010). The interactions between cells and particles without any targeting ligand are poorly understood and remain a challenge for the future.

3.6 Conclusions

Lipid vesicles are one of the most favoured tools in a variety of scientific fields. There are hundreds of papers covering this topic. Among the most recent experimental studies where lipid vesicles are becoming a useful tool are nanobiology, nanomedicine, nanotoxicology, etc. The already available products of these new technologies have definitely established the position of NPs in modern life, and likewise have established new nano-inspired research fields.

The aims of bio-nano studies are multiple. Firstly, it is successful application of new products in medicine, pharmacy, and everyday life products. Secondly, this knowledge may help to characterize the membrane disruption potential of NPs as an intrinsic property and next, to link the biological potential of NPs and their toxic effects. Understanding NP-induced defects in biological membranes is among the major challenges of bio-nano related fields of research. In the future, research on NP–membrane interactions needs to advance towards understanding the mechanism(s) of interaction, hopefully leading to less hazardous nanotechnologies. Some of the most frequently used methods in vesicle studies and some less known and newer are ones presented in the next chapter. Time will tell which applications of NPs will prove to be successful and safe enough, and which not.

Chapter 4

Some Experimental Techniques for Studying the Structure and Properties of Lipid Vesicles and Other Lipid Self-Assembled Structures

Techniques for studying the structure and properties of lipid vesicles and some other lipid self-assembled structures range from direct visualization (optical, electron, or atomic force microscopy) to scattering techniques, among them light scattering (LS), small angle neutron scattering (SANS), and small angle X-ray scattering (SAXS) (Rappolt et al., 2004; Rappolt and Pabst, 2008).

A variety of techniques are available for imaging lipid vesicles. These include light microscopy, electron microscopy (EM), and atomic force microscopy (AFM). A very promising technique for direct imaging of the dynamics of lipid bilayer morphological alterations is optical (video) microscopy (Diguet et al., 2012; Haluska et al., 2006). Standard 2-D light or electron microscopy provides an image of the cross-section of the object that may not capture many of its features. Image processing to extract the 3-D shape of the object is a considerable challenge. For such purposes

---

Nanostructures in Biological Systems: Theory and Applications
Aleš Iglič, Veronika Kralj-Iglič, and Damjana Drobne
Copyright © 2015 Pan Stanford Publishing Pte. Ltd.
ISBN 978-981-4267-20-5 (Hardcover), 978-981-4303-43-9 (eBook)
www.panstanford.com

confocal laser microscopy has been the method of choice for many years (Sakashita et al., 2012).

The plethora of techniques for imaging liposomes and other lipid bilayer structures (vesicles) were reviewed by Bibi et al. (2011). Light microscopy is among the most frequently used techniques for imaging larger lipid vesicles such as multilamellar and giant unilamellar lipid vesicles. However, the more detailed physical properties of lipid vesicles need to be investigated by other microscopy techniques like fluorescence and confocal microscopy and various electron microscopy techniques such as transmission (TEM), cryo, freeze-fracture, and environmental scanning electron microscopy (SEM).

4.1 Light Microscopy

Phase contrast microscopy is based on the phase shifts in light passing through a transparent specimen and reveals many structures that are not visible with a simpler bright field microscope. Phase-contrast light microscope is a very convenient tool for observing the size and shape of lipid vesicles (Fig. 4.1) (Zupanc et al., 2012).

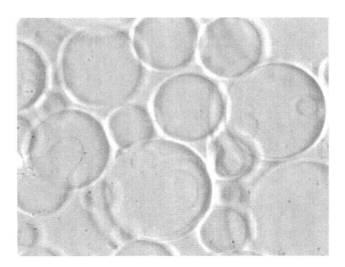

Figure 4.1 Phase-contrast optical microscopy of POPC lipid vesicles.

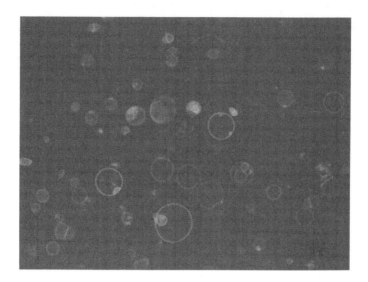

Figure 4.2 Fluorescent microscopy of GUVs.

New light microscopy approaches, such as two-photon microscopy, allow a more detailed visualization of lipid vesicles. This is a fluorescence imaging technique that allows imaging in depth. High-resolution fluorescence imaging using two dyes may provide direct information on the coupling between the inhomogeneous lateral distribution of membrane components (i.e., local membrane composition) and the local membrane curvature of the membrane of lipid vesicles (Baumgart et al., 2003).

For investigating lipid vesicles by electron microscopy, TEM and SEM are frequently used (Figs. 4.3, 4.4). In these measurements the selection of the method of sample preparation plays a very important role. For example, in the case of TEM investigation the lipid vesicles may be spread over a copper grid coated with carbon (Chakraborty et al., 2008) and negatively stained with 2% (v/v) phosphotungstic acid (PTA) and investigated by TEM at 80 kV and/or 200 kV with a resolution of 0.2 nm.

For SEM investigation of lipid vesicles, fixation is usually performed by incubation in a solution of a buffered chemical fixative, such as glutaraldehyde, sometimes in combination with formaldehyde and other fixatives, and optionally followed by

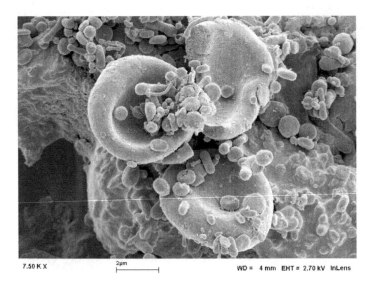

Figure 4.3 Scanning electron microscopy of blood plasma.

postfixation with osmium tetroxide (Drobne, 2013). The fixed tissue is then dehydrated. The dry specimen is mounted on a specimen stub using electrically conductive double-sided adhesive tape, and sputter coated with gold or gold–palladium alloy before examination in the microscope.

4.2 Atomic Force Microscopy

Atomic force microscopy (AFM) (Reviakine and Brisson, 2000) has also been frequently used for investigating the properties of lipid vesicles. AFM or scanning force microscopy (SFM) is a very high-resolution type of scanning probe microscopy. Among other information AFM measurements may provide the 3-D surface profile of lipid vesicles. The outstanding advantage of using AFM in lipid vesicle research is that it allows investigation *in situ* and in real time processes of vesicles formation or transformation. In addition, samples viewed by AFM do not require any special treatment that would affect the sample surface. Most AFM devices may operate in ambient air or even in a liquid environment.

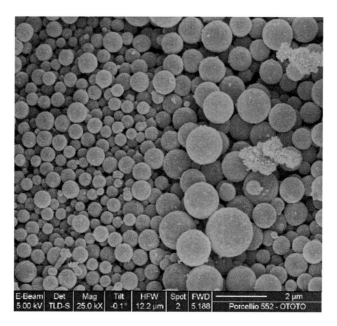

Figure 4.4 Scanning electron microscopy of vesicles secreted by digestive gland cells (Photo courtesy: F. Tatti, FEI, Italy).

4.3 Small-Angle X-Ray Scattering

Small angle X-ray scattering belongs to the family of X-ray scattering techniques used in the characterization of different organic materials (Rappolt et al., 2004; Rappolt and Pabst, 2008; Yaghmur et al., 2010; Yaghmur and Rappolt, 2012; Zupanc et al., 2012). SAXS is not a direct imaging technique, but may still provide detailed information on the shape and size of organic macromolecules, information on characteristic distances of partially ordered self-assembled organic–biological structures up to 150 nm, data on pore size in different lipid structures and structural information about biological macromolecules in the range between 5 and 25 nm. In the application of SAXS in lipid research, elastic scattering of X-rays of wavelength 0.1–0.2 nm is utilized to study the physical and structural properties of the lipid vesicles (Fig. 4.5) and to detect inhomogeneities in the nanometer range at very low angles of scattered X-rays (typically 0.1–10 degrees).

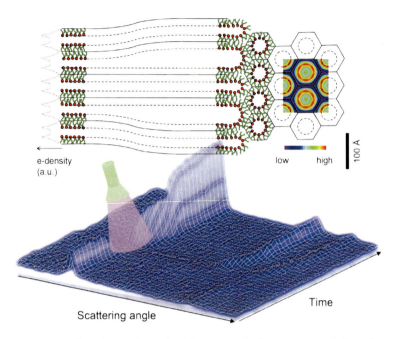

Figure 4.5 Optothermally induced structural changes in multilamellar vesicles loaded with hydrophilic gold nanoparticles. Synchrotron time-resolved SAXS experiments combined with UV light source irradiation demonstrated that the structural pathway from the fluid lamellar phase (L_α) to an inverted hexagonal phase (H_{II}) passes through an intermediate state of uncorrelated membranes. The electron density profile of the L_α-phase is shown at the far left, and the electron density map of the H_{II}-phase is shown on the far right. For the H_{II}-phase, the electron density values are colour coded. Reprinted with permission from Yaghmur, A., Paasonen, L., Yliperttula, M., Urtti, A., and Rappolt, M. Structural elucidation of light activated vesicles. *J. Phys. Chem. Lett.*, 1, pp. 962–996. Copyright 2010 American Chemical Society.

Chapter 5

Mathematical Description of the Curvature of Biological Nanostructures

Biological surfaces may in the first approximation be considered as smooth surfaces that can be described by two principal radii (inverse curvatures) at each point of the surface. In the following, the mathematical definition of the two principal curvatures C_1 and C_2 is be briefly described.

The position of an arbitrary point P on the surface (Fig. 5.1) is determined by position vector $\mathbf{r}$, which is a function of two parameters u and v:

$$\mathbf{r}(u, v) = (x_1(u, v), x_2(u, v), x_3(u, v)) \qquad (5.1)$$

where, $x_i(u, v)$ are the coordinates of the vector $\mathbf{r}$. Partial derivatives of $\mathbf{r}(u, v)$ with respect to u and v (the vectors $\mathbf{r}_u$ and $\mathbf{r}_v$) define the tangential plane at the point P on the surface:

$$\mathbf{r}_u(u, v) = \partial \mathbf{r}/\partial u, \qquad (5.2)$$

$$\mathbf{r}_v(u, v) = \partial \mathbf{r}/\partial v. \qquad (5.3)$$

At every point P on the surface, one can also find a vector normal to the surface ($\mathbf{n}$) and the corresponding normal plane, which contains the normal vector $\mathbf{n}$ (Fig. 5.1). The cross-section

---

Nanostructures in Biological Systems: Theory and Applications
Aleš Iglič, Veronika Kralj-Iglič, and Damjana Drobne
Copyright © 2015 Pan Stanford Publishing Pte. Ltd.
ISBN 978-981-4267-20-5 (Hardcover), 978-981-4303-43-9 (eBook)
www.panstanford.com

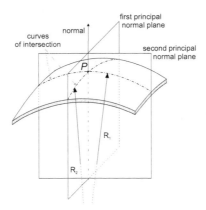

Figure 5.1 A schematic figure of the two principal normal planes and the corresponding two principal curvature radii R_1 and R_2, which define the two principal curvatures $C_1 = 1/R_1$ and $C_2 = 1/R_2$. Figure adapted from Perutková et al. (2009).

of the surface with the normal plane defines the curve called the normal cut. The curvature of this curve is called the curvature of the normal cut and is denoted by $C = 1/R$, where, R is the radius of curvature. The curvature of the normal cut is determined by the fraction (Korn and Korn, 1968):

$$1/R = \frac{L du^2 + 2M du dv + N dv^2}{E du^2 + 2F du dv + G dv^2}, \qquad (5.4)$$

where E, F, and G are the coefficients of the first fundamental form (Korn and Korn, 1968):

$$E = \mathbf{r}_u \cdot \mathbf{r}_u, \qquad (5.5)$$

$$F = \mathbf{r}_u \cdot \mathbf{r}_v, \qquad (5.6)$$

$$G = \mathbf{r}_v \cdot \mathbf{r}_v, \qquad (5.7)$$

while L, M, and N are the coefficients of the second fundamental form (Korn and Korn, 1968):

$$L = (\mathbf{r}_{uu}, \mathbf{r}_u, \mathbf{r}_v)/W, \qquad (5.8)$$

$$M = (\mathbf{r}_{uv}, \mathbf{r}_u, \mathbf{r}_v)/W, \qquad (5.9)$$

$$N = (\mathbf{r}_{vv}, \mathbf{r}_u, \mathbf{r}_v)/W, \qquad (5.10)$$

where

$$\mathbf{r}_{uu} = \partial^2 \mathbf{r}/\partial u^2, \tag{5.11}$$

$$\mathbf{r}_{uv} = \partial^2 \mathbf{r}/\partial u \partial v, \tag{5.12}$$

$$\mathbf{r}_{vv} = \partial^2 \mathbf{r}/\partial v^2, \tag{5.13}$$

and

$$W = \sqrt{EG - F^2}. \tag{5.14}$$

It can be seen from Eq. 5.4 that the curvature of the normal cut depends on differentials du and dv, that is, on the direction in which the surface is cut by the normal plane. There are an infinite number of normal planes containing the same surface point P, but only two orthogonal normal planes contain the curves of intersection having maximal and minimal curvature (Fig. 5.1, Korn and Korn, 1968). These two curvatures are defined as the two principal curvatures C_1 and C_2 of the surface at the given point P.

In the following, we briefly describe the mathematical procedure for determining the normal planes corresponding to the *maximal* and *minimal* curvature of the normal cut (Fig. 5.1). First, Eq. 5.4 is rewritten by introducing the variables $\tilde{\alpha}$ and $\tilde{\beta}$ as follows:

$$1/R = L\tilde{\alpha}^2 + 2M\tilde{\alpha}\tilde{\beta} + N\tilde{\beta}^2, \tag{5.15}$$

where

$$\tilde{\alpha} = du/ds \tag{5.16}$$

and

$$\tilde{\beta} = dv/ds. \tag{5.17}$$

The variables $\tilde{\alpha}$ and $\tilde{\beta}$ are not independent but are connected through the relation

$$E\tilde{\alpha}^2 + 2F\tilde{\alpha}\tilde{\beta} + G\tilde{\beta}^2 - 1 = 0. \tag{5.18}$$

which follows directly from

$$ds^2 = E\,du^2 + 2F\,dudv + G\,dv^2 \tag{5.19}$$

and Eqs. 5.16 and 5.17.

The minimization problem of finding the extrema of curvature $1/R$ (Eq. 5.15) which obeys the constraint 5.18 is stated by constructing a function:

$$\mathcal{L}(\tilde{\alpha}, \tilde{\beta}) = L\tilde{\alpha}^2 + 2M\tilde{\alpha}\tilde{\beta} + N\tilde{\beta}^2 - C(E\tilde{\alpha}^2 + 2F\tilde{\alpha}\tilde{\beta} + G\tilde{\beta}^2 - 1), \quad (5.20)$$

where C is the Lagrange multiplier. The Lagrange multiplier C can be shown to be equal to $1/R$. The function $\mathcal{L}(\tilde{\alpha}, \tilde{\beta})$ attains its stationary point when its partial derivatives with respect to $\tilde{\alpha}$ and $\tilde{\beta}$ are equal to zero:

$$\partial \mathcal{L}/\partial \tilde{\alpha} = 0, \quad (5.21)$$

$$\partial \mathcal{L}/\partial \tilde{\beta} = 0. \quad (5.22)$$

From Eqs. 5.21 and 5.20, it follows:

$$L\tilde{\alpha} + M\tilde{\beta} - C(E\tilde{\alpha} + F\tilde{\beta}) = 0, \quad (5.23)$$

while Eqs. 5.22 and 5.20 yields

$$M\tilde{\alpha} + N\tilde{\beta} - C(F\tilde{\alpha} + G\tilde{\beta}) = 0. \quad (5.24)$$

Equations 5.23 and 5.24 form a system of two homogeneous linear equations for two unknowns $\tilde{\alpha}$ and $\tilde{\beta}$. The trivial solution of this system of equations $\tilde{\alpha} = \tilde{\beta} = 0$ cannot satisfy the conditions 5.18. A non-trivial solution exists exactly in the case when (Korn and Korn, 1968):

$$(EG - F^2)C^2 - (EN + GL - 2FM)C + (LN - M^2) = 0. \quad (5.25)$$

Equation 5.25 has two real solutions for $C = 1/R$: $C_1 = 1/R_1$ and $C_2 = 1/R_2$, which are defined as the principal curvatures (Fig. 5.1), where R_1 and R_2 are the corresponding principal radii, which may also attain negative values (Fig. 5.2).

The sum and the product of the two principal curvatures define the mean curvature H and the Gaussian curvature K:

$$C_1 + C_2 = \frac{EN + GL - 2FM}{EG - F^2} = 2H, \quad (5.26)$$

$$C_1 C_2 = \frac{LN - M^2}{EG - F^2} = K. \quad (5.27)$$

The mean curvature H and the Gaussian curvature K are defined uniquely at every point on the surface. In the special case of a shape with rotational symmetry around the y-axis, we express the coordinates x_1, x_2, and x_3 via parameters $u \equiv x$ in $v \equiv \varphi$:

$$x_1 = x \cos \varphi, \quad x_2 = x \sin \varphi, \quad x_3 = y(x); \quad \varphi \in [0, 2\pi]. \quad (5.28)$$

The position vector can be then expressed as (see also Eq. 5.1):

$$\mathbf{r}(x, \varphi) = \left(x \cos \varphi, x \sin \varphi, y(x) \right) \quad (5.29)$$

Taking into account Eqs. 5.5–5.14, we can solve the system of Eqs. 5.26 and 5.27 to get the principal curvatures C_1 and C_2 in the form:

$$C_1 = -\frac{y''}{(1 + y'^2)^{3/2}}, \quad (5.30)$$

$$C_2 = \frac{1}{y(1 + y'^2)^{1/2}}, \quad (5.31)$$

where $y' = dy/dx$ and $y'' = d^2y/dx^2$. Due to axial symmetry the principal radii of curvature R_1 and R_2 point along the meridians and parallels: $C_1(x)$ is the principal curvature along the meridians and $C_2(x)$ the principal curvature along the parallels. The signs of the principal curvatures are chosen so that the principal curvatures of the sphere is positive.

In a tensor notation, both principal curvatures can be written as a diagonalized curvature tensor:

$$\underline{C} = \begin{bmatrix} C_1 & 0 \\ 0 & C_2 \end{bmatrix}. \quad (5.32)$$

Within the theory of membrane elasticity, the membrane curvature at a given point is usually described by the mean (H) and the Gaussian curvature (K), that are invariants of the curvature tensor $\underline{C}$ (Eq. 5.32). The mean curvature H is related to the trace of the curvature tensor $\underline{C}$, and the Gaussian curvature K is the determinant of $\underline{C}$ (Seddon and Templer, 1995):

$$H = \frac{C_1 + C_2}{2}, \quad (5.33)$$

$$K = C_1 C_2. \quad (5.34)$$

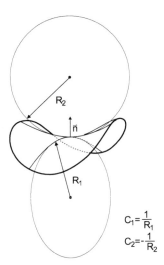

Figure 5.2 Schematic illustration of the two principal curvatures $C_1 > 0$ and $C_2 < 0$ of a saddle-like membrane surface.

For planar and spherical surfaces the two principal curvatures are equal, while for saddle-like (Fig. 5.2) and cylindrical planes the principal curvatures are different. High anisotropy in the curvature (i.e., a large difference between the two principal curvatures) has been revealed in numerous membrane systems, for example, in phospholipid bilayer nanotubes (see Iglič et al., 2003; Kralj-Iglič et al., 2001a; Kralj-Iglič, 2002; Mathivet et al., 1996), torocytic endovesicles of erythrocyte membranes (Bobrowska-Hägerstand, 1999; Fošnarič et al., 2002), phospholipid bilayer membrane pores (Fošnarič et al., 2003; Kandušer et al., 2003), and narrow necks of phospholipid bilayers connecting buds to the parent membrane (Kralj-Iglič et al., 2006). Instead of the Gaussian curvature, to explain the stability of these structures, another invariant is advantageous in description of the membrane free energy, namely the curvature deviator D (Kralj-Iglič et al., 2006):

$$D = |C_1 - C_2|/2. \tag{5.35}$$

The invariants, H, K, and D are inter-connected through the relation:

$$H^2 = D^2 + K, \tag{5.36}$$

meaning that the description using H and K is mathematically equivalent to the description with H and D.

Chapter 6

Lipid Nanostructures

6.1 Polymorphism of Lipid Nanostructures and Intrinsic Shapes of Lipid Molecules

Phospholipid molecules can be described as composed of two parts: a multipolar headgroup and two carbohydrate $(CH_2)_n$–CH_3 tails. The two tails may be of different lengths and may also contain double bonds between the carbon atoms (for a thorough description of different phospholipid molecules, (see Cevc and Marsh, 1987; Israelachvili, 1997). When mixed with water or electrolyte solution, above a certain threshold concentration the phospholipid molecules self-assemble into different lipid structures/aggregates (Fig. 6.1) so that the tails are hidden from the water, while the hydrophilic parts of the molecules (phospholipid headgroups) are in contact with the water or electrolyte solutions (Cevc and Marsh, 1987; Israelachvili, 1997). In this way the least number of hydrogen bonds between the water molecules are broken due to the presence of phospholipid molecules. Among the possible objects that may be formed by aggregation of lipid molecules, spherical aggregates of single-chained lipids (surfactants) (Fig. 6.1A) are the smallest. Double-chained lipids can aggregate into unilammellar lipid bilayers (Fig. 6.1C) that may be closed into vesicles (Fig. 6.6) and separate

---

Nanostructures in Biological Systems: Theory and Applications
Aleš Iglič, Veronika Kralj-Iglič, and Damjana Drobne
Copyright © 2015 Pan Stanford Publishing Pte. Ltd.
ISBN 978-981-4267-20-5 (Hardcover), 978-981-4303-43-9 (eBook)
www.panstanford.com

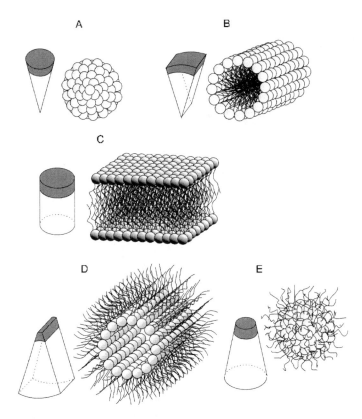

Figure 6.1 Schematically depicted polymorphism of phospholipid aggregates. Aggregated forms with the corresponding isotropic and anisotropic shapes of phospholipid molecules: a spherical micelle (A), a cylindrical micelle (B), a bilayer (C), an inverted cylinder (D), and an inverted spherical micelle (E) (Perutková et al., 2009).

an internal compartment from the continuous phase of the solution. Multilamellar lipid bilayers (Fig. 6.3) and vesicles can also be formed by a number of lipids.

The curvature of lipid aggregates/structures depends on the intrinsic shape of the phospholipid molecules (Fig. 6.1). Hence, non-cylindrically shaped phospholipid molecules self-assemble in water solution into non-planar structures.

For a lipid monolayer of finite thickness the following convention was adopted (see Seddon and Templer, 1995). When the pivotal

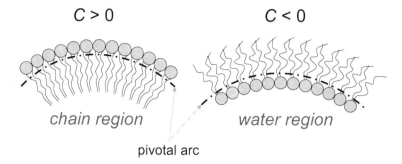

Figure 6.2 Sign convention of the curvature $C = C_1 \cos^2 \beta + C_2 \sin^2 \beta$ of the normal cut of a lipid monolayer, where, C_1 and C_2 are the two principal curvatures (see Fig. 5.2). The curvature C is positive when the monolayer is bent towards the chain region and negative when the monolayer is bent towards the water region. The angle β describes the orientation of the normal cut with respect to the principal direction, corresponding to the largest curvature (see Fig. 5.1) (Perutková et al., 2009).

plane (defined as the plane whose area does not change upon bending deformation; see Leikin et al., 1996) bends towards the chain region the monolayer curvature is considered positive $C > 0$), whereas when the pivotal plane bends towards the water region the monolayer curvature is considered negative ($C < 0$) (Fig. 6.2). According to this convention the mean curvature H can be positive or negative, that is, the monolayer can be regular or inverted. For positive values of the Gaussian curvature, K the monolayers are naturally convex or concave to form closed shells, micelles or inverted micelles. On the other hand, when K is negative the principal curvatures have opposite sign, that is, the monolayer has a saddle-like shape (see Seddon and Templer, 1995).

The tendency for the shape of the monolayer to bend without any external torques and forces is called the spontaneous (intrinsic) curvature (see Mouritsen, 2005). The definition of the principal intrinsic curvatures that define the intrinsic shape of lipid molecules (see Fig. 7.1) is very similar to the description of membrane curvature. The principal *intrinsic* curvatures are defined as

$$C_{1m} = \frac{1}{R_{1m}}, \tag{6.1}$$

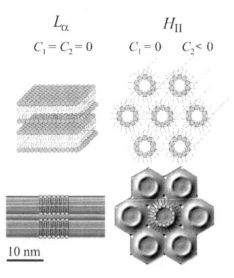

Figure 6.3 Schematic diagram and the corresponding electron density map of the lamellar fluid (L_α) phase (left) and of the inverted hexagonal (H_{II}) phase (right). The configurations of the lipid molecules are indicated. In the L_α phase both principal curvatures are equal to zero, while in the H_{II} phase one of the principal curvatures is equal to zero and the other one is negative. The data for the electron density reconstructions are taken from Rappolt et al. (2003). The maps depict POPE–water structures at the phase transition temperature of 74°C (compare also Table 7.1). Reprinted with permission from Mareš, T., Daniel, M., Perutková, Š., Perne, A., Dolinar, G., Iglič, A., Rappolt, M., and Kralj-Iglič, V. Role of Phospholipid Asymmetry in the Stability of Inverted Hexagonal Mesoscopic Phases. *J. Phys. Chem. B.*, 112(51), pp. 16575–16584. Copyright 2008, American Chemical Society.

and

$$C_{2m} = \frac{1}{R_{2m}}, \quad (6.2)$$

where R_{1m} and R_{2m} are the principal radii of a monolayer that would completely fit the molecule (see also Iglič and Kralj-Iglič, 2003; Kralj-Iglič et al., 2004). Written in tensor notation:

$$\underline{C}_m = \begin{bmatrix} C_{1m} & 0 \\ 0 & C_{2m} \end{bmatrix}, \quad (6.3)$$

where $\underline{C}_m$ is defined as the intrinsic curvature tensor (see Kralj-Iglič et al., 2004, 2006).

In a similar way to the mean curvature H and to curvature deviator D we can define the mean intrinsic curvature:

$$H_m = \frac{C_{1m} + C_{2m}}{2} \tag{6.4}$$

and the intrinsic curvature deviator of the molecule:

$$D_m = \frac{|C_{1m} - C_{2m}|}{2}, \tag{6.5}$$

which are related to the molecular shape. If the intrinsic principal curvatures are different ($C_{1m} \neq C_{2m}$) the membrane constituents are anisotropic. If the intrinsic curvatures are equal ($C_{1m} = C_{2m}$), the membrane constituents are isotropic (see Fig. 7.1). Isotropic constituents with zero intrinsic curvatures ($C_{1m} = C_{2m} = 0$) tend to form planar monolayers, while constituents having an inverted wedge shape ($C_{1m} = 0, C_{2m} < 0$) favour the formation of an inverted hexagonal structure (see Israelachvili, 1997; Perutková et al., 2009) (see also Fig. 6.1). The intrinsic principal curvatures account for the geometrical shape of the lipid molecule and the local interactions of the molecule with its surroundings, including hydration effects (see Kozlov et al., 1994).

The curvature of different monolayer and bilayer lipid structures (Fig. 6.1) depends to a great extent on the intrinsic shape of the phospholipid molecules, which in turn depends on the temperature, degree of hydration, presence of specific enzymes, pH, etc. (see Mouritsen, 2005).

Flat lipid bilayers are formed preferentially when the lipid molecules have cylindrical shapes (Fig. 6.1C), whereas cylindrical monolayers are formed when the lipid molecules are wedge shaped (as depicted in Fig. 6.1B). Conical and inverted conical shapes of lipids favour spherical (Fig. 6.1A) and inverted spherical (Fig. 6.1E) micellar shapes, respectively (see also Israelachvili, 1997).

The inverted hexagonal phase (H_{II}) (Fig. 6.3) is one of the lipid mesophases that are important for many biological processes in nature. Understanding the mechanisms of their formation and stability, and their physical properties may help us to elucidate their biological functions.

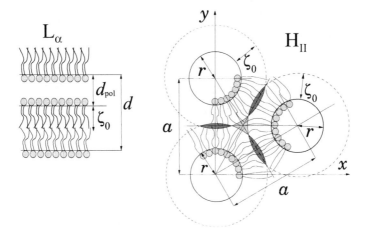

Figure 6.4 Geometry of the lamellar and inverted hexagonal phases. One bilayer and one neighbouring monolayer are depicted for the lamellar phase. The lattice unit of the lamellar phase (d) and the distance between the polar regions of the two bilayers (d_{pol}) are denoted. For the inverted hexagonal phase three cylinders of radius r at the distance a are depicted. ζ_0 denotes the equilibrium length of the hydrocarbon chains. The formation of H_{II} phase requires stretching or compressing some of the hydrocarbon chains as shown schematically. Reprinted with permission from Mareš, T., Daniel, M., Perutková, Š., Perne, A., Dolinar, G., Iglič, A., Rappolt, M., and Kralj-Iglič, V. Role of phospholipid asymmetry in the stability of inverted hexagonal mesoscopic phases. *J. Phys. Chem. B.*, 112(51), pp. 16575–16584. Copyright 2008, American Chemical Society.

6.2 Relevance of some Non-Lamellar Phases in Biological Systems

The bicontinuous cubic phase, the inverse hexagonal phase, and the inverse micellar cubic phase belong to the group of biologically most relevant non-lamellar mesophases. These mesophases resist excess of water and thus, they can be stable under certain conditions in biological systems (see Luzzati, 1997; Rappolt, 2006).

It is known that a wide range of phospholipids which occur in biological organisms may self-assemble into non-lamellar structures when they are extracted from cells and rehydrated in aqueous solution. However, despite the fact that many non-lamellar phases have undoubtedly been identified in various biological systems (see Hyde et al., 1997), still little is understood concerning their function.

The formation of non-planar mesophases might play a role in the regulation of protein function. Also membrane fusion in endocytosis and exocytosis is thought to be dependent on such highly curved lipid structures. It is also supposed that interbilayer tight junctions host non-bilayer structures. Direct evidence for the formation of the stable H_{II} phase was found in the paracrystalline inclusions of the retina (see Corless and Costello, 1981).

The non-lamellar structures of phospholipids are also common in some species of bacteria. It was suggested that the bilayers of bacteria are close to the transition from a lamellar to a non-lamellar structure (see Mouritsen, 2005). Many different types of bacteria can enzymatically change the intrinsic curvature of phospholipids, and consequently, they can prefer non-lamellar phases (see Mouritsen, 2005).

6.3 Inverted Hexagonal Phase

The lipids in the inverted hexagonal phase are self-assembled in long tubes arranged in a hexagonal lattice. Figure 6.4 shows the geometry of the H_{II} phase: two neighbouring tubes with diameter r are located at the distance a. The phospholipid chains point outward from the cylinder surface defined as the pivotal plane, while the headgroups form polar nanotubes filled with aqueous solution. Experiments revealed high anisotropy in the curvature (one principal curvature is equal to the negative inverse value of the radius of the tube and the second principal curvature is equal to zero) of tubes of the H_{II} phase.

It can be seen in the Fig. 6.4 that in inverted hexagonal phase there are triangular regions (called voids) between neighbouring tubes that are energetically expensive. One possible way to abolish voids for the lipid chains with tips in the void regions to stretch beyond their average length ζ_0 so that all the lipid tails in the hexagonal lattice do not have the same length as shown schematically in Fig. 6.4. In theoretical studies of the stability of inverted hexagonal phases an energy term which accounts for the stretching of the hydrocarbon chains in void regions was taken into account (see Kozlov et al., 1994; Malinin and Lentz, 2004; Mareš et al., 2008; Perutková et al., 2011; Siegel, 1988, 1999).

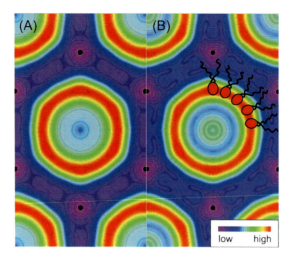

Figure 6.5 Electron density maps of (A) DOPE at 20°C and (B) SOPE at 68°C with measured lattice spacings (unit cell parameter), a, of 7.58 and 7.42 nm, respectively. The positions of the lipid head groups are coded in red, the water core regions in light blue and the hydrocarbon chain regions are highlighted in violet to black. Reproduced from Perutková, Š., Daniel, M., Rappolt, M., Pabst, G., Dolinar, G., Kralj-Iglič V., and Iglič, A. (2011), Elastic deformations in hexagonal phases studied by small angle X-ray diffraction and simulations. *Phys. Chem. Chem. Phys.*, 13, pp. 3100–3107, with permission from the PCCP Owner Societies.

Different experimental and theoretical studies showed that the cross-section of the tubes in the inverted hexagonal phase is not precisely circular but is rather an intermediate between a circle and a hexagon (Fig. 6.5) (see also Malinin and Lentz, 2004; Perutková et al., 2011; Turner and Gruner, 1992). Nevertheless, in Section 7.4 of this book we assume, for sake of simplicity, that the cross-section is circular.

6.4 Phospholipid Nanotubes

It was previously observed (see Mathivet et al., 1996) that the giant unilamellar phospholipid vesicles, immediately after preparation by the electroformation method (see Angelova et al., 1992) are usually rigid and spherical. It was further indicated (see Mathivet et al.,

1996) (but not observed) that the vesicles are connected by thin tubular membraneous structures. These indications were drawn from an experiment (Mathivet et al., 1996) where a few percent of fluorescent phospholipid NBD-PC was mixed with the unlabelled phospholipid rendering the vesicles fluorescent. A laser beam was applied to the vesicles and suppressed the fluorescence in the affected part of the sample. However, after a very short time (about 2 min.) the fluorescence reappeared. Such quick restoration of fluorescence was unlikely due to transport of phospholipid through the water solution, therefore it was suggested that the vesicles must be connected by very thin and fragile membraneous structures (see Mathivet et al., 1996). Until recently (see Fig. 12.2), these tubular connections have not been directly observed.

When the vesicles are made of the phospholipid POPC and observed under an optical microscope they undergo a slow spontaneous shape transformation in which the difference between the outer and inner membrane layers decreases (Kralj-Iglič et al., 2001a). The mechanism of the shape transformation is not known; suggested possibilities are the inequality of the chemical potential of the phospholipid molecules in the vesicle membrane and in the solution causing a slow but continuous loss of phospholipid molecules from the outer membrane layer into the solution, the drag of the phospholipid molecules from the outer solution of the vesicles by the glass walls of the chamber, the slight evaporation of the liquid caused by imperfect sealing of the chamber by grease, the chemical modification of the phospholipid molecules and their flip-flop (see Kralj-Iglič et al., 2001a). Consequently, the tubular protrusion(s) of vesicles, if present, would become shorter and thicker with time. It was assumed that after a certain period of time the tubular structures (if present) would become thick enough to be visible under the optical microscope. These assumptions proved to be correct. Some time after the solution containing the vesicles was placed into the observation chamber (usually about half an hour) long myelin-like structures appeared attached to the spherical part of the vesicle at one end with the other end usually free. A small number of myelin-like vesicles with a very low volume to area ratio could also be observed. These myelin-like structures are derived from the remnants of the nanotubular network (Fig. 12.2) created during the vesicle formation phase in the electroformation chamber; the network is partially torn when the vesicles are rinsed from the chamber. A description of the experiments proving the existence of phospholipid nanotubes and the results is given below.

6.4.1 Nanotubes of Giant Phospholipid Vesicles

Giant phospholipid vesicles can be prepared at room temperature by the method of electroformation (see Angelova et al., 1992; Heinrich and Waugh, 1996; Kralj-Iglič et al., 2001a). In this procedure 20 µl of phospholipid (or a mixture of phospholipid and fluorescent probe) dissolved in a 2:1 chloroform–methanol mixture was applied to a pair of Pt electrodes. The solvent was allowed to evaporate in a low vacuum for two hours. The electrodes were placed 4 mm apart in the electroformation chamber which was filled with 2 ml of 0.2 M sucrose solution (or with 2 ml of pure water). An AC electric field (1 V/mm, frequency 10 Hz) was applied for two hours. Then, the AC field was reduced to 0.75 V/mm, 5 Hz, and applied for 15 min, to 0.5 V/mm, 2 Hz, and applied for 15 min, and to 0.25 V/mm, 1 Hz, and applied for 30 min. The contents of the chamber were poured into a plastic beaker. The chamber was then filled with 2 ml 0.2 M glucose solution (or with 2 ml of pure water) that contained no phospholipid. This solution was also poured into the solution that was already in the plastic beaker. The contents of the plastic beaker were gently mixed by turning the beaker upside down. Immediately after its preparation, the solution containing the vesicles was placed in the observation chamber made by a pair of cover glasses and sealed by vacuum grease. The vesicles were observed with a phase contrast microscope and with a fluorescence microscope.

After being placed in the observation chamber, the vesicles appeared spherical and had different sizes. Myelin-like protrusions were not visible, nor were long-wavelength shape fluctuations. Short-wavelength shape fluctuations were barely visible. After a certain period of time (of the order of about half an hour) long thin myelin-like protrusions became visible under the fluorescence microscope (Fig. 6.6) and later also under the phase contrast microscope (Fig. 6.8A). Usually, when recognized, the myelin-like shapes appeared as very thin long tubes connected to the vesicle

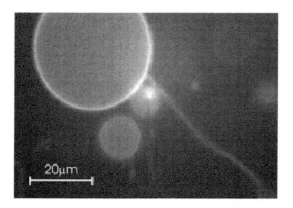

Figure 6.6 A fluorescence microscope image of a vesicle made of POPC and 1.5% NBD-PC. The length of the myelin-like protrusion was several diameters of the spherical part. The fluorescence measurements were made by an inverted optical microscope (IMT-2, Olympus, Japan), using the IMT2-RFL reflected light fluorescence attachment. The dichroic mirror unit (IMT-DMB) allowed excitation from 405 to 490 nm and observation of fluorescence at wavelengths higher than 515 nm. Reprinted from *Colloids and Surfaces A: Physicochemical and Engineering Aspects*, 181(1–3), Veronika Kralj-Iglič, Gregor Gomišček, Janja Majhenc, Vesna Arrigler, Saša Svetina, Myelin-like protrusions of giant phospholipid vesicles prepared by electroformation, pp. 315–318, Copyright 2001, with permission from Elsevier.

surface at one end, while the movement of the myelin-like shapes indicated that they were otherwise free.

In order to obtain a well-focused view of the vesicle and of the protrusions, the vesicles should be prepared in sugar solution (see Kralj-Iglič et al., 2001a). Thus, the vesicles should be grown in sucrose solution and be rinsed out of the electroformation chamber with a glucose solution. The two solutions should be equiosmolar, but as sucrose has larger molecular weight than glucose, the density of the solution inside the vesicles is higher than the density of the surrounding solution and the vesicles sink to the bottom of the observation chamber with the protrusion aligned with it. Thereby, sharp focus can be obtained simultaneously on the spherical part and on the protrusion (see Kralj-Iglič et al., 2001a).

It was considered possible that the chirality of the vesicle membrane constituents might be essential in determining the stable tubular shape of the protrusion. Namely, a theory was proposed (see Selinger et al., 1996) where a stable tubular shape was explained on the basis of chirality. It was shown in Selinger et al. (1996) that the stable tubular shape corresponds to the minimum of membrane free energy obtained by expansion over the curvature and nematic fields. For a nonzero chirality parameter, stable tubes were obtained by orientational ordering of bilayer constituents and also by a periodic helical variation in orientational ordering within stripe-like domains. Further, the proposed theory described modulation of the degree of twist of the ribbons formed by dimeric surfactants associated with chiral counterions (see Oda et al., 1999). It was thus of interest to investigate whether chirality of the bilayer constituents is a prerequisite factor that is responsible for the stability of the thin tubular structures of the phospholipid membrane (see Kralj-Iglič et al., 2001a). The POPC molecules are not chiral, but chirality of the constituents may develop due to their association with ions or glucose from the adjacent solution (Kralj-Iglič, 2002; Oda et al., 1999). In order to clarify this issue, vesicles were prepared and rinsed from the electroformation chamber with pure water. Figure 6.7A shows a first sight of the vesicle with protrusion in pure water. The protrusion is barely visible. The parent sphere is floating in the solution while the protrusion is wobbling, so that it is difficult to obtain a focus on the mother sphere and the protrusion at the same time, or even to obtain a sharp picture of the protrusion. The line in Fig. 6.7B is drawn to help in locating the protrusion. As stable tubular structures were also found in systems containing pure water (see Kralj-Iglič, 2002), this experiment supports the notion that chirality is not a prerequisite mechanism for the stability of phospholipid nanotubes.

From the observations described (Figs. 6.6 and 6.7) (see Kralj-Iglič et al., 2001a; Kralj-Iglič, 2002), we cannot determine the radius of the protrusion. The radius may be much smaller than the width of the shadow seen in the pictures. Further, the direction of the slow shape transformation indicates that the protrusion exists before it becomes visible and is therefore then even thinner. The possibility should be considered that the radius of the tubular protrusion immediately after its formation is very small—of the order of the phospholipid bilayer thickness.

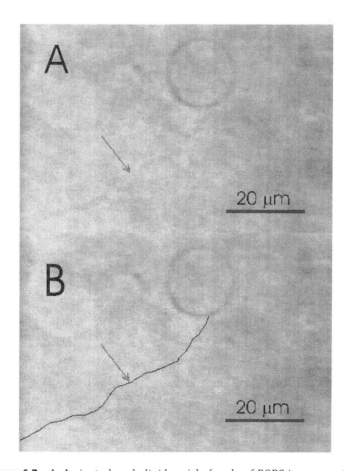

Figure 6.7 A: A giant phospholipid vesicle (made of POPC in pure water) with a long thin tubular protrusion. The vesicle was observed in a closed chamber made of cover glasses, several hours after the preparation. The figure shows the barely visible protrusion, as observed in the beginning of the process. B: A duplicate of the same picture with a line drawn to help in locating the protrusion. The vesicles were observed under an inverted Zeiss IM 35 microscope with phase contrast optics. Reproduced with permission from Kralj-Iglič, V., Iglič, A., Gomišček, G., Sevšek, F., Arrigler, V., and Hägerstrand, H. (2002), Microtubes and nanotubes of a phospholipid bilayer membrane. *J. Phys. A: Math. Gen.*, 35, pp. 1533–1549. Copyright IOP Publishing. doi:10.1088/0305-4470/35/7/305.

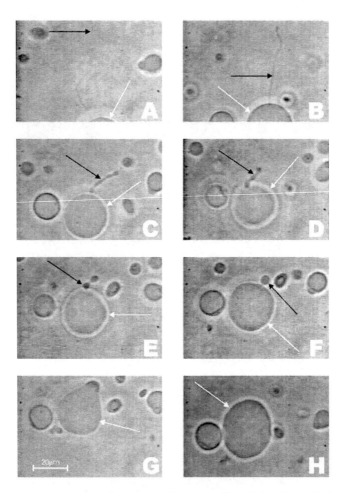

Figure 6.8 Shape transformation of a giant phospholipid vesicle (made of POPC and 1.5% NBD-PC) with time. The times after preparation of the vesicles are A: 3 h, B: 3 h 20 min, C: 4 h, D: 4 h 2 min, E: 4 h 4 min 30 s, F: 4 h 8 min 15 s, G: 4 h 14 min 25 s, H: 4 h 14 min 30 s. The black arrows indicate the protrusion while the white arrows indicate the mother vesicle. The vesicles were observed under an inverted Zeiss IM 35 microscope with phase contrast optics. Reprinted from *Colloids and Surfaces A: Physicochemical and Engineering Aspects*, 181(1–3), Veronika Kralj-Iglič, Gregor Gomišček, Janja Majhenc, Vesna Arrigler, Saša Svetina, Myelin-like protrusions of giant phospholipid vesicles prepared by electroformation, pp. 315–318, Copyright 2001, with permission from Elsevier.

6.4.2 Shape Transformation of the Vesicle with Tubular Protrusion

Vesicles were chosen and followed for several hours. A typical time course of the shape transformation can be seen in Fig. 6.8. The sequence started from a spherical parent vesicle with a long thin myelin-like protrusion that appeared as a cylinder (A). The barely visible protrusion was perceived about three hours after the solution containing the vesicles was placed in the observation chamber. By the time the myelin-like protrusion thickened and shortened (B,C), the undulations of the cylinder became noticeable and more pronounced. The mother vesicle remained more or less spherical. In the shortened myelin-like protrusion, the necks seemed to persist while exhibiting oscillations in their width, making the final phases of the process look-like as if the beads were integrated stepwise into the mother vesicle (D–F). Finally, the neck of the only remaining daughter vesicle opened (G) yielding a globular vesicle (H). Before opening, the neck widened and shrunk several times. The subsequent transformation of the vesicle into a pear shape and further into a prolate shape was completed in seconds (Fig. 6.8F–H).

The long wavelength fluctuations of the mother vesicle increased with shortening of the myelin-like protrusion and became vigorous when the myelin-like protrusion was completely incorporated into the membrane of the mother vesicle.

Chapter 7

Physics of Lipid Micro- and Nanostructures

7.1 Single-Lipid Molecule Energy

Starting from the single molecule energy and applying the methods of statistical mechanics, the free energy of a lipid monolayer (bilayer) is derived in this section (Fournier, 1996; Kralj-Iglič, 2002; Kralj-Iglič et al., 1999, 2006). The local bending energy of a laterally homogeneous monolayer (bilayer) (see Canham, 1970; Helfrich, 1973; Landau and Lifshitz, 1997; Petrov and Derzhanski, 1976) is obtained, and an additional contribution due to average orientational ordering of lipid molecules—that is, the contribution of the deviatoric bending (Fischer, 1992, 1993)—is derived (Kralj-Iglič, 2002; Kralj-Iglič et al., 1999, 2006). The average orientational ordering of anisotropic phospholipids lowers the free energy of the system; the effect is more pronounced for lipid molecules of larger anisotropy and stronger membrane curvature anisotropy (see Kralj-Iglič et al., 2006).

In the lipid monolayer lipid molecules are closely packed to form a sheet-like continuum (Fig. 6.2). A local curvature can be ascribed to this continuum at each chosen point (Fig. 6.2). As there is no

---

Nanostructures in Biological Systems: Theory and Applications
Aleš Iglič, Veronika Kralj-Iglič, and Damjana Drobne
Copyright © 2015 Pan Stanford Publishing Pte. Ltd.
ISBN 978-981-4267-20-5 (Hardcover), 978-981-4303-43-9 (eBook)
www.panstanford.com

apparent evidence for local symmetry of this structure with respect to the axis perpendicular to the membrane, it is generally considered to be anisotropic.

We assume that the lipid molecule, owing to its structure and local interactions, would energetically prefer a local curvature that is described by the two *intrinsic* principal curvatures C_{1m} and C_{2m} (see also Fig. 5.2). The intrinsic principal curvatures are in general not identical (see Fig. 7.1). If they are identical ($C_{1m} = C_{2m}$), the average in-plane orientation of the inclusion is immaterial. Such a lipid molecule is called isotropic. If $C_{1m} \neq C_{2m}$, the lipid molecule is called anisotropic (Fig. 7.1). The average orientation of the lipid molecule is important for its free energy. It is assumed that the lipid molecule spends on average more time in the orientation that is energetically more favourable than in any other orientation.

The energy of a single lipid molecule is assumed to depend on the mismatch between curvature tensors $\underline{C}_m$ (Eq. 6.3) and $\underline{C}$ (Eq. 5.32). In general, the curvature tensors $\underline{C}_m$ and $\underline{C}$ have different orientations, that is, they are rotated by an angle ω with respect to each other. To express the mismatch between $\underline{C}_m$ and $\underline{C}$ we introduce the mismatch tensor $\underline{M}$:

$$\underline{M} = \underline{R}\,\underline{C}_m\underline{R}^{-1} - \underline{C}, \qquad (7.1)$$

where $\underline{R}$ is the transformation matrix for rotation,

$$\underline{R} = \begin{bmatrix} \cos\omega & -\sin\omega \\ \sin\omega & \cos\omega \end{bmatrix}. \qquad (7.2)$$

The single molecule energy at a given point of the membrane should be a scalar quantity, hence it may by expressed by two invariants of the tensor $\underline{M}$, trace and determinant:

$$E = \frac{K_1}{2}(\mathrm{Tr}(\underline{M}))^2 + K_2 \mathrm{Det}(\underline{M}), \qquad (7.3)$$

where K_1 and K_2 are constants (see Kralj-Iglič et al., 2006). Eq. 7.3 can be rewritten as

$$E = (2K_1 + K_2)(H - H_m)^2 - K_2(D^2 - 2DD_m\cos(2\omega) + D_m^2), \qquad (7.4)$$

where H is the mean curvature of the membrane (Eq. 5.33), H_m is the mean intrinsic (spontaneous) curvature of the molecule (Eq. 6.4), D and D_m are the curvature deviators of the membrane and

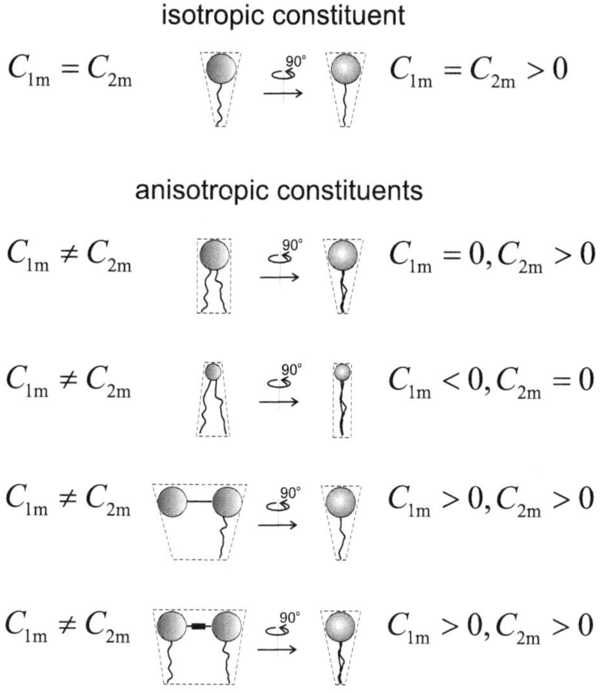

Single-Lipid Molecule Energy | 101

isotropic constituent

$C_{1m} = C_{2m}$ $C_{1m} = C_{2m} > 0$

anisotropic constituents

$C_{1m} \neq C_{2m}$ $C_{1m} = 0, C_{2m} > 0$

$C_{1m} \neq C_{2m}$ $C_{1m} < 0, C_{2m} = 0$

$C_{1m} \neq C_{2m}$ $C_{1m} > 0, C_{2m} > 0$

$C_{1m} \neq C_{2m}$ $C_{1m} > 0, C_{2m} > 0$

Figure 7.1 Schematic representation of the different intrinsic shapes of some isotropic and anisotropic lipids and detergents. Front and side views are shown.

the molecule (Eqs. 5.35 and 6.5), respectively (see Kralj-Iglič et al., 2006). In the following we introduce the definitions:

$$(2K_1 + K_2) = \frac{\xi}{2} \quad \text{and} \quad K_2 = -\frac{(\xi + \xi^*)}{4}. \quad (7.5)$$

Constants ξ and ξ^* describe the strength of intermolecular interactions. Using the definitions of ξ and ξ^*, Eq. 7.4 can be rewritten in the form:

$$E(\omega) = \frac{\xi}{2}(H - H_m)^2 + \frac{\xi + \xi^*}{4}(D^2 - 2DD_m \cos(2\omega) + D_m^2). \quad (7.6)$$

It is obvious that the energy expressed by Eq. 7.6 reaches its minimum when $\cos(2\omega) = 1$ and its maximum when $\cos(2\omega) = -1$. In the first case, the systems of tensors $\underline{C}_m$ and $\underline{C}$ are aligned ($\omega = 0$) or rotated by an angle $\omega = \pi$ with respect to each other:

$$E_{\min} = \frac{\xi}{2}(H - H_m)^2 + \frac{\xi + \xi^*}{4}(D^2 + D_m^2) - \frac{\xi + \xi^*}{2}DD_m, \quad (7.7)$$

while in the second case the systems are rotated by an angle $\omega = \pi/2$ or $\omega = 3\pi/2$ with respect to each other:

$$E_{max} = \frac{\xi}{2}(H - H_m)^2 + \frac{\xi + \xi^*}{4}(D^2 + D_m^2) + \frac{\xi + \xi^*}{2}DD_m. \quad (7.8)$$

The energy states at $\omega = 0, \pi$ and at $\omega = \pi/2, 3\pi/2$, respectively, are degenerate.

The free energy of a single lipid molecule (f_i) can be derived if all possible orientations of the molecule are taken into account. In this case the partition function of a single lipid molecule is (see Fournier, 1996; Kralj-Iglič et al., 1999):

$$Q_1 = \frac{1}{\omega_0} \int_0^{2\pi} \exp\left(-\frac{E(\omega)}{kT}\right) d\omega, \quad (7.9)$$

where ω_0 is an arbitrary angle quantum and the energy E is defined by Eq. 7.6. Taking into account that

$$\int_0^{2\pi} \exp\left(\frac{(\xi + \xi^*)DD_m \cos(2\omega)}{2\,kT}\right) d\omega = I_0\left(\frac{(\xi + \xi^*)DD_m}{2kT}\right), \quad (7.10)$$

and $f_i = -kT \ln Q_1$, it follows from Eq. 7.10 that (Kralj-Iglič et al., 1999, 2006):

$$f_i = \frac{\xi}{2}(H - H_m)^2 + \frac{\xi + \xi^*}{4}(D^2 + D_m^2) - kT \ln\left(I_0\left(\frac{(\xi + \xi^*)DD_m}{2kT}\right)\right), \quad (7.11)$$

where I_0 is the modified Bessel function.

Within the *two-energies state model* (E_{min} and E_{max}), that is, considering only orientations $\omega = 0, \pi/2, 3\pi/2, \pi$, the single molecule free energy (f_i) can be derived from the partition function:

$$Q_1 = 2\exp(-E_{min}/kT) + 2\exp(-E_{max}/kT), \quad (7.12)$$

where the orientations 0 and π and orientations $\pi/2$ and $3\pi/2$ are considered to be indistinguishable. The corresponding free energy of a single lipid molecule can then be obtained by the expression

$$f_i = -kT \ln Q_1 = \frac{\xi}{2}(H - H_m)^2 + \frac{\xi + \xi^*}{4}(D^2 + D_m^2)$$
$$-kT \ln[\cosh((\xi + \xi^*)DD_m/2kT)], \quad (7.13)$$

where we omitted the constant terms.

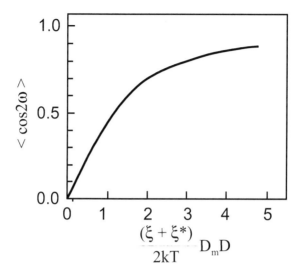

Figure 7.2 Average orientation of a single lipid molecule described by $\langle\cos(2\omega)\rangle$ as a function of $(\xi + \xi^*)DD_m/2kT$ (see Iglič et al., 2000).

Note that the third terms in Eqs. 7.13 and 7.11 are very similar and also give the same limit values for large or small arguments. In the limit of small $(\xi + \xi^*)DD_m/2kT$, Eqs. 7.13 and 7.11 reduce to the ordinary Helfrich Hamiltonian (Helfrich, 1973). However, in the limit of large $(\xi + \xi^*)DD_m/2kT$ Eqs. 7.13 and 7.11 transform into:

$$f_i \cong \frac{\xi}{2}(H - H_m)^2 + \frac{\xi + \xi^*}{4}(D^2 + D_m^2) - \frac{\xi + \xi^*}{2}DD_m, \qquad (7.14)$$

where, $D = (H^2 - C_1C_2)^{1/2}$, which cannot be written in the form of a Helfrich Hamiltonian.

The average orientation of the lipid molecule may be given by $\langle\cos(2\omega)\rangle$,

$$\langle\cos(2\omega)\rangle = \frac{I_1\left(\left|\frac{(\xi+\xi^*)D_m D}{2kT}\right|\right)}{I_0\left(\frac{(\xi+\xi^*)D_m D}{2kT}\right)}. \qquad (7.15)$$

where I_1 is the modified Bessel function (see Iglič et al., 2000). Figure 7.2 shows the average orientation of a single anisotropic lipid molecule as a function of $(\xi + \xi^*)DD_m/2kT$. For small $(\xi + \xi^*)DD_m/2kT$, the lipid molecules are randomly oriented. The average orientational ordering increases $(\xi + \xi^*)DD_m/2kT$.

7.2 Bending Energy of the Anisotropic Lipid Monolayer

To derive the bending energy of the whole, in general anisotropic lipid monolayer, the membrane monolayer is divided into small patches, each containing a sufficiently large number of lipid molecules in order to apply the methods of statistical mechanics (see Kralj-Iglič et al., 2006). The principal curvatures C_1 and C_2 are taken to be constant over the patch and phospholipid molecules are considered to be equal and independent. Considering a simple two-energy state model (Eqs. 7.7 and 7.8), there are M equivalent molecules within the patch. Each molecule can exist in a state of lower energy E_{min} or higher energy E_{max}, just like in the description of a two-orientation model of non-interacting magnetic dipoles in an external magnetic field (see Hill, 1986). In our model, the external magnetic field is represented by the curvature deviator D (see Kralj-Iglič et al., 2006). N molecules are assumed to be in the state with maximal energy E_{max} and $(M - N)$ molecules are in the state with minimal energy E_{min}:

$$E_D = NE_{max} + (M - N)E_{min}, \qquad (7.16)$$

where E_D is the deviatoric bending energy of the membrane patch. Introducing Eqs. 7.7 and 7.8 into Eq. 7.16 gives:

$$E_D = ME_q - \left(\frac{M}{2} - N\right) kT d_{eff}, \qquad (7.17)$$

where

$$E_q = \frac{\xi}{2}(H - H_m)^2 + \frac{\xi + \xi^*}{4}(D^2 + D_m^2) \qquad (7.18)$$

and

$$d_{eff} = \frac{(\xi + \xi^*) D_m D}{kT}. \qquad (7.19)$$

The parameter d_{eff} is called the effective curvature deviator (see Kralj-Iglič et al., 2006).

Another contribution to the bending energy is that due to direct interactions between the phospholipid molecules. At most the molecules interact with their nearest neighbours. It is assumed that if the actual shape of the membrane is attuned to the local curvature field, the tails of the molecules move closer together and this leads to lowering of the energy. On the other hand, if the molecules are oriented less favourably, the chain packing is less dense. This causes an increase in energy. It is considered that this effect is proportional to d_{eff} (Eq. 7.19). Direct interaction energy of N molecules that exhibit less favourable packing is taken into account by the expression:

$$E_N = \tilde{k} N d_{\text{eff}}, \qquad (7.20)$$

while the direct interaction energy of molecules that exhibit more favourable packing (negative contribution) is described by

$$E_{M-N} = -\tilde{k}(M - N)d_{\text{eff}}, \qquad (7.21)$$

where $\tilde{k}$ is the interaction constant (see Kralj-Iglič et al., 2006). The total energy caused by direct interaction is given by summation of Eqs. 7.20 and 7.21 divided by 2 so as to avoid counting each molecule twice:

$$E_i = -\tilde{k}\left(\frac{M}{2} - N\right)d_{\text{eff}}. \qquad (7.22)$$

The total bending energy of the patch is thus

$$E^P = E_D + E_i, \qquad (7.23)$$

where E_D is the contribution of the mutual orientation of the local curvature tensor and intrinsic curvature tensor (deviatoric bending), and E_i is the contribution of the direct interaction between the neighbour molecules.

We consider all the patches to have a constant area A^P, a constant number of molecules M and a constant temperature T of the system. The phospholipid molecules within the system are treated as indistinguishable. We assume that the system is in thermodynamic equilibrium and only two energy states of the single molecule are possible. The canonical partition function $Q^P(M, T, D)$ of M molecule in the patch of the membrane is therefore

$$Q^P = \sum_{N=0}^{M} \frac{M!}{N!(M-N)!} \exp\left(-\frac{E^P}{kT}\right), \qquad (7.24)$$

where the energy of the patch E^P is defined by Eq. 7.23. Using Eqs. 7.17–7.24 gives

$$Q^P = q^M \sum_{N=0}^{M} \frac{M!}{N!(M-N)!} \exp\left(d_{\text{eff}}\left(1 + \frac{\tilde{k}}{kT}\right)\left(\frac{M}{2} - N\right)\right), \qquad (7.25)$$

where by considering Eq. 8.22:

$$q = \exp\left(-\frac{E_q}{kT}\right). \tag{7.26}$$

Using the binomial (Newton) formula for summation of the finite series in Eq. 7.25 yields:

$$Q^{\mathrm{p}} = \left(2q \cosh\left(\frac{d_{\mathrm{eff}}(1 + \tilde{k}/kT)}{2}\right)\right)^M. \tag{7.27}$$

The Helmholtz free energy of the patch is $F^{\mathrm{P}} = -kT \ln Q^{\mathrm{P}}$. Combining Eqs. 7.25–7.27 yields the free energy of the patch:

$$F^{\mathrm{P}} = M\frac{\xi}{2}\left[(H - H_{\mathrm{m}})^2 + D^2 + D_{\mathrm{m}}^2\right] \tag{7.28}$$
$$-kT\, M \ln\left[2\cosh\left(\frac{(1 + \tilde{k}/kT)\xi D_{\mathrm{m}} D}{kT}\right)\right].$$

where we used the relation $D^2 = H^2 - C_1 C_2$ (Eq. 5.36) and assumed $\xi = \xi^*$ (which yields $K_1 = -K_2$).

The bending energy of the monolayer is then obtained by summing the contributions of all the patches of the monolayer, that is, F^{P} (Eq. 7.28) is integrated over the whole monolayer area A (Kralj-Iglič et al., 2006):

$$F_{\mathrm{b}} = \int_A \frac{n_0 \xi}{2}\left((H - H_{\mathrm{m}})^2 + D^2 + D_{\mathrm{m}}^2\right) \mathrm{d}A$$
$$- n_0 kT \int_A \ln\left(2\cosh\left(\frac{\xi(1 + \tilde{k}/kT)D_{\mathrm{m}} D}{kT}\right)\right) \mathrm{d}A, \tag{7.29}$$

where n_0 is the area density of the lipid molecules (Kralj-Iglič et al., 2006) and $\mathrm{d}A$ is the area element of the lipid monolayer.

Being aware of diverse contributions to the direct interaction between the phospholipid molecules, we attempt only to give a rough estimate of its order of magnitude. We can estimate the energy $\tilde{k}/kT$ by van der Waals interactions between the tails of orientationally ordered and disordered nearest neighbours of a given molecule. We assume that the phospholipid molecules are distributed in a quadratic lattice and take into account the nearest tails of the neighbouring molecules. The tail of a phospholipid molecule is described as a cylinder. The energy of the van der Waals interaction between two cylinders with aligned geometrical axes is $w_W(\delta) = A_H L\sqrt{r_0}/24\delta^{3/2}$, where A_H is the Hamaker constant (see Israelachvili, 1997), L is the length of the cylinders, δ is the distance between the cylinders and r_0 is the radius of the cylinders. For hydrocarbons, $A_H = 3\,kT/4$ (see Israelachvili, 1997) while we take for lipid molecules $L = 1.5$ nm, $r_0 = 3.5$ nm and $\delta = 0.3$ nm. The estimated energy is $\tilde{k}/kT = 2\,w_W(\delta)/kT \simeq 1$ (Kralj-Iglič et al., 2006).

In the simplest case where only isotropic phospholipid molecules within the lipid monolayer are taken into account ($D_m = 0$), our general expression for the monolayer bending energy (Eq. 7.29) transforms into the Helfrich expression for the local bending energy of a lipid monolayer (see Helfrich, 1973):

$$F_b = \int_A \left(\frac{k_c}{2}(2H - C_0)^2 + k_G K \right) dA , \qquad (7.30)$$

where f_b is the area density of the Helfrich local bending energy. The bending constants k_c and k_G are:

$$k_c = \frac{\xi n_0}{2}, \qquad (7.31)$$

$$k_G = -\frac{\xi n_0}{2}, \qquad (7.32)$$

while the expression for the spontaneous (intrinsic) curvature C_0 is equal to the intrinsic mean curvature of a single lipid molecule:

$$C_0 = H_m . \qquad (7.33)$$

7.3 Comparison between Planar, Inverted Spherical and Inverted Cylindrical Monolayer Nanostructures

As already mentioned, due their amphiphilic character (i.e., polar head groups and non-polar hydrocarbon chains in one molecule) the lipid molecules in aqueous solution undergo a self-assembling process and form various structures such as cylindrical, spherical, inverted spherical, and hexagonal (inverted cylindrical) micelles (Fig. 6.1). Biologically important lipid–water systems are known for their rich polymorphism (Seddon and Templer, 1995). The driving force for this process is predominantly the hydrophobic effect where the hydrophilic (polar) surfaces are in contact with water solution, while the hydrophobic (non-polar) parts composed of lipid headgroups are hidden from water (Chandler, 2002, 2005).

The most common and biologically the most relevant phase is the fluid lamellar lipid bilayer phase (L_α). Nevertheless, non-lamellar model membranes are a subject of increasing interest (Cullis et al., 1986; Luzzati, 1997; Luzzati et al., 1968; Perutková et al., 2011; Seddon and Templer, 1995), due to their importance in living organisms and due to their promising technical applications such as in drug delivery (see Larsson and Tiberg, 2005; Yaghmur et al., 2007), gene transport and nanotechnology (Attard et al., 1995).

To shed light on the role of the deviatoric bending energy (Eq. 7.29) in the stability of different lipid nanostructures, in this section the bending (free) energy per lipid molecule in three different geometries with constant principal curvatures (see Fig. 6.1), that is, planar (corresponding to the lamellar L_α phase), spherical (corresponding to the inverted micellar M_{II} phase) and cylindrical (corresponding to the inverted hexagonal H_{II} phase) is compared in Fig. 7.3.

In the planar system, $H = D = 0$, in the spherical system, $H = -1/r_s$ and $D = 0$, while in the inverted cylindrical system $H = -D = -1/2r$, where r_s is the radius of the sphere and r is the radius of the cylinder. The free (bending) energy per lipid molecule in the lipid monolayer with constant curvature is calculated by using Eq. 7.29:

$$F = \frac{F_b}{n_0 A} = \frac{\xi}{2}\left((H - H_m)^2 + D^2 + D_m^2\right)$$
$$-kT \ln\left(2 \cosh\left(\frac{(1 + \tilde{k}/kT)\xi D_m D}{kT}\right)\right). \quad (7.34)$$

Here, $n_0 A$ is the total number of lipid molecules in the membrane of area A. The value of interaction constant ξ was estimated from the monolayer bending constant $\xi = 2k_c a_0$, where for POPE $k_c = 11\,kT$ is the bending constant (Laggner et al., 1991) and $a_0 = 1/n_0 = 0.65 \cdot 10^{-18}$ m^2 is the area per phospholipid molecule (Rappolt et al., 2003).

Figure 7.3 shows the equilibrium bending energy per lipid molecule as a function of mean intrinsic curvature $H_m = (C_{1m} + C_{2m})/2$

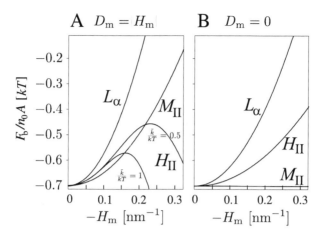

Figure 7.3 The equilibrium bending energy per lipid molecule $F = F_b/n_0 A$ (Eq. 7.34) as a function of the intrinsic mean curvature H_m for the L_α, M_{II} and H_{II} phases. A: a system composed of anisotropic molecules ($D_m = |H_m|$) and B: a system composed of isotropic molecules ($D_m = 0$). Reprinted with permission from Mareš, T., Daniel, M., Perutkova, Š., Perne, A., Dolinar, G., Iglič, A., Rappolt, M., and Kralj-Iglič, V. Role of phospholipid asymmetry in the stability of inverted hexagonal mesoscopic phases. *J. Phys. Chem. B.*, 112(51), pp. 16575–16584. Copyright 2008, American Chemical Society.

for anisotropic wedge-like molecules (with $C_{1m} < 0$, $C_{2m} = 0$ or $C_{2m} < 0$, $C_{1m} = 0$) having $|H_m| = D_m$ (panel A) and isotropic molecules (with $C_{2m} = C_{1m}$), for which $D_m = |C_{2m} - C_{1m}|/2 = 0$ (panel B) (see also Fig. 7.1). For small $|H_m| = D_m$, the bending energy increases with increase in $|H_m|$ in all three geometries (panel A). In the M_{II} and L_α phases which are isotropic with respect to curvature (i.e., having $D = |C_2 - C_1|/2 = 0$), there is no orientational ordering of the molecules and the bending energy monotonously increases also for larger $|H_m| = D_m$. In the H_{II} phase, however, the non-zero values of both, the intrinsic curvature deviator D_m and the curvature deviator D give rise to a negative energy contribution of the deviatoric bending energy (last term in Eq. 7.34). Therefore, the equilibrium free energy reaches a maximum upon increase in D_m (which for this particular choice of molecules is equal to $|H_m|$), but then decreases at a certain threshold, and such that the H_{II} phase becomes energetically the most favourable.

Summing up, for small $D_m = |H_m|$, the M_{II} phase has the lowest bending energy, while at larger $D_m = |H_m|$, the H_{II} phase becomes the most favourable due to the average orientational ordering of phospholipid molecules. The effect is stronger for higher values of the constant $\tilde{k}$ (see Eq. 7.21) describing the direct interaction between phospholipid tails (see Fig. 7.3A).

Figure 7.3B shows that for isotropic molecules (having $D_m = 0$, i.e., $C_{1m} = C_{2m}$, see also Fig. 7.1), the M_{II} phase is always favoured, that is, the calculated energy per lipid $F_b/n_0 A$ in the M_{II} phase is equal to the reference value and is the smallest compared to the energy of the L_α and the H_{II} phases. We note that for isotropic molecules there can be no energy lowering due to the average orientational ordering of the molecules since all orientations of the lipid molecules are energetically equivalent.

The deviatoric bending of anisotropic molecules may thus alone explain the stability of the H_{II} phase at higher temperatures. At lower temperatures, the M_{II} phase is energetically favoured except for $D_m = |H_m| = 0$, where the L_α phase is the stable phase. At small $D_m = |H_m|$, however, the equilibrium radii of the simulated M_{II} phase are so large that this case would correspond to flat membrane systems. For some intermediate $|H_m| = D_m$ the simulated M_{II} phase consists of aggregated micelles of a given size, but such configurations were actually not observed (Delacroix et al., 1996; Seddon et al., 2000).

To obtain better agreement with experimental observations also in the intermediate range of $D_m = |H_m|$, we include the effect of the void-filling energy (already discussed in a previous chapter) using a simple model where the void-filling energy is considered constant for a given geometry (see also Kozlov et al., 1994). Figure 7.4 shows the minimal free energy $F/n_0 A = F_b/n_0 A + F_i/n_0 A$ as a function of the intrinsic mean curvature $|H_m|$ for the L_α, H_{II} and M_{II} phases. Here, F_i is the interstitial (void-filling) energy (see Mareš et al., 2008). Since the energy contribution of voids is smaller in the system of close packed inverted cylinders than in the system of close-packed inverted spheres, the value of the void-filling energy per lipid molecule $F_i/n_0 A$ was taken to be lower for cylinders than for spheres. It was estimated from the results of Kozlov et al. (1994) that $F_i/n_0 A$ should be of the order of kT, therefore it was taken

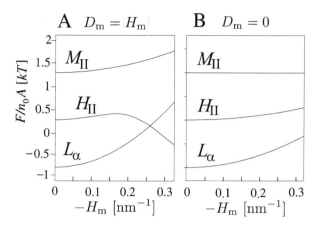

Figure 7.4 The equilibrium free energy per lipid molecule $F/n_0 A = F_b/n_0 A + F_i/n_0 A$ consisting of the contribution of bending (F_b) and (constant) void-filling energy (F_i), calculated per lipid molecule as a function of the intrinsic mean curvature $|H_m|$ for the L_α ($F_i/n_0 A = 0$), H_{II} ($F_i/n_0 A = 1kT$) and M_{II} ($F_i/n_0 A = 2kT$) phases. A: $D_m = |H_m|$ and B: $D_m = 0$, $\tilde{k}/kT = 1$. Reprinted with permission from Mareš, T., Daniel, M., Perutkova, Š., Perne, A., Dolinar, G., Iglič, A., Rappolt, M., and Kralj-Iglič, V. Role of phospholipid asymmetry in the stability of inverted hexagonal mesoscopic phases. *J. Phys. Chem. B.*, 112(51), pp. 16575–16584. Copyright 2008, American Chemical Society.

for the H_{II} phase that $F_i/n_0 A = 1kT$ and for the M_{II} phase that $F_i/n_0 A = 2kT$.

In Figs. 7.4(A) and 7.4(B), the curves corresponding to the H_{II} and M_{II} phases (see Fig. 7.3) are shifted up by different constants $F_i/n_0 A$, respectively, and the overall picture is now more realistic. As a consequence, it can be seen in Figs. 7.4(A) and 7.4(B) that for small $D_m = |H_m|$ the L_α phase is energetically the most favourable, since it requires no void-filling energy F_i. For anisotropic molecules (Fig. 7.4(A)) at a certain threshold $D_m = |H_m|$ the H_{II} phase becomes energetically the most favourable due to the average orientational ordering of the lipid molecules. In the isotropic case (Fig. 7.4(B)), all the curves monotonously increase, but the curve corresponding to the L_α phase increases faster and therefore it would eventually intersect with the curve corresponding to the H_{II} phase. However, the value of H_m where the intersection would take place would be very high (out of the range given in Fig. 7.4), where the maximal value 0.4 nm^{-1} already corresponds to a cylinder with a radius of 1.25 nm.

To conclude, the effects shown in Fig. 7.4(A) indicate that in the simple model where the interstitial energy is taken to be constant within a phase (Kozlov et al., 1994; Mareš et al., 2008; Perutková et al., 2009), an increase in $D_m = |H_m|$, caused by the increase in temperature can induce the transformation from L_α to H_{II} lipid phase. The interstitial energy for small $|H_m|$ (lower temperature) renders the L_α phase energetically the most favourable. However at a certain threshold, $D_m = |H_m|$ (higher temperature) the H_{II} phase becomes energetically the most favourable in accordance with experimental results.

Having eliminated the M_{II} phase due to high packing frustration (see Fig. 7.4), in the following section we compare only the L_α and H_{II} phases using an improved model for the void-filling energy, where stretching of the lipid tails in the actual hexagonal geometry is taken into account (Fig. 6.4 and Eq. 7.42).

7.4 A Detailed Study of the Stability of the Inverted Hexagonal Phase

Transition of the lamellar to inverted hexagonal phase and the mechanisms that drive this transition are the main subjects of this section. To interpret the experimental data and to contribute to a better understanding of the underlying mechanisms, different models have been put forward (Kachar and Reese, 1982; Kozlov et al., 1994; Rappolt et al., 2003, 2008; Siegel, 1988).

The majority of theoretical models of the formation of the inverted hexagonal phase have in common the assumption that nucleation starts with a line defect. Based on freeze-fracture electron micrograph experiments, a deformation pair of intramembrane cylinders embedded in a tight junction was proposed (Kachar and Reese, 1982), and also monolayer-embedded lipid tubes formed via the coalescence of a "string-of-pearls" of inverted micellar intermediates (IMI), as suggested by Hui et al. (1983). In 1986 Siegel further elaborated this model of the L_α–H_{II} transition (Siegel, 1988).

He proposed a three-step process with formation of intermediates driven by changes in temperature and lipid composition. The first step is formation of IMI, which form between two sufficiently close opposed bilayers. The IMI can diffuse within the plane of the membrane and form an IMI coalescence representing the second step. Two possible ways of IMI coalescence were suggested. Two spherical micelles can fuse into a single rod-shaped micelle and form rod-like micellar intermediates (RMI) or they can separate within the coalescence intermediate and form line defects (LD) (Siegel, 1988).

Temperature affects the configuration of phospholipid molecules in the head-group and in the tail regions (Israelachvili, 1997). The motion of the hydrocarbon chain increases with increase in temperature, consequently there is an increasing relative number of "gauche" C–C bond configurations which require more space in the lateral (in-plane) direction of the monolayer. Since there are two tails, they effectively spread in the direction of their alignment, thereby also increasing the anisotropy of the tail region (Rappolt et al., 2008). In fact, a simple molecular wedge shape model which was applied to interpret experimental X-ray data in the inverted hexagonal phase of a PE–water system demonstrates clearly that the wedge angle increases monotonously as a function of temperature (see Rappolt et al., 2008, and Fig. 7.5(B)).

Based on the temperature-dependent experimental results from differential scanning calorimetry and small-angle X-ray scattering, another view of the L_α–H_{II} transition is given by Rappolt et al. (2003, 2008). The hypothesis of the growth mechanism of the first few rods is connected with spontaneous creation of the line defect (water core) at the transition temperature. The first rod is created due to the spontaneous monolayer curvature, which induces the formation of new water cores. The pivotal plane arrangement corresponding to the first few steps of the transition was proposed in Rappolt et al. (2008) (see Fig. 7.6). The first cylinder of the H_{II} phase formed from the first line defect is created between two bilayers. Thus, a system of one cylinder, two monolayers and bulbous closures on both sides of the cylinder is introduced. The bulbous closures are created from neighbouring disjunct layers as a consequence of reducing the water cores. The two outer monolayer leaflets follow the contours of the

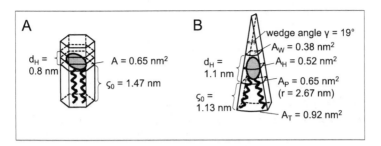

Figure 7.5 Simplest space filling molecular models for the fluid lamellar (A) and the inverted hexagonal phase (B). The models are derived from structural data on POPE at $T = 74\,°C$, at which the L_α phase coexists with the H_{II} phase (Rappolt et al., 2003). (A) The steric length of the lipid molecule of 2.27 nm can be divided into the head-group extension, d_H (0.8 nm), and the hydrocarbon chain length, ζ_0 (1.47 nm). The area per lipid was determined to be 0.65 nm^2. (B) The simplest anisotropic molecular model for PE lipids in the inverted hexagonal phase. The different molecular areas are defined graphically, comprising the lipid–water, the head-group, the pivotal, and the terminal interface, respectively. Explicit values for the areas are given, the area per lipid at the head-group position $A_H = 0.52$ nm^2. Figure adapted from Perutková et al. (2009) and Rappolt et al. (2008).

cylinder and the bulbous closures. This configuration is the smallest geometrical unit appropriate to study the nucleation of the H_{II}–L_α transition.

In general, solving the stability conditions for different lipid phases, as well as conditions for the transition between lipid phases, is the problem of defining the free energy of the system and its minimization. In the following a brief overview of theoretical models of the L_α to H_{II} phase transition and the corresponding expression for the free energy of the system are described.

Kozlov et al. (1994) studied the energy of the hexagonal phase in the H_{II}–L_α–H_{II} re-entrant phase transition of dioleoylphosphatidylethanolamine (DOPE) upon changes in hydration and temperature. Combining osmotic stress and X-ray diffraction experiments, the spontaneous curvature (R_0^{-1}) and the monolayer bending constant (k_c) of the H_{II} phase were determined. Further, they considered a theoretical model describing the stability of hexagonal and lamellar lipid phases by minimization of the free

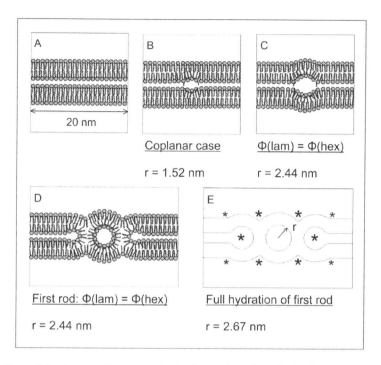

Figure 7.6 Intermediate steps in the formation of a cylinder between two bilayers. The structural schemes are based on structural data for POPE recorded at the transition temperature $T = 74\,°C$ (see Rappolt et al., 2003). Pivotal interfaces are outlined by full lines and for ease of interpretation lipid molecules are superimposed in the first four panels. (A) The fluid lamellar phase can be decomposed into a steric monolayer of thickness 2.27 nm and a free water layer of thickness 0.27 nm. (B) By spontaneous splay of lipid molecules a line defect may form, which is integrated in the stack of bilayers in a coplanar fashion. (C) If one sets the water concentration per lipid in the line defect, Φ_{hex}, to be equal to the water concentration given in the fluid lamellar phase, Φ_{lam}, then the radius of the pivotal plane increases from $r = 1.52$ nm to 2.44 nm. (D) This panel shows the formation of a first rod under the condition $\Phi_{lam} = \Phi_{hex}$. (E) Finally, full hydration of the first cylinder between two bilayers increases the pivotal plane radius to $r = 2.67$ nm. Loci for the formation of new cylinders are marked with stars (Perutková et al., 2009; Rappolt et al., 2008). Reprinted from *Chemistry and Physics of Lipids*, 154(1), Michael Rappolt, Aden Hodzic, Barbara Sartori, Michel Ollivon, Peter Laggner. Conformational and hydrational properties during the L_β- to L_α- and L_α- to H_{II}-phase transition in phosphatidylethanolamine, pp. 46–55, Copyright 2008, with permission from Elsevier.

energy composed of elastic, hydration, interstitial and van der Waals energies.

In the model of Kozlov and colleagues, the free energy of the hexagonal phase was approximated by the elastic energy of the local bending deformation (Helfrich, 1973):

$$F^H = N_l^H \frac{1}{2} k_c a_0 \left(\frac{1}{R} - \frac{1}{R_0} \right)^2, \qquad (7.35)$$

where N_l^H is the number of lipid molecules, k_c is the bending elasticity of the lipid monolayer, a_0 is the area per lipid molecule, $1/R$ is the curvature of the pivotal plane of the lipid monolayer and $1/R_0$ is the spontaneous curvature in the fully hydrated (unstressed) state. For convenience, it was assumed that the free energy of the fully hydrated hexagonal phase is 0 ($1/R = 1/R_0$) (Kozlov et al., 1994).

The free energy of the lamellar phase was assumed to be of the form:

$$F^L = N_l^L \frac{1}{2} P_0 \lambda a_0 \exp\left(-\frac{d_w}{\lambda}\right) - N_l^L a_0 \frac{A_H}{24\pi d_w^2} + N_l^L a_0 \frac{1}{2} k_c \frac{1}{R_0^2} - N_l^L g_i, \qquad (7.36)$$

where N_l^L is the number of lipid molecules in the lamellar phase and d_w is the thickness of the water layer separating the bilayers. The first term is the energy of hydration repulsion between the bilayers (P_0 and λ are the pre-exponential factor and the characteristic length of the repulsion, respectively). The second term is the leading term in the energy of the van der Waals interaction between the bilayers, where A_H is the Hamaker constant (Israelachvili, 1997). The last two terms describe the difference between the free energies in the fully hydrated hexagonal and lamellar phases and form a constant contribution independent of the distance between the bilayers. The third term is the energy of "unbending" the lipid monolayer to flatness according to Eq. 7.35 and the last term represents the energy associated with voids in the hexagonal lattice. For simplicity, $g_i > 0$ was referred to as the curvature-independent part of the interstitial energy (the curvature-dependent part is accounted for within the elastic energy of the inverted hexagonal phase F^H (Eq. 7.35)) (Kozlov et al., 1994).

Kozlov et al. assumed that all the parameters in Eqs. 7.35 and 7.36 except the intrinsic curvature R_0 are independent on temperature. By assuming a negligible dependence of g_i on temperature and equating the free energies in the hexagonal and lamellar phases in excess water at the temperature for the re-entrant transition ($T_H = 10°C$) we obtain (Kozlov et al., 1994):

$$g_i = \frac{1}{2}k_c a_0 \frac{1}{[R_0(T_H)]^2} + \frac{1}{2}P_0 a_0 \lambda \exp\left(-\frac{d_{wmax}}{\lambda}\right) - \frac{a_0 A_H}{24\pi (d_{wmax})^2}, \tag{7.37}$$

where N_l^L and N_l^H are taken to be equal and the free energy of the inverted hexagonal lipid phase is assumed to be $F^H = 0$ (i.e., $1/R = 1/R_0$), d_{wmax} represents the equilibrium spacing in the lamellar phase in the absence of osmotic stress and T_H is the temperature of the hexagonal-lamellar re-entrant transition in excess water. The energy g_i was computed by substituting the measured parameters into Eq. 7.37 and is a positive constant for this case.

In summary, Kozlov et al. described a model of the L_α–H_{II}–L_α re-entrant transition. On the basis of experiments, they derived the structural parameters and all of the force constants defining the energetic terms of the H_{II} and L_α lipid phases. They found an expression for the interstitial energy of the inverted hexagonal phase as the constant difference between the H_{II} and L_α phases at the transition point.

Another study on the hexagonal phase was performed by Rand et al. (1990). In this work two types of energy contributions to the free energy of the lipid monolayer were taken into account:

$$G_{H_{II}} = \frac{1}{2}k_c a_0 \left(\frac{1}{R} - \frac{1}{R_0}\right)^2 + \Pi V_w. \tag{7.38}$$

The first term in Eq. 7.38 introduces the local bending energy and the second term is the osmotic energy, where k_c is the bending modulus, a_0 is the area per lipid molecule, R and R_0 are the actual local radius of curvature and the intrinsic radius of curvature at the pivotal plane, respectively. Π is the the difference in osmotic pressure between the outer and inner solution of the H_{II} cylinder and V_w is the volume of water per lipid inside the cylinder (Rand et al., 1990).

Without consideration of the energy of interstices, Rand et al. (1990) made two approximations. The first approximation was that the water cylinders are perfectly circular in cross-section (see Fig. 7.7(A)). Second, the interstitial energy is supposed to be independent of the size of the hexagonal unit cell (Rand et al., 1990).

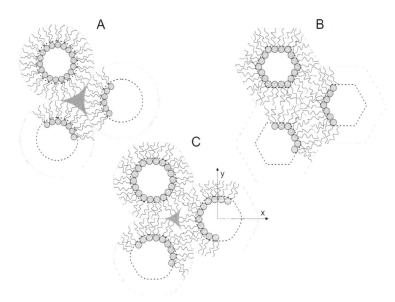

Figure 7.7 Schemes of the approaches by different authors to the geometry of the inverted hexagonal phase: (A) a circular cross-section (Rand et al., 1990; Siegel, 1993), (B) hexagonal cross section (Hamm and Kozlov, 1998), (C) intermediate between circular and hexagonal cross section (Malinin and Lentz, 2004; Perutková et al., 2009).

Two different approaches exist to express the interstitial (void) energy of the inverted hexagonal phase. In the first approach the rods of the inverted hexagonal phase are assumed to be circular in cross-section and the interstitial energy is assumed to be proportional to some imaginary surface of the voids between hexagonally packed cylinders (Siegel, 1993 and Fig. 7.7A). In the second approach the interstitial energy was accounted to in terms of the tilt and splay deformation of the phospholipid chains which have to fill the hexagonal unit cell, while the cross-section of the neutral plane of the lipid rods is assumed to be hexagonal (Hamm and Kozlov, 1998 and Fig. 7.7B). Both approaches result in a proportionality constant on equating the free energies of the lamellar and inverted hexagonal phases at the transition temperature.

Malinin and Lentz (2004) later improved the model of Rand and co-workers (1990) and Eq. 7.38 by including the energy cost due to voids (interstitial energy) (see Fig. 6.4). To calculate the interstitial energy, they assumed that the cross-section of the pivotal plane is intermediate between circular and hexagonal geometry (see Fig. 7.7C), and thus, they parameterized the shape of the cross-section:

$$y = \sqrt{d_p^2 - x^2} + \delta_o \left(1 - \frac{4x^2}{d_p^2}\right)^2, \qquad (7.39)$$

where x, y are coordinates of the pivotal plane, d_p is the distance from the axis of a rod to the pivotal plane in the interaxial direction and δ_o is the maximal deviation from circular cylindrical geometry. Using Eq. 7.39, they computed the volumes of water, voids, and the total unit cell volume. By assuming that the interstitial energy of the inverted hexagonal phase is proportional to the volume of voids, the total free energy per lipid molecule was then derived as:

$$g = w_b + K_v V_v + \Pi V_w, \qquad (7.40)$$

where w_b is the bending energy per lipid molecule, K_v is a proportionality coefficient representing the free energy of a unit of void volume, V_v and V_w are the volumes of the void and of water, respectively (Malinin and Lentz, 2004). The interstitial energy in Eq. 7.40 was assumed to be proportional to the volume of the voids in the hexagonal lattice.

Kozlov et al. (1994) showed that the free energy of the phospholipid monolayer in the inverted hexagonal phase may be expressed in terms of bending, interstitial, hydration, and van der Waals energy contributions. It was pointed out that the contribution of the hydration energy in excess water conditions is insignificant. Also the van der Waals energy contributes only slightly to the total free energy.

In the contrast to the above described models of interstitial energies in Eq. 7.37 and in Eq. 7.40, in the the model described in this section (see also Mareš et al., 2008; Perutková et al., 2011) the interstitial (void-filling) energy (Eq. 7.41) explicitly depends on the stretching of the phospholipid chains so that the tips of the phospholipid chains fill the voids in the inverted hexagonal phase. In addition, a new formalism describing the role of the anisotropy of the phospholipid molecules is also considered in this model. A new bottom-up approach concerning the description of monolayer bending and packing frustration in the inverted hexagonal phase is outlined. The expression for the total free energy of the phospholipid system in the inverted hexagonal phase is assumed to involve two main energy terms: the interstitial energy (void-filling energy) and the bending energy which also involves a deviatoric term (i.e., a logarithmic term in Eq. 7.29), which takes into account the temperature-dependent anisotropic (wedge-like) shape of the lipid molecules (see Fig. 7.5). On the basis of minimization of the system free energy, the optimal geometry and physical conditions for the stability of the inverted hexagonal phase may be theoretically predicted (see Mareš et al., 2008; Perutková et al., 2011). Using the Monte Carlo simulations annealing method, the first step in the L_α–H_{II} phase transition is also described (see Mareš et al., 2008; Perutková et al., 2011). Insight into the nature of the mechanisms that determine the stability of the inverted hexagonal lipid phases (see Kozlov et al., 1994; Malinin and Lentz, 2004; Mareš et al., 2008; Perutková et al., 2011; Seddon and Templer, 1995) may contribute to better understanding of different biologically important processes involving the formation of inverted hexagonal phases within biomembranes.

In the following, an expression for the interstitial energy due to "voids" in the inverted hexagonal phase is described in which the specific packing of lipids in the inverted hexagonal phase is taken into account (Figs. 6.4 and 7.7). In the lamellar phase L_α, the monolayers have constant thickness and there are no voids in the mid-plane of the bilayer. On the other hand, in the inverted hexagonal phase the distance between two adjacent monolayers varies over the monolayer surface. To avoid water pockets in the voids (Fig. 6.4), the hydrocarbon tails of lipid molecules have to stretch appropriately. The void-filling energy contribution due to lipid stretching can be expressed on the basis of Hook's law (Duesing et al., 1997; May, 2000):

$$f_d = \tau(\zeta - \zeta_0)^2, \qquad (7.41)$$

where ζ is the actual length of the lipid fatty acid chain, ζ_0 the optimal length of the lipid chain (see Fig. 6.4 and τ is the stiffness

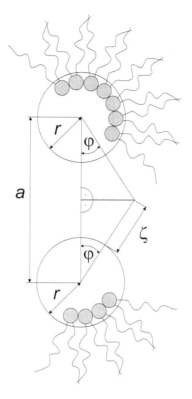

Figure 7.8 Scheme of two neighbouring inverted lipid tubes in a hexagonal lattice. The lipid tails have to stretch in order to fill voids in the hydrocarbon region. The symbol a denotes the H_{II} phase lattice constant and r denotes the radius of the pivotal plane of the H_{II} phase. The actual length of hydrocarbon tails (ζ) depends on the angle φ (Perutková et al., 2009).

(stretching modulus) of the chain. The total contact energy is then given as:

$$F_i = Y\tau n_0 \int_l (\zeta - \zeta_0)^2 dl, \quad (7.42)$$

where n_0 is the area density of phospholipid molecules ($n_0 = 1/a_0$), $dl = rd\varphi$ is the length element of the curve corresponding to the phospholipid monolayer in the projection of the hexagonal phase (see Fig. 7.8) and Y is the length of the inverted hexagonal tube.

To estimate the actual length of the hydrocarbon chain ζ, cylindrical coordinates are introduced. The length of hydrocarbon chains may be estimated from the hexagonal geometry of the lattice. From the right-angled triangle depicted in Fig. 7.8 it follows:

$$\zeta = \frac{a}{2\cos\varphi} - r. \qquad (7.43)$$

Because of hexagonal symmetry, Eq. 7.43 is valid for the contact region of two adjacent lipid cylinders, that is, for 1/12 of the area of one lipid cylinder. The values of the angle φ are therefore, defined in the range of $\varphi \in \left[0, \frac{\pi}{6}\right)]$. If $\varphi = 0$, the length of hydrocarbon chains ζ is equal to $\frac{a}{2} - r$. At the upper limit of the range of φ, the length of the hydrocarbon chain is equal to $a/\sqrt{3} - r$.

The total free energy per lipid molecule in the inverted hexagonal (H_{II}) phase can be expressed as the sum of the bending energy (Eq. 7.34) and interstitial energy (Eq. 7.42) as follows (Mareš et al., 2008):

$$F = \frac{F_b + F_i}{2\pi n_0 Y r} = \frac{\xi}{2}\left((H - H_m)^2 + D^2 + D_m^2\right)$$
$$- kT \ln\left(2\cosh\left(\frac{(1 + \tilde{k}/kT)\xi D_m D}{kT}\right)\right)$$
$$+ \frac{6}{\pi}\tau\left(\frac{a^2\sqrt{3}}{12} - a(r + \zeta_0)\ln\sqrt{3} + \frac{\pi}{6}(r + \zeta_0)^2\right), \qquad (7.44)$$

where $A = 2\pi r Y$ is the total area of one lipid cylinder in the inverted hexagonal phase. The first two terms in Eq. 7.44 represent the Helfrich and deviatoric bending energy contributions and the third term is the interstitial energy contribution (Eq. 7.42) to the free energy.

In order to determine the free energy of different configurations of lipid monolayers, the values of the model constants should be estimated. The value of interaction constant ξ was already estimated.

The reference (non-stretched) length of the phospholipid tails ζ_0 (Fig. 6.4) was taken to be 1.30 nm (Rappolt et al., 2003). In calculation of the interstitial energy the lipid stretching modulus τ was taken to be in the range from 0.95 kT nm^{-2} to 95 kT nm^{-2} (May, 2000). For the sake of simplicity we assumed that the molecules favour cylindrical geometry, that is, $|H_m| = D_m$ corresponding to a wedge-like molecular shape (see Fig. 7.5).

The effect of the temperature was simulated by increase in the intrinsic curvatures $|H_m|$ and D_m with increase in temperature; this is consistent with increased spreading of the phospholipid tails while the head-group extensions in POPE remain relatively unchanged. The range of magnitude of the intrinsic curvatures was taken to be from 0 to 0.4 nm^{-1}, corresponding to curvature radii down to 1 nm. To study the effect of deviatoric bending, the hypothetical case where the molecules are isotropic ($D_m = 0$) was also considered.

To test the importance of the interstitial (stretching) energy written in the form of Eq. 7.42, we compare the energies per lipid molecule (Eq. 7.44) in two different geometries of lipid monolayers: in the planar L_α phase and in the inverted cylindrical H_{II} phase.

In Figure 7.9, the total free energy per molecule is calculated for anisotropic ($|H_m| = D_m$) and isotropic ($D_m = 0$) phospholipid molecules (see also Figs. 6.1, 7.1 and 7.5) as a function of the mean intrinsic curvature H_m. Three curves corresponding to the inverted hexagonal phase with different stiffness constants τ, and one curve corresponding to the lamellar phase are given.

Increasing the value of the stretching modulus τ considerably increases the free energy (see Figs. 7.9A and 7.9B). With increase in τ the void-filling energy becomes more important relative to the bending energy. As there is no void-filling contribution to the free energy in the L_α phase, increase in τ increases the free energy of the H_{II} phase with respect to the free energy in the L_α phase. Accordingly, for smaller τ, the H_{II} phase is already preferred at smaller $|H_m|$ (Fig. 7.9B). For stiff hydrocarbon chains (i.e., high values of τ), the lamellar phase has lower energy than the inverted hexagonal phase. Isotropic lipid molecules in the inverted hexagonal phase also exhibit the lowest energy for less stiff hydrocarbon chains.

To promote and stabilize the H_{II} phase with increasing temperature, the energy difference between the L_α and the H_{II} phase should be larger than the energy of thermal shape fluctuations. It is not likely that the system will remain in a state of high energy; rather the configuration will adjust such that the free energy is minimized. Further, it is important to stress that the anisotropy of the phospholipid molecules contributes to a steeper increase in the

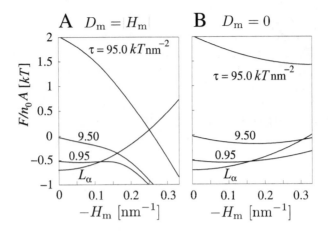

Figure 7.9 Free energy per lipid molecule $F/n_0 A$ comprising bending and interstitial contributions as a function of the intrinsic mean curvature of lipid molecules $|H_m|$ in the L_α and H_{II} phase for various values of τ and $\tilde{k}/kT = 1$ (see Eq. 7.44). The values of the intrinsic curvature deviator $D_m = -H_m$ and $H_m < 0$ correspond to inverted wedge-like lipid shapes (A) (see also Fig. 7.5 and Fig. 6.1D), while $D_m = 0$ and $H_m < 0$ correspond to inverted conical lipid shapes (Fig. 6.1E). Reprinted with permission from Mareš, T., Daniel, M., Perutkova, Š., Perne, A., Dolinar, G., Iglič, A., Rappolt, M., and Kralj-Iglič, V. Role of phospholipid asymmetry in the stability of inverted hexagonal mesoscopic phases. *J. Phys. Chem. B.*, 112(51), pp. 16575–16584. Copyright 2008, American Chemical Society.

absolute value of the energy difference between the L_α and the H_{II} phase with temperature (compare panels (A) and (B) in Fig. 7.9) and therefore, greatly promotes and stabilizes the H_{II} phase.

For a more detailed study of the H_{II} phase, Fig. 7.10 shows the dependence of the unit parameter a (panel A) and of the effective radius of the pivotal surface in the H_{II} phase r (panel B) on the intrinsic mean curvature H_m for anisotropic molecules ($D_m = |H_m|$). Figure 7.10 shows the dependence of the cylinder radius r (i.e., the effective radius of the pivotal surface) and of the distance between the centres of the lipid cylinders a, respectively, (Fig. 6.4), on the intrinsic curvature $|H_m|$ for three values of constant τ of anisotropic lipid molecules. The increase in $|H_m|$ causes a decrease in both a and r, that is, the H_{II} phase is composed of lipid cylinders with small radius r and small separation a for lipids of large mean

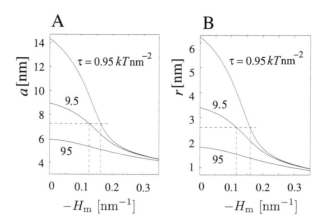

Figure 7.10 Structural parameters of the H$_{II}$ phase for inverted wedge-like shaped lipids with $D_m = |H_m|$ (see Figs. 6.1D and 7.5). The optimal unit cell parameter a (A) and the optimal pivotal plane radius r (B) are plotted versus the absolute value of the mean curvature H_m for different lipid chain rigidities τ and $\tilde{k}/kT = 1$. The two horizontal dashed lines mark realistic values for a and r, respectively (Table 7.1). For definitions of a and r see Fig. 6.4. Reprinted with permission from Mareš, T., Daniel, M., Perutkova, Š., Perne, A., Dolinar, G., Iglič, A., Rappolt, M., and Kralj-Iglič, V. Role of phospholipid asymmetry in the stability of inverted hexagonal mesoscopic phases. *J. Phys. Chem. B.*, 112(51), pp. 16575–16584. Copyright 2008, American Chemical Society.

intrinsic curvature. Decreasing the absolute value of the mean intrinsic curvature $|H_m|$ increases both the radius of the H$_{II}$ cylinders and the lattice length. However, cylinders of large radii increase the void space and the corresponding stretching of hydrocarbon chains. Therefore, the maximum radii of the cylinders are limited by the energy of the interface region between the cylinders. If the hydrocarbon chains are stiff enough (large value of τ), the creation of voids is energetically unfavourable. In this case, small radii of the cylinders are preferred as they provide small void spaces (Fig. 7.10A). On the other hand, if the stretching of hydrocarbon chains does not require much energy (small τ), larger radii of the hydrocarbon chains are permitted.

It is instructive to compare the theoretical predictions with experimental data (see Rappolt et al., 2003, 2008, and Fig. 7.10, dashed lines). First, it shows us that realistic values of the stretching

Table 7.1 Geometrical parameters of the L_α and H_{II} phases at $T = 74°C$

	L_α (74°C)	H_{II} (74°C)
d, a [nm]	4.99	7.24
d_{pol}, r [nm]	2.5	2.67
ζ_0 (ζ_{min}, ζ_{max}) [nm]	1.47	1.13 (0.95, 1.51)
a_0 [nm^2]	0.65	0.65
H [nm^{-1}]	0	0.187

Note: The structural parameters are defined in Figs. 6.4 and 7.8. The experimental values are taken from Rappolt et al. (2003)

moduli τ most probably lie between 0 and 20 kT nm^{-2} (for large enough τ, for example, $\tau = 95$ kT nm^{-2} no realistic dimensions of the H_{II} lattice can be predicted). Second, realistic magnitudes of the intrinsic mean curvature $|H_m|$ lie probably in the range of 0.1–0.2 nm^{-1}. Note that this comes close to the value of the mean curvature of the POPE–water system (Table 7.1) and is also in good agreement with the values of intrinsic curvatures of lipids important in the membrane fusion process (Churchward et al., 2008) and references therein) where structures similar to inverted hexagonal phases are formed. The effect of the contact (stretching) energy in stabilization of the hexagonal phase becomes important if the value of τ is large enough. A large diameter of the lipid cylinder with radius r produces larger voids that are energetically unfavourable (see also Figs. 6.4 and 7.8).

7.5 Nucleation in the Lamellar (L_α) to Inverted Hexagonal (H_{II}) Phase Transition

In order to describe the L_α–H_{II} phase transition we can follow a simple scenario, in which a configuration is imagined consisting of an inverted central phospholipid cylinder embedded in two adjacent lipid bilayers (see Fig. 7.6). The two inner lamellar monolayers are fused, exhibiting bulb-like closures on both sides of the cylinder, while the outer monolayer leaflets follow the contours of the cylinder and of the bulb-like closures (see Fig. 7.11). The chosen configuration is considered to be the smallest unit to follow the

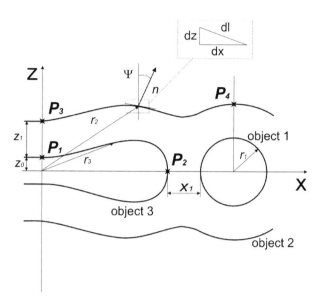

Figure 7.11 Parametrization of the pivotal surface. A bulb-like closure (object 3) is placed between adjacent bilayers (objects 2) is a cylinder (object 1). The geometry of the system is symmetrical with respect to the x-axis. Reprinted with permission from Mareš, T., Daniel, M., Perutková, Š., Perne, A., Dolinar, G., Iglič, A., Rappolt, M., and Kralj-Igliš, V. Role of phospholipid asymmetry in the stability of inverted hexagonal mesoscopic phases. *J. Phys. Chem. B.*, 112, 51, pp. 16575–16584. doi: 10.1021/jp805715r. Copyright 2008 American Chemical Society.

nucleation process of the H_{II} hexagonal phase in the L_α phase and is based on experimental results (see also Rappolt et al., 2003, 2008).

As the temperature increases, D_m and $|H_m|$ change (see also Fig. 7.5) thereby affecting the equilibrium configuration. The nucleation configuration is considered to be stable when the free energy per molecule of the configuration with a bulb-like closure is lower than the free energy per molecule of the all-planar lipid configuration.

To estimate the overall optimum configuration (the shape of the neighbouring closures, the radius of the central cylinder and the shapes of the neighbouring enclosing monolayers), the minimum of the free energy of the system was determined. For this purpose an original approach was developed which combines the solution of the Euler–Lagrange differential equations and the Monte Carlo simulation annealing numerical method described below.

Following Rappolt's nucleation model of the L_α–H_{II} transition (see Rappolt et al., 2003, 2008), the surface of the monolayer forming a closure is described by the radius vector $\mathbf{r} = (x, y, z(x))$ (Figs. 7.6 and 7.11), from which the mean (see also Chapter 5):

$$2H = \frac{-\frac{\partial^2 z}{\partial x^2}}{(1 + (\frac{\partial z}{\partial x})^2)^{3/2}} \tag{7.45}$$

and the Gaussian curvatures:

$$K = C_1 C_2 = 0. \tag{7.46}$$

are derived. The surface is given in terms of the arc length l, so that $\sin \psi = -\,dz/dl$ and $\cos \psi = dx/dl$. Considering the above definitions, the mean curvature is expressed as $2H = 2D = d\psi/dl$, while the area element is $dA = dl\,dy$. For reason of symmetry, only the part of the contour above the x-axis is considered in determination of the equilibrium shape of the closure.

The coordinates, the area, the area element and the bending energy are written in dimensionless form. Normalizing the curvatures and distances by an arbitrary unit of length z_0 (for the sake of simplicity we set $z_0 = 1$ nm) gives dimensionless (reduced) curvatures $h = z_0 H$, $d = z_0 D$, $h_m = z_0 H_m$, $d_m = z_0 D_m$ and a dimensionless arc length $\tilde{l} = l/z_0$. The area element is normalized to yz_0. The bending energy (Eq. 7.29) is normalized to $n_0 \xi y / 2z_0$:

$$f_b = \int (\zeta - \zeta_m)^2 d\tilde{l} + \int (d^2 + d_m^2) d\tilde{l} \tag{7.47}$$

$$-\kappa \int \ln(2\cosh((1+\tilde{k}/kT)\vartheta 2 d_m d)) d\tilde{l},$$

where $\kappa = 1/\vartheta = 2kT z_0^2/\xi$. To minimize the bending energy (Eq. 7.48) the functional

$$L = \left(\frac{1}{2}\frac{d\psi}{d\tilde{l}} - \zeta_m\right)^2 + \frac{1}{4}\left(\frac{d\psi}{d\tilde{l}}\right)^2 - \kappa \ln(2\cosh((1+\tilde{k}/kT)\vartheta 2 d_m d))$$

$$-\lambda\left(\cos\psi - \frac{dx}{d\tilde{l}}\right) - \nu\left(\sin\psi + \frac{dz}{d\tilde{l}}\right) \tag{7.48}$$

is substituted in a system of Euler–Lagrange equations (see Mareš et al., 2008):

$$\frac{\partial L}{\partial \psi} - \frac{d}{d\tilde{l}}\left(\frac{\partial L}{\partial \psi_{\tilde{l}}}\right) = 0, \tag{7.49}$$

$$\frac{\partial L}{\partial x} - \frac{d}{d\tilde{l}}\left(\frac{\partial L}{\partial x_{\tilde{l}}}\right) = 0, \qquad (7.50)$$

$$\frac{\partial L}{\partial z} - \frac{d}{d\tilde{l}}\left(\frac{\partial L}{\partial z_{\tilde{l}}}\right) = 0, \qquad (7.51)$$

where $\psi_{\tilde{l}} = d\psi/d\tilde{l}$, $x_{\tilde{l}} = dx/d\tilde{l}$ and $z_{\tilde{l}} = dz/d\tilde{l}$. By introducing the variable $\Upsilon = x d\psi/d\tilde{l}$, the system of equations (7.49–7.51) yields (see Mareš et al., 2008)

$$\frac{d\Upsilon}{d\tilde{l}} = \frac{\Upsilon}{x}\cos\psi + \frac{(\lambda\sin\psi - \nu\cos\psi)x}{1 - \frac{\kappa\tilde{\vartheta}^2 d_m^2}{\cosh^2(\frac{\tilde{\vartheta} d_m \Upsilon}{x})}}, \qquad (7.52)$$

$$\lambda = \text{const}, \quad \nu = \text{const}, \qquad (7.53)$$

where λ and ν are local Lagrange multipliers and $\tilde{\vartheta} = \vartheta(1 + \tilde{k}/kT)$. The system of Eqs. 7.52–7.53 was solved numerically by using the Merson method (Mareš et al., 2008) to yield the equilibrium contour map of the pivotal plane of the bulb-like closure as shown in Fig. 7.11.

The configuration of monolayers adjacent to the central cylinder representing a nucleation line for the L_α–H_{II} phase transition is described by the radius of the central cylinder and a set of N angles, $\psi_i = 1, 2, \ldots N$, describing the bulb-like closure and the surrounding monolayers (see Fig. 7.11), which were divided into N sufficiently small parts. Boundary conditions were introduced to reflect connections within the different parts of the system. Due to symmetry, this unit includes a quarter of the cylinder, half of the bulb-like closure, and one neighbouring monolayer.

Minimization of the free energy of the system was performed by the Monte Carlo simulation annealing sampling strategy. The method was introduced by Kirkpatrick et al. in 1983 as an adaptation of the Metropolis–Hastings algorithm, which constitutes the Monte Carlo method (Metropolis et al., 1953).

Solving the equilibrium configuration of the system with an inverted cylinder surrounded by two monolayers and two bulb-like closures yielded the results depicted in Figs. 7.12 and 7.13.

In Figure 7.12, snapshots of the equilibrium configurations for anisotropic phospholipids (setting $D_m = |H_m|$) and different values of model parameters are displayed. The top row presents the L_α

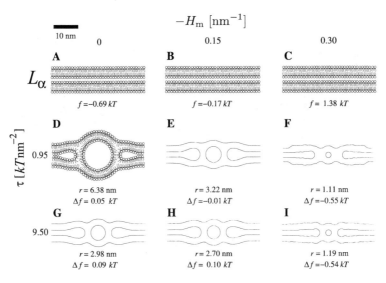

Figure 7.12 Configuration of a system of two monolayers, a cylinder of H_{II} phase and two bulb-like closures representing a nucleation line in the L_α–H_{II} transition for different intrinsic curvatures H_m and different stretching moduli of the phospholipid chains τ. We assume that phospholipid molecules are anisotropic corresponding to $D_m = |H_m|$. The free energy per lipid molecule and the radius of the central cylinder are given for each configuration. Reprinted with permission from Mareš, T., Daniel, M., Perutkova, Š., Perne, A., Dolinar, G., Iglič, A., Rappolt, M., and Kralj-Iglič, V. Role of phospholipid asymmetry in the stability of inverted hexagonal mesoscopic phases. *J. Phys. Chem. B.*, 112(51), pp. 16575–16584. Copyright 2008, American Chemical Society.

phase with values of the free energy per lipid molecule of the pure L_α phase. The next two rows show the equilibrium configuration of the system with the first cylinder of the H_{II} phase embedded between two monolayers. The energy of these structures is described by the energy difference $\Delta f = f_{H_{II}} - f_{L_\alpha}$, where $f_{H_{II}}$ is the energy per lipid molecule in the hexagonal phase and f_{L_α} is the energy per lipid molecule in the lamellar phase at the given values of model constants. From top to bottom, the stretching modulus of the phospholipid chains is increased: $\tau =$ (0.95, 9.50 and 95.00) $kT\,\text{nm}^{-2}$. From left to right the lipid intrinsic mean curvature $|H_m|$ is increased: $|H_m| = (0, 0.15, 0.3)\,\text{nm}^{-1}$.

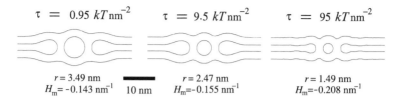

Figure 7.13 Nucleation configurations for different values of the stretching modulus of phospholipid tails (τ) at the transition point from L_α to H_{II} phase where $\Delta f = 0$. Anisotropic case ($D_m = |H_m|$). Reprinted with permission from Mareš, T., Daniel, M., Perutkova, Š., Perne, A., Dolinar, G., Iglič, A., Rappolt, M., and Kralj-Iglič, V. Role of phospholipid asymmetry in the stability of inverted hexagonal mesoscopic phases. *J. Phys. Chem. B.*, 112(51), pp. 16575–16584. Copyright 2008, American Chemical Society.

The configuration with the cylinder and bulb-like closures becomes energetically more favourable than the L_α phase at high enough values of $D_m = |H_m|$. This is in agreement with the fact that formation of the H_{II} phase is promoted with increasing temperature.[6] In the model, increase in temperature is simulated by increasing $D_m = |H_m|$ (see also Fig. 7.5). For higher $D_m = |H_m|$ the energy difference Δf decreases thereby favouring the configuration with the cylinder. This phenomenon is in accordance with experimental results showing that the formation of the H_{II} phase is promoted by increasing temperature (Perutková et al., 2011; Rappolt et al., 2003). The difference between the configurations C and F in Fig. 7.12 is -1.39 kT per lipid molecule in favour of the configuration with the cylinder, which is considerable.

It is evident from Fig. 7.12 that the radius of the central cylinder r decreases with increase in stretching modulus of the phospholipid chains τ and decrease in $D_m = |H_m|$ which is in agreement with the results presented in Fig. 7.10. Formation of a cylinder in the lamellar phase disturbs the adjacent lipid layers less as the radius of the cylinder r decreases.

For high enough values of τ there is a negligible effect of $D_m = |H_m|$ on the equilibrium radius of the central cylinder r because the stretching modulus τ plays a decisive role in the energy balance, and also because the contact energy is much higher than the bending energy. On the other hand, small τ means a low contact (stretching) energy that cannot compete with the bending energy. Consequently, for larger $D_m = |H_m|$ and small τ the radius r is determined mainly by the bending energy, which is the lowest when r comes close to $|1/H_m|$ (see Fig. 7.12). With the increasing contribution of the interstitial energy, the shape of the curved monolayers is mainly determined by avoiding stretching of the lipid tails.

To resume, when the free energy of the presented configuration is calculated and compared to the energy of the pure lamellar system, the configurations of anisotropic molecules with high enough intrinsic curvatures and low enough stretching moduli have a lower energy than the L_α phase and promote the formation of the H_{II} phase.

The transition from the L_α to H_{II} phase in the described nucleation model (Mareš et al., 2008) occurs at the energy difference $\Delta f = 0$, that is, when the energy of the H_{II} phase is equal to the energy of the L_α phase for $|H_m| = D_m$, (see Fig. 7.13). By comparison of three different configurations of H_{II} nucleation corresponding to different values of phospholipid chain stiffness, one can see that for low τ the L_α-H_{II} transition takes place for smaller $|H_m|$ and the predicted radius of the initial cylinder does not have a realistic value ($r = 3.49$ nm), that is, it is much larger than the experimental values (Rappolt et al., 2003, 2008). However, for larger values of τ the calculated r corresponds to the experimental values much better. At $|H_m| = 0.155$ nm^{-1} the nucleation cylinder radius is 2.47 nm, which agrees well with data obtained from X-ray experiments (Laggner et al., 1991; Rappolt et al., 2003). As the decrease of free energy with increase in $|H_m|$ is more pronounced in the pure hexagonal phase (Fig. 7.9) than in the nucleation configuration (Fig. 7.13), values of τ around $9.5\,kT/\text{nm}^2$ would lead to stabilization of the H_{II} phase at higher temperatures. For large $\tau = 95\,kT/\text{nm}^2$, the predicted nucleation transition is again less realistic since the predicted value of $r = 1.49$ nm is too small.

To conclude, the stability of the inverted hexagonal phase depends on the energy balance between different contributions to the system free energy, hence the main problem in the theoretical description of the lamellar to inverted hexagonal phase transition and in explanation of the stability of the H_{II} lipid phase consists in finding an appropriate expression for the free energy of the system.

Most contemporary theoretical models of the free energy of the inverted hexagonal phase showed that in addition to the bending energy term, it is necessary to consider the energy term, which depends on the dimensions of the "voids" in the hexagonal lattice, the so-called interstitial energy (Kozlov et al., 1994; Malinin and Lentz, 2004). In one study (Mareš et al., 2008; Perutková et al., 2011), this assumption was followed and the interstitial energy taken into account. In our model the interstitial energy is expressed by the stretching energy of the phospholipid chains (Duesing et al., 1997; May, 2000). In addition, description of the bending energy was improved by taking into account deviatoric bending due to the average orientational ordering of lipid molecules which may in general be anisotropic (see Mareš et al., 2008; Perutková et al., 2011; Rappolt et al., 2008) and also Fig. 7.5.

It is noteworthy that both the deviatoric contribution as well as the stretching energy of the chains are necessary to explain the stability of the L_α and the L_α to H_{II} phase transition for the model constants estimated from experimental data (Rappolt et al., 2003). In a first approach the effect of the stretching of the chains was considered constant (as in Kozlov et al., 1994), while in a second approach the model was improved (Mareš et al., 2008) by introducing the conformational free energy of the individual hydrocarbon chains in the hexagonal lattice (the stretching energy of the hydrocarbon chains). Assuming solely the isotropic bending and stretching energy of the chains leads to quite high intrinsic curvatures of the phospholipid molecules in comparison to the curvature of the cylinders in the stable inverted hexagonal phase, whereas if the stretching energy of the chains is neglected the stability of the lamellar phase for low intrinsic curvatures of the lipids cannot be predicted, as observed in real lyotropic mesophases (Mareš et al., 2008; Perutková et al., 2011; Seddon and Templer, 1995).

Models based on isotropic elasticity described the L_α–H_{II} phase transition by showing that at a certain temperature, the free energy of the system is lowered as it converts from the L_α phase to the H_{II} phase (see Kirk et al., 1984). However, the energy difference was found to be lower than 0.1 kT (Kozlov et al., 1994). The results presented in this section follow the general conclusions of previous models. However, the energy difference obtained becomes much larger at elevated temperatures if the average orientational ordering of anisotropic lipid molecules on the highly curved surfaces of the H_{II} phase is taken into account (i.e., if the anisotropic elasticity of the lipid monolayer is considered). This energy difference is sufficient for the stability of a single cylinder within the lamellar stack and therefore supports previously suggested nucleation models, which are based on line defects (Marrink and Mark, 2004; Rappolt et al., 2003, 2008; Siegel, 1986).

Our results therefore indicate that deviatoric bending can explain the stability of the H_{II} phase at higher temperatures. However, for the L_α-H_{II} transition, tuning of the deviatoric bending energy by the isotropic bending energy and the interstitial energy is needed. In spite of the many simplifications introduced into the present theoretical description, the results of our modelling and simulations are in good agreement with the experimental results (Mareš et al., 2008; Rappolt et al., 2003, 2008). Among other things it is shown that with increasing absolute values of the intrinsic curvatures of lipid molecules C_1 and C_2 (which are assumed to increase with increase in temperature), the L_α-H_{II} phase transition occurs beyond a certain threshold temperature. Further, we could also reproduce realistic structures in good agreement with the experimental results. The results presented (see also Mareš et al., 2008; Perutková et al., 2011) thus, show that deviatoric bending plays an important role in the stability of the inverted hexagonal phase and in the L_α-H_{II} phase transition.

In this theoretical analysis we did not take into account the dependence of the chain stretching modulus τ on temperature (see Boal, 2002), which is based on the elasticity of lipid chains. We expect that neglecting the temperature dependency of τ results in the slope of the energy dependence of $D_m = |H_m|$ being less pronounced (see Fig. 7.9). Another simplification introduced in our theoretical model is the assumption of circular cross-sections of lipid tubes in the H_{II} phase. A non-circular cross-section of lipid tubes would lower the stretching energy of phospholipid chains (Perutková et al., 2011), but would also contribute to higher bending of the monolayer.

Recently, the non-circular cross-section of the polar–apolar interface of the H_{II} phase was studied in minute detail by analysing small angle X-ray diffraction data (Perutková et al., 2011). On this structural basis Monte Carlo simulated annealing (MC) variation of the free energy was carried out, both on the formation of the H_{II}-phase and on the particular shape of the cross-section in the H_{II}-phase. Equilibrium in the H_{II}-phase pivotal-plane contour and the corresponding values of the mean intrinsic curvature (H_m) and the hydrocarbon chain stiffness (τ) were determined from the MC calculations (Perutková et al., 2011). Comparing the measured structural data with predictions from the MC calculations, including lipid anisotropy, and accounting for the elastic deformations of the pivotal plane allowed determination of a relation between bending deformation and stretching of the hydrocarbon chains (Perutková et al., 2011).

7.6 Bending Energy of Anisotropic Lipid Bilayer

As in the previous sections, it is assumed that a single phospholipid molecule represents the building unit of the phospholipid bilayer, and that in the phospholipid bilayer there are two opposing surfaces that are in close contact. As before it is considered that the phospholipid molecules, due to their structure, are anisotropic with respect to the axis pointing in the direction of the normal to the bilayer (Fig. 7.1). They are free to rotate within the plane of the bilayer, but at a given site of the molecule (a given local curvature of the layer) it could be expected that different orientational states would have different energies and that the molecule would on average spend more time in the configuration with lower energy. It is therefore appropriate to use Eq. 7.11 to calculate the contribution of a single phospholipid molecule to the free energy of the bilayer.

In the first approximation, the free energy of the phospholipid bilayer is obtained by summing the contributions of individual phospholipid molecules (f_i) of both layers:

$$F_b = \int n_{out} f_i(C_1, C_2) dA + \int n_{in} f_i(-C_1, -C_2) dA, \quad (7.54)$$

where n_{out} and n_{in} are the area densities of lipid molecules in the outer and the inner layer, respectively. Integration is performed over the whole bilayer area A. Note that the principal curvatures in the inner layer have the opposite sign to the sign of the principal curvatures of the outer layer due to the specific configuration of the phospholipid molecules within the layers touching by the tails.

If we assume for simplicity that the area densities are constant over the respective layers and also equal $n_{out} = n_{in} = n_0 = 1/a_0$, where a_0 is the area per lipid molecule, and substitute the expression for the single-unit energy (Eq. 7.11) in Eq. 7.54, we obtain (Kralj-Iglič, 2002):

$$F_b = n_0 \xi \int H^2 dA + n_0 \frac{\xi + \xi^*}{2} \int D^2 dA \qquad (7.55)$$
$$- 2n_0 kT \int \ln\left(I_0\left(\frac{\xi + \xi^*}{2kT} D D_m\right)\right) dA,$$

where constant terms are omitted. In integrating, the differences in the areas of the inner and the outer layer were disregarded, so that the contributions proportional to the intrinsic mean curvature H_m of the inner and the outer layer cancelled and there is no spontaneous curvature for the bilayer vesicles composed of a single species of molecules. It follows from Eq. 7.55 that the free energy of the phospholipid bilayer can be expressed by two first-order invariants of the curvature tensor (Eq. 5.32)—trace $(2H)$ and deviator (D). Taking into account the relation $D^2 = H^2 - C_1 C_2$ we can rewrite Eq. 7.55 in the form $F_b = \int f_b \, dA$, where the area energy density f_b is

$$f_b = \frac{(3\xi + \xi^*)}{8} n_0 (2H)^2 - \frac{(\xi + \xi^*) n_0}{2} C_1 C_2 \qquad (7.56)$$
$$- 2n_0 kT \ln\left(I_0\left(\frac{\xi + \xi^*}{2kT} D D_m\right)\right).$$

If we consider surfaces with small curvature deviators D or lipid molecules with small D_m, we can substitute the term $\ln(I_0)$ in Eq. 7.56 by the first term in the Taylor expansion: $\ln(I_0(x)) \cong \ln(1+x^2/4) \cong x^2/4$. Thus, the above general expression for the area density of the local bilayer bending energy (Eq. 7.56) transforms into the area density of the Helfrich local (isotropic) bending energy (Helfrich, 1973):

$$f_b = \frac{k_c}{2}(2H)^2 + k_G K, \qquad (7.57)$$

where the constants k_c and k_G are:

$$k_c = \frac{(3\xi + \xi^*)n_0}{4} - \frac{(\xi + \xi^*)^2 D_m^2 n_0}{16kT}, \qquad (7.58)$$

$$k_G = -\frac{(\xi + \xi^*)n_0}{2} + \frac{(\xi + \xi^*)^2 D_m^2 n_0}{8kT}. \qquad (7.59)$$

In the simplest case, where only isotropic phospholipid molecules within the lipid monolayer are taken into account ($D_m = 0$), the constants are defined as:

$$k_c = \frac{(3\xi + \xi^*)n_0}{4}, \qquad (7.60)$$

$$k_G = -\frac{(\xi + \xi^*)n_0}{2}. \qquad (7.61)$$

However, in the limit of large $(\xi + \xi^*)DD_m/2kT$ it follows from Eq. 7.55 (or Eq. 7.56):

$$f_b \cong n_0 \xi H^2 + \frac{(\xi + \xi^*)n_0}{2} D^2 - n_0(\xi + \xi^*)DD_m \qquad (7.62)$$

$$= \frac{k_c}{2}(2H)^2 + k_G K - n_0(\xi + \xi^*)DD_m.$$

which cannot be rewritten in the form of the Helfrich Hamiltonian, and k_c and k_G are given by Eqs. 7.60 and 7.61. Note that $D = (H^2 - C_1 C_2)^{1/2}$. Eq. 7.62 can be also rewritten (up to the constant term) in the form (see also Fischer, 1992, 1993):

$$f_b \cong n_0 \xi H^2 + \frac{(\xi + \xi^*)n_0}{2}(D - D_m)^2. \qquad (7.63)$$

7.7 Stability of Phospholipid Nanotubes Determined by the Anisotropic Properties of Lipid Molecules

It is assumed that the stable shape of the phospholipid vesicle is determined by the minimum in the free energy of the phospholipid bilayer. This represents a variational problem in which it is required that the variation of the free energy (Eq. 7.55) with respect to the curvature field vanish at given constraints. The principal curvatures as functions of the position are the relevant extremal. A rigorous solution of the variational problem would be obtained by stating and solving the corresponding Euler–Lagrange equations (Deuling and Helfrich, 1976). However, in the present state of knowledge it is more appropriate to estimate the behaviour of the system by applying an adjustable parametric ansatz for the shape. As in this contribution we focus on the general properties of the system and not on the details of the shape, we do not in this section consider the rigorous solution of the variational problem but rather follow the method based on the parametric model.

The equilibrium shape is determined by the minimum of the bilayer membrane free energy (Eq. 7.55). The relevant geometrical constraints are taken into account: the bilayer area A and the enclosed volume V are fixed,

$$A = \int dA, \qquad (7.64)$$

$$V = \int dV. \qquad (7.65)$$

Considering the bilayer couple principle (Evans, 1974; Helfrich, 1974; Sheetz and Singer, 1974), another constraint requires that the difference between the two membrane layer areas ΔA is fixed (Svetina et al., 1982),

$$\Delta A = \delta \int (2H) dA, \qquad (7.66)$$

where δ is the distance between the two layer neutral areas. In expression (7.66) it is assumed that δ is small with respect to $1/H$. The quantity ΔA is assumed to reflect the conditions in which vesicle formation took place and is determined, for example, by the number of phospholipid molecules that constitute the respective layers.

To determine the equilibrium shape, for the sake of simplicity we compare two shapes that represent the limits of the class of shapes with a long thin protrusion. In the first case the protrusion consists of equal small spheres (see Fig. 7.14A), while in the second case the protrusion consists of a cylinder closed by hemispherical caps (see Fig. 7.14B). It is expected that these two limiting shapes are continuously connected by a sequence of shapes with decreasingly exhibited undulations of the protrusion. As we focus on the general

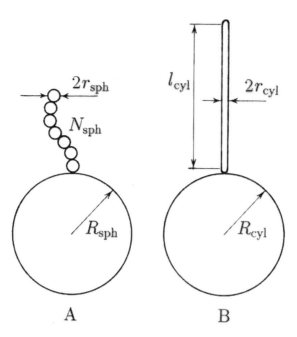

Figure 7.14 Schematic representation of a shape composed of the mother sphere and a protrusion composed of small spheres connected by infinitesimal necks (A), and of a shape composed of the mother sphere and a thin cylinder closed by hemispherical caps (B).

behaviour of the system we do not consider the intermediate shapes explicitly.

Each of these two limiting cases can be described by three geometrical model parameters (see Fig. 7.14). In the shape with small spheres these parameters are the radius of the spherical mother vesicle R_{sph}, the radius of the small spheres r_{sph} and the number of small spheres N_{sph} (see Fig. 7.14A). As in long thin protrusions N_{sph} is expected to be large, any real number is allowed for the parameter N_{sph}. In the shape with the cylindrical protrusion these parameters are the radius of the spherical mother vesicle R_{cyl}, the radius of the cylinder and the closing hemispheres r_{cyl}, and the length of the cylinder l (see Fig. 7.14B). The geometrical parameters of the shape in both cases can be determined from the

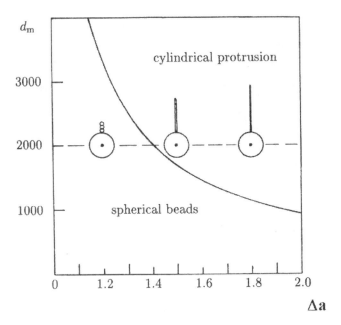

Figure 7.15 A phase diagram of calculated equilibrium vesicle shapes with bead-like or tubular protrusions in the space of the relative (reduced) intrinsic curvature deviator $d_m = RD_m$ and the relative (reduced) area difference $\Delta a = \Delta A/8\pi\delta R$. Regions where the vesicle shapes with the respective kind of protrusions (bead-like or tubular) are energetically more favourable are marked. The sequence of vesicle shapes shown in the figure indicates the process of diminishing Δa at constant v that could be observed experimentally (Fig. 6.8). For simplicity we assume $\xi = \xi^*$ therefore $\xi \simeq k_c/n_0$. The values of model parameters are: $a_0 = 0.6$ nm^2, $R = (A/4\pi)^{1/2} = 10^{-5}$ m, $k_c = 20\ kT$, while $v = (36\pi V^2/A^3)^{1/2} = 0.95$ and $a = A/4\pi R^2 = 1$. The shapes corresponding to different Δa are depicted with the centre of the spherical part at the respective Δa values. Reproduced with permission from Kralj-Iglič, V., Iglič, A., Gomišček, G., Sevšek, F., Arrigler, V., and Hägerstrand, H. (2002). Microtubes and nanotubes of a phospholipid bilayer membrane. *J. Phys. A: Math. Gen.*, 35, pp. 1533–1549. Copyright IOP Publishing. doi:10.1088/0305-4470/35/7/305.

geometrical constraints for the relative area, the relative volume v and the relative area difference Δa (see Fig. 7.15) (Kralj-Iglič, 2002).

In considering the deviatoric energy (third term in Eqs. 7.55 and 7.56), it can be assumed that there is no deviatoric contribution in the shape composed of spheres connected by infinitesimal necks.

At the spherical parts there is no deviatoric contribution as the local curvature deviator D is equal to zero. In the infinitesimal neck, the curvature deviator is very large, but the area of the neck is very small. Numerical calculations of the membrane free energy of the shape sequence leading to two spheres connected by an infinitesimal neck showed that as the limit shape is approached, the deviatoric contribution of the neck diminishes (Kralj-Iglič et al., 1999; Kralj-Iglič, 2002). In the shape with a cylindrical protrusion we considered the deviatoric contribution of the cylindrical part. There is no deviatoric contribution from the neck connecting the mother sphere and the protrusion, the spherical caps of the protrusion and the mother sphere.

Figure 7.15 shows a phase diagram exhibiting the regions corresponding to calculated stable shapes composed of the spherical mother vesicle and a tubular protrusion and to stable shapes composed of the spherical mother vesicle and a protrusion consisting of small spheres connected by infinitesimal necks.

For tubular protrusions the deviatoric contribution (third term in Eq. 7.55) is large enough to compensate for the less favourable isotropic local bending energy of the cylinder. The corresponding deviatoric energies are larger than the estimated energy of thermal fluctuations. On the other hand, for lower $\Delta a = \Delta A/8\pi \delta R$ (where $R = (A/4\pi)^{1/2}$), the protrusion of the same membrane area and enclosed volume is shorter and broader, so that its mean curvature is lower. The corresponding deviatoric term of the cylinder is too small to be of importance and the shape with the bead-like protrusion(s) has lower free energy. At a chosen intrinsic anisotropy of lipids, the calculated shapes with small spheres are energetically more favourable below a certain Δa, while above this threshold the shapes with cylinders are favoured.

The sequence of shapes shown in Fig. 7.15 roughly simulates the transformation observed experimentally (Fig. 6.8). Initially, Δa is large and the shape is composed of the mother sphere and a long thin nanotube. Assuming that the volume of the vesicle remains constant, the number of phospholipid molecules in the outer layer diminishes with time, therefore Δa decreases and the tubular protrusion becomes thicker and shorter. In the experiment (Kralj-Iglič et al., 2001a), undulations of the protrusion became increasingly noticeable with time. Our theoretical results shown in Fig. 7.15 exhibit a discontinuous transition from a tubular protrusion to a protrusion composed of small spheres connected by infinitesimal necks as we consider only the limits of the given class of shapes. Therefore, the phase diagram and the sequence (see Fig. 7.15) should be viewed only as an indication of the tendency to the shape transition and not of the details of the shape.

It follows from the above described analysis (Kralj-Iglič, 2002) that the deviatoric contribution to the membrane free energy (third term in Eq. 7.55) is considerable only in those regions of the vesicle membrane with a large absolute value of the difference between the two principal curvatures (i.e., for the values of $1/D$ of the order of a micrometer or smaller). Elsewhere the deviatoric contribution (third term in Eq. 7.56) is negligible.

It should also be stressed that within the Helfrich elasticity theory (Eq. 7.57) of the isotropic bilayer membrane (where the third term in Eq. 7.56 is neglected), the calculated shape with a protrusion composed of small spheres that are connected by infinitesimal necks would always be favoured over the shape with a tubular protrusion. Therefore, this theory is unable to explain stable tubular protrusions (see also Kralj-Iglič, 2002).

The mechanism of spontaneous shape transformation that was observed in experiments (Kralj-Iglič et al., 2001a) remains largely obscure. The tubular character of the protrusions may persist even when the protrusions become thicker, while more peculiar shapes with undulating protrusions can also be found (see Fig. 7.16). Also, the timing of the transformation may vary from minutes to hours, as the protrusions are initially of very different lengths (see Fig. 7.16). If the tubular protrusion becomes thicker in the process of spontaneous shape transformation, the curvature decreases and the deviatoric contribution may become negligible, unless the protrusion develops necks that may also produce minima in the free energy dependence on Δa (Kralj-Iglič et al., 1999). Indeed, oscillations of the neck width with time were observed, indicating increased stability of the necks (not shown). A similar effect— persistence of the neck connecting a spherical daughter vesicle and a mother vesicle—was also observed in the opening of the neck induced by cooling, while formation of the neck by heating was quick

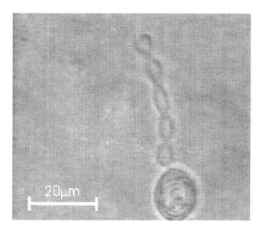

Figure 7.16 A giant phospholipid vesicle (made of POPC in pure water). Note the undulations of the protrusion and a multi-lamellar structure inside the globular part. The vesicle was observed several hours after the solution containing the vesicles was placed in the observation chamber. Reproduced with permission from Kralj-Iglič, V., Iglič, A., Gomišček, G., Sevšek, F., Arrigler, V., and Hägerstrand, H. (2002). Microtubes and nanotubes of a phospholipid bilayer membrane. *J. Phys. A: Math. Gen.*, 35, pp. 1533–1549. Copyright IOP Publishing. doi:10.1088/0305-4470/35/7/305.

and took place at higher temperature, indicating hysteresis (Käs and Sackmann, 1991). The undulations of the protrusion producing narrow but finite necks could therefore, provide a mechanism that through shapes of lower Δa would keep the membrane curvature deviator as high as possible and therefore the membrane free energy as low as possible.

It was suggested already by Fischer (1992, 1993) that phospholipid molecules with two hydrocarbon chains are in general anisotropic, despite the motion of their segments within the membrane layer. Based on decomposition of the elastic continuum into isotropic and deviatoric bending, he proposed an expression for the membrane local free energy

$$F_b = 2B_s \int (H - C_0/2)^2 dA + 2B_a \int (D - \theta)^2 dA, \qquad (7.67)$$

where B_s and B_a are the constants of local isotropic and deviatoric bending, respectively, C_0 is the spontaneous curvature of the membrane and θ is the spontaneous warp. As evident, Fischer's Eq. 7.67

is actually consistent with the limit expression of Eq. 7.55 for large $(\xi + \xi^*)DD_\mathrm{m}/2kT$ given by Eqs. 7.62 and 7.63, where C_0 is assumed to be zero due to symmetry of the lipid monolayers. As claimed by Fischer the spontaneous warp (equivalent to our intrinsic (spontaneous) curvature deviator D_m) should originate from the anisotopy of the constituent molecules as also postulated in this chapter. However, Fischer then claimed that the spontaneous warp is negligible for a one component phospholipid membrane due to the fact that the membrane of such a vesicle, as observed in experiments, is locally flat. He argued that for a non-zero spontaneous warp the membrane would be corrugated. Experimental results for shapes with tubular protrusions (Kralj-Iglič et al., 2001a; Kralj-Iglič, 2002) show that the membrane is usually not flat. However, the bilayer is rather organized in a few longer protrusions than in numerous shorter folds. This seems to be energetically more favourable taking into account that the beginning and the end of the protrusion have a high local bending energy of the isotropic continuum. It must also be considered that the shape of the vesicle is subject to constraints regarding the membrane area, enclosed volume and the numbers of molecules constituting both layers. A shape with folds would have a considerably lower relative volume and a higher difference between the two membrane layer areas than a smooth shape of roughly equal appearance, therefore the two shapes would be rather far apart in the phase diagram of possible shapes. Shifting from one point to the other may involve processes required to overcome energy barrier(s), for example, due to the local bending energy of the isotropic continuum (Kralj-Iglič et al., 1999). Further, it was shown theoretically that the deviatoric effect is usually not uniformly distributed over the area of the vesicle, so that in this respect a description by spontaneous warp (Eq. 7.67) is oversimplified. Nevertheless, the theory of deviatoric elasticity of the lipid bilayer (Kralj-Iglič, 2002) presented in this section supports the general ideas of deviatoric elasticity proposed by Fischer.

Some models of the phospholipid bilayer membrane consider that the area per molecule may be different in the two membrane layers, but equal within each layer (Evans and Skalak, 1980; Helfrich, 1974). This effect is referred to as the relative stretching of the two layers. Considering the relative stretching of the two layers, an additional non-local term appears in the expression for the Helfrich–Evans bending energy of a closed isotropic membrane bilayer (Evans and Skalak, 1980; Helfrich, 1974; Stokke et al., 1986):

$$F_{\text{tot}} = \frac{k_c}{2} \int (2H - \bar{C}_0)^2 \, dA + k_G \int C_1 C_2 \, dA + 2k_r A(\langle H \rangle)^2, \quad (7.68)$$

where

$$\langle H \rangle = \frac{1}{A} \int H \, dA, \quad (7.69)$$

is the average mean curvature and k_r is the non-local bending constant (Evans and Skalak, 1980). The effective spontaneous curvature of the bilayer $\bar{C}_0$ (Helfrich, 1974; Miao et al., 1994; Mukhopadhyay et al., 2002) may derive from bilayer asymmetry due to the different environments on the two sides of the bilayer, due to their different compositions and due to the different numbers of molecules in the two constituent monolayers (Evans and Skalak, 1980; Helfrich, 1974). Equation 7.68 can be rewritten in the equivalent form:

$$F_{\text{tot}} = \frac{k_c}{2} \int (2H)^2 \, dA + k_G \int C_1 C_2 \, dA + 2k_r A(\langle H \rangle - H_0)^2, \quad (7.70)$$

where the spontaneous average mean curvature H_0 is proportional to the parameter $\bar{C}_0$. Using the relation between ΔA and $\langle H \rangle$ (Eqs. 7.66 and 7.69), the energy F_b can also be expressed by the area difference ΔA and the effective area difference $\overline{\Delta A_0} = 2A\delta H_0$ (Miao et al., 1994; Mukhopadhyay et al., 2002; Stokke et al., 1986). Therefore much later the above model of membrane bilayer elasticity was also named the area-difference-elasticity (ADE) model, (see, e.g., Käs and Sackmann, 1991). The parameters $\overline{\Delta A_0}$ and H_0 depend on asymmetry in composition, environment and the number of molecules with respect to the two monolayers. In accordance with previous considerations (Helfrich, 1974; Miao et al., 1994), it was established that these effects should not enter the expression for the bending energy of a closed isotropic membrane bilayer (Eqs. 7.68 and 7.70) independently but only in the form of the (effective) spontaneous curvature of the bilayer $\bar{C}_0$, or alternatively in the form of the spontaneous average mean curvature H_0 (or effective relaxed area difference $\overline{\Delta A_0}$) (Mukhopadhyay et al., 2002).

However, in determining the equilibrium shape of a phospholipid vesicle with protrusion the estimated effect of the non-local bending (relative stretching of the two membrane layers) on the calculated stable shape was found to be negligible in the region of long thin protrusions (Kralj-Iglič, 2002).

If the tube radius were only several nanometres, the thickness of the membrane itself ($\simeq 5$ nm) is comparable to the radius of the protrusion. Therefore, the expression for the area difference (Eq. 7.66) should be reformulated (Szleifer et al., 1990) by considering that the membrane thickness is not very small compared to the dimensions of the protrusion.

The crude model of elasticity of the lipid bilayer presented in this chapter nevertheless shows that deviatoric elasticity offers a possible explanation for the stability of the phospholipid nanotubes attached to giant spherical phospholipid vesicles and for the observed shape transformation of the protrusion from the cylinder-like to the bead-like shape.

7.8 Shape Equation and Budding Transition of Phospholipid Vesicles

Budding of a bilayer membrane is a process that is vitally important for cells (Greenwalt, 2006; McMahon and Gallop, 2005). Accordingly, it is of interest to understand the mechanisms that are involved in the budding process (Božič et al., 2006; Laradji and Kumar, 2004; Miao et al., 1994; Sens and Gov, 2007; Sens and Turner, 2004). An important role of membrane budding has been found in immune response and pathological conditions (Farsad and De Camilli, 2003; Greenwalt, 2006). It was shown that membrane skeleton-detached, laterally mobile membrane lipids and integral membrane protein components, or their small complexes (membrane nanodomains) may be differentiated into highly curved spherical or tubular regions of cell membranes depending on their intrinsic shape and/or the direct interactions between them (see Farsad and De Camilli, 2003; Hägerstrand et al., 2006; Holopainen et al., 2000; Huttner and Zimmerberg, 2001; Iglič et al., 2007c). Clustering of membrane components or membrane nanodomains in highly

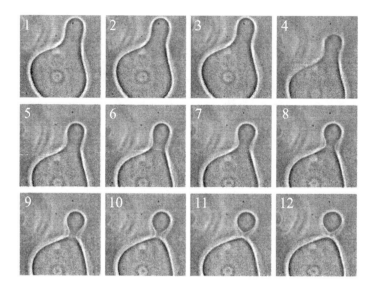

Figure 7.17 Budding process of the POPC-cardiolipin-cholesterol vesicle (GUV) induced by increasing the temperature. With kind permission from Springer Science+Business Media: Urbanija, J., Babnik, B., Frank, M., Tomšič, N., Rozman, B., Kralj-Iglič, V., and Iglič, A. (2008a). Attachment of β_2-glycoprotein I to negatively charged liposomes may prevent the release of daughter vesicles from the parent membrane. *Eur. Biophys. J.*, 37, pp. 1085–1095.

curved membrane regions therefore plays an important role in generation and stabilization of spherical and tubular membrane protrusions (Farsad and De Camilli, 2003; Huttner and Zimmerberg, 2001; Veranič et al., 2008).

In order to understand the basic physical properties of membrane budding (Fig. 7.17), the budding process has been studied in a simple system of bilayer membrane vesicles composed of a single or several phospholipid species (Lipowsky, 1991; Miao et al., 1994; Sackmann, 1994; Urbanija et al., 2008a) where changes of temperature may cause changes in the vesicle shapes and may in certain conditions induce formation of buds from the membrane bilayer surface (Käs and Sackmann, 1991; Urbanija et al., 2008a).

In the budding transition of a POPC-cardiolipin-cholesterol vesicle the initial pear-like shape was observed to continuously (smoothly) transform into a limiting shape composed of a larger spheroidal parent cell and a smaller spheroidal daughter vesicle which are connected by a thin neck (see Fig. 7.17). In general temperature-induced budding of liposomes observed previously was continuous or discontinuous (Käs and Sackmann, 1991). It was noticed that the vesicles formed from charged lipids can undergo continuous transitions to an outside budded state via the pear shape, while in pure vesicles made from POPC or DMPC the budding seems to be discontinuous in the vicinity of the limiting shapes (Käs and Sackmann, 1991). The so-called ADE model (defined in the previous Section 7.7) based on minimization of the local and non-local bending energy (Eq. 7.70) (Evans and Skalak, 1980; Stokke et al., 1986), cannot explain the above mentioned continuous shape transitions and/or discontinuity in the vicinity of limiting shapes (Miao et al., 1994). Namely, according to the predictions of the ADE model, a discontinuous shape transition from a cigar type shape to a vesiculated shape composed of a larger spheroidal parent vesicle and a smaller spheroidal daughter vesicle is possible. But the observed discontinuous shape transition from a weak pear to a vesiculated shape composed of two spheres is not a possibility within the ADE model (Miao et al., 1994).

The results of some previous studies suggested that the continuous transition and the discontinuity in the vicinity of the limiting shape could be explained by taking into account the average orientational ordering and the direct interactions between oriented lipids (Urbanija et al., 2008a). The intrinsic properties of membrane lipids and the interactions between them are thus assumed to influence the macroscopic features such as the equilibrium shape of the vesicle and/or the budding process of the membrane (Kralj-Iglič et al., 2006; Urbanija et al., 2008a).

Taking into account the two-state energy model for the average orientational ordering of lipid molecules and the direct interaction between lipids, the free energy of a one-component lipid bilayer may be written in the form (see Eq. 7.56 for comparison) (Kralj-Iglič et al., 2006):

$$F_b = \frac{(3\xi + \xi^*)}{8} n_0 \int (2H)^2 dA - \frac{(\xi + \xi^*) n_0}{2} \int C_1 C_2 dA$$
$$- 2n_0 kT \int \ln \cosh(d_{\text{eff}}(1 + \tilde{k}/kT)/2) dA, \qquad (7.71)$$

where the constant terms are omitted and the parameter $d_{\text{eff}} = (\xi + \xi^*)D_m D/kT$ (Eq. 7.19). The second term in Eq. 7.71 is not further considered since according to the Gauss–Bonnet theorem it is constant for the closed surfaces that are considered in this section. Therefore, in what follows we consider the expression for the free energy F_b:

$$F_b = \frac{k_c}{2} \int (2H)^2 dA - 2n_0 kT \int \ln \cosh(d_{\text{eff}}(1 + \tilde{k}/kT)/2) dA. \tag{7.72}$$

where $k_c = (3\xi + \xi^*)n_0/4$. The first term in Eq. 7.72 yields the local bending energy of a closed lipid bilayer vesicle (Helfrich, 1973), while the second term accounts for the average orientational ordering of lipid molecules. In order to consider also the non-local bending energy as well, the final expression for the free energy of a lipid bilayer should be (see Eq. 7.70) (Urbanija et al., 2008a):

$$F_{\text{tot}} = F_b + 2 k_r A (\langle H \rangle - H_0)^2. \tag{7.73}$$

The second term accounts for the non-local isotropic bending elasticity of the lipid bilayer membrane (Evans and Skalak, 1980; Miao et al., 1994).

The equilibrium configuration of a closed bilayer membrane corresponding to the minimum of F_{tot} can be determined as follows. First, the equilibrium shape of the closed bilayer membrane corresponding to the minimum of F_b (F_{min}) is found for different values of $\langle H \rangle$. Second, the shape corresponding to the minimal value of F_{tot} (Eq. 7.73) is determined by minimization of $F_{\text{tot}} = F_{\text{min}}(\langle H \rangle) + 2k_r A (\langle H \rangle - H_0)^2$ with respect to $\langle H \rangle$ (Urbanija et al., 2008a).

The equilibrium configuration of a closed lipid bilayer membrane (i.e., the equilibrium shape and the corresponding distribution of the average quadrupolar lipid ordering) corresponding to minimal F_b (F_{min}) is sought by variation of F_b (Eq. 7.72):

$$\delta F_b = 0, \tag{7.74}$$

under the relevant geometrical constraints. We require that the membrane area A (Eq. 7.64), the enclosed volume V (Eq. 7.65) and the average mean curvature $\langle H \rangle$:

$$\langle H \rangle = \frac{1}{A} \int H dA, \tag{7.75}$$

are fixed.

The variation $\delta F_b = 0$ is performed in dimensionless form. We introduce dimensionless (reduced) curvatures $c_1 = RC_1$, $c_2 = RC_2$, $h = RH$, $d = RD$, $d_m = RD_m$, the relative (reduced) area $a = A/4\pi^2 R = 1$, the relative (reduced) volume $v = (36\pi V^2/A^3)^{1/2}$, the relative (reduced) average mean curvature $\langle h \rangle = R\langle H \rangle = \Delta a = \int h\, da$, where $R = (A/4\pi)^{1/2}$ is chosen as the unit of length. The bending free energy of the phospholipid bilayer F_b (Eq. 7.72) is normalized relative to $(3\xi + \xi^*)2\pi n_0$:

$$f_b = \frac{1}{4}\int (c_1 + c_2)^2 da - \kappa \int \ln\cosh(d_{\text{eff}}/2)\, da, \qquad (7.76)$$

where $\kappa = 4kT R^2/(3\xi + \xi^*)$.

In the following we consider only axisymmetric shapes. The geometry of the shape is described in terms of the arc length l. We use the coordinates $\rho(l)$ and $z(l)$ where ρ is the perpendicular distance between the symmetry axis and a certain point on the contour and z is the position of this point along the symmetry axis. The principal curvatures are

$$c_1 = \frac{\sin\psi}{\rho}, \quad c_2 = \frac{d\psi}{dl} \equiv \psi_l, \qquad (7.77)$$

where ψ is the angle between the normal to the surface and the symmetry axis. The dimensionless area element is $da = \rho\, dl/2$ and the dimensionless volume element is $dv = 3\rho^2 \sin\psi\, dl/4$. Using the above coordinates, the dimensionless free energy (Eq. 7.76) is:

$$f_b = \int \frac{1}{8}\left(\frac{\sin\psi}{\varrho} + \psi_l\right)^2 \rho\, dl - \int \frac{\kappa\rho}{2}\ln\cosh\left(\vartheta\left(\frac{\sin\psi}{\varrho} - \psi_l\right)\right) dl. \qquad (7.78)$$

where

$$\vartheta = \frac{(\xi + \xi^*)D_m}{4kT R}\left(1 + \frac{\tilde{k}}{kT}\right), \qquad (7.79)$$

while the dimensionless global constraints for reduced area, reduced volume, and reduced average mean curvature are

$$\int \frac{1}{2}\rho\, dl = 1, \qquad (7.80)$$

$$\int \frac{3}{4}\rho^2 \sin\psi\, dl = v \qquad (7.81)$$

and
$$\int \frac{1}{4}(\sin\psi + \psi_l)dl = \langle h \rangle. \tag{7.82}$$

Also, we must consider a local constraint between the chosen coordinates,
$$\frac{d\rho}{dl} = \cos\psi. \tag{7.83}$$

A functional is constructed
$$G = \int \mathcal{L} dl, \tag{7.84}$$

where
$$\mathcal{L} = \frac{1}{8}\left(\frac{\sin\psi}{\varrho} + \psi_l\right)^2 \rho - \frac{\kappa\rho}{2}\ln\cosh\left(\vartheta\left(\frac{\sin\psi}{\varrho} - \psi_l\right)\right)$$
$$+\lambda_a \frac{\rho}{2} + \lambda_v \frac{3}{4}\rho^2 \sin\psi + \lambda_{\langle h \rangle}\frac{1}{4}\left(\frac{\sin\psi}{\varrho} + \psi_l\right)\rho + \lambda(\rho_l - \cos\psi), \tag{7.85}$$

λ_a, λ_v and λ_h are the global Lagrange multipliers and λ is the local Lagrange multiplier. The above variational problem is expressed by a system of Lagrange–Euler differential equations:
$$\frac{\partial \mathcal{L}}{\partial \rho} - \frac{d}{dl}\left(\frac{\partial \mathcal{L}}{\partial \rho_l}\right) = 0, \tag{7.86}$$

$$\frac{\partial \mathcal{L}}{\partial \psi} - \frac{d}{dl}\left(\frac{\partial \mathcal{L}}{\partial \psi_l}\right) = 0. \tag{7.87}$$

It follows from Eqs. 7.86 and 7.85 that
$$\frac{d\lambda}{dl} = \frac{1}{8}\left(\frac{\chi^2 - \sin^2\psi}{\rho^2}\right) + \frac{\lambda_a}{2} + \frac{3}{2}\lambda_v \varrho \sin\psi + \frac{1}{4}\lambda_{\langle h \rangle}\frac{\chi}{\rho}$$
$$-\frac{\kappa}{2}\ln\cosh\left(\vartheta\left(\frac{\sin\psi - \chi}{\varrho}\right)\right)$$
$$+\frac{\kappa\vartheta}{2\rho}\sin\psi \tanh\left(\vartheta\left(\frac{\sin\psi - \chi}{\varrho}\right)\right), \tag{7.88}$$

while it follows from Eqs. 7.87 and 7.85 that
$$\frac{d\chi}{dl} = \frac{\mathcal{A}}{\mathcal{B}}, \tag{7.89}$$

where

$$B = \left(1 - \frac{2\kappa\vartheta^2}{\cosh^2\left(\vartheta\left(\frac{\sin\psi - \chi}{\varrho}\right)\right)}\right), \quad (7.90)$$

$$A = \frac{\sin\psi\cos\psi}{\rho}\left(1 + \frac{2\kappa\vartheta^2}{\cosh^2\left(\vartheta\left(\frac{\sin\psi - \chi}{\varrho}\right)\right)}\right)$$
$$- \frac{4\kappa\vartheta^2\chi\cos\psi}{\rho\cosh^2\left(\vartheta\left(\frac{\sin\psi - \chi}{\varrho}\right)\right)} + 3\lambda_v\varrho^2\cos\psi + 4\lambda\sin\psi$$
$$- 4\kappa\vartheta\cos\psi\tanh\left(\vartheta\left(\frac{\sin\psi - \chi}{\varrho}\right)\right), \quad (7.91)$$

and

$$\psi_l = \frac{\chi}{\rho}. \quad (7.92)$$

At the poles $\psi_l = \sin\psi/\rho$. The system of Eqs. 7.83 and 7.88–7.92 can be solved numerically. Integration over the arc length l is performed from both poles so that the relative area of the calculated shape is equal to 1. Then, the validity of the constraints is tested and new initial values of the above quantities are set. The procedure is repeated until the constraints and the smoothness of the variables at the meeting point are fulfilled up to the prescribed accuracy. The contour of the cell shape is determined using the relation

$$\frac{dz}{dl} = -\sin\psi. \quad (7.93)$$

The equilibrium vesicle shapes corresponding to minimal F_{tot} as a function of the normalized spontaneous average mean curvature $h_0 = R_s H_0$ are calculated for a given relative cell volume v as described above. Fig. 7.18 shows the equilibrium value of the normalized average mean curvature $\langle h \rangle = R_s \langle H \rangle$ as a function of h_0. Case A corresponds to the ADE model, where the free energy consists of the local and non-local isotropic bending energy terms only ($d_{\text{eff}} \equiv 0$), while in cases B–D we also took into account the averaged quadrupolar ordering of lipid molecules ($d_{\text{eff}} \neq 0$) (see Eqs. 7.72 and 7.73).

Within the so-called ADE model, the absolute minimum of the membrane free energy may, by an appropriate choice of the

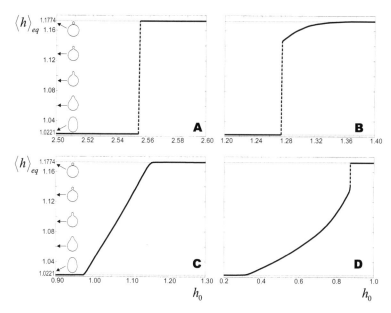

Figure 7.18 Calculated normalized average mean curvature corresponding to the minimum of the membrane energy ($\langle h \rangle_{eq} = R_s \langle H \rangle_{eq}$) as a function of h_0 for pear-shaped axisymmetric vesicle shapes with the relative volume $v = 0.95$ and $k_r/k_c = 2$ (see Hwang and Waugh, 1997). Figure A shows the corresponding dependence of $\langle h \rangle_{eq}$ within the ADE model where the orientational ordering of interacting lipid molecules is not taken into account. The calculated dependence in Figures B–D take into account the orientational ordering of lipids and direct interactions between oriented lipids, where: $(\xi + \xi^*)D_m/4kT R_s = 1.5 \cdot 10^{-4}$, $4kT R_s^2/(3\xi + \xi^*) = 7 \cdot 10^6$ (see Kralj-Iglič et al., 2006) and $\tilde{k}/kT = 0.67$ (B), 0.8 (C) and 1.0 (D). The figure also shows some characteristic vesicle shapes corresponding to different values of $\langle h \rangle$. Reprinted with kind permission from Springer Science+Business Media: Urbanija, J., Babnik, B., Frank, M., Tomšič, N., Rozman, B., Kralj-Iglič, V., and Iglič, A. (2008a). Attachment of b2-glycoprotein I to negatively charged liposomes may prevent the release of daughter vesicles from the parent membrane. *Eur. Biophys. J.*, 37, pp. 1085–1095.

parameters k_r/k_c and H_0, be shifted to the limit shape of a pear-shaped vesicle (composed of two spheres connected by an infinitesimal neck). However, a considerably higher value of k_r/k_c than the experimentally estimated one (Hwang and Waugh, 1997) is needed to obtain this effect (Miao et al., 1994) or alternatively the values of H_0 should be larger than any $\langle h \rangle$ within the sequence of pear shapes (see Fig. 7.18A). This gives a significant increase of the membrane free energy and of the lateral tension within the membrane. It seems unlikely that the vesicle (GUV) would favour a high lateral membrane tension within the membrane as it may develop processes to relax it, such as transient pore formation (Holopainen et al., 2000; Raphael and Waugh, 1996).

In outline, we have shown in this section that a decrease in the free energy due to orientational ordering of phospholipid molecules and direct interactions between lipid molecules may complement the non-local isotropic bending in stabilizing pear vesicle shapes, including shapes with thin neck(s). It should also be noted that the calculated equilibrium vesicle shapes determined by minimization of the membrane free energy given by Eq. 7.73 can also have a wider neck(s) (see Fig. 7.18C), corresponding to a deep minimum of the membrane free energy that would exceed the energies of thermal fluctuations. Minimization of the membrane free energy given by Eq. 7.73 predicts a continuous transition between pear-shaped liposomes (see Fig. 7.18C), or a discontinuity in the vicinity of limiting shapes composed of a spherical parent cell and a spherical daughter vesicle (see Fig. 7.18D). This is not possible within the ADE model (Käs and Sackmann, 1991; Miao et al., 1994) where only the discontinuous shape transition between a cigar type shape to a vesiculated pear type shape is possible (see Fig. 7.18A).

To conclude, including the average orientational ordering of lipids and their direct interactions in calculation of equilibrium liposome shapes may result in a minimum of the liposome membrane free energy close to the shape with a narrow neck even for low values of h_0. Contrary to the predictions of the ADE model, both, continuous shape transitions and discontinuous shape transitions in the vicinity of limiting shapes are possible for realistic values of model parameters.

Chapter 8

Membrane Nanodomains

Membrane nanodomains are important functional building blocks of biological membranes. As an addition to the pure lipid bilayer, they can significantly increase the complexity and alter the physical properties of biological membranes.

Flexible membrane nanodomains are small complexes composed of proteins and lipids, where the proteins are often chain-like biopolymers that cross the membrane bilayer several times (see Fig. 8.1A and Hägerstrand et al., 2006). Membrane raft elements of biological membranes may also fall into this category. Membrane nanodomains (inclusions) may also be induced by a single rigid globular membrane protein, which can be described in the first approximation as a rigid object of a simple geometrical shape (see Fig. 8.1B and Gruler, 1975). Some membrane-embedded peptides may induce such nanodomains. The single-nanodomain energy is derived in this chapter.

In this chapter, we present a theoretical approach to the study of membrane nanodomains. We derive the contribution to the free energy of the membrane bilayer including nanodomains which are in general flexible. For flexible membrane nanodomains the phenomenological interaction constants that appear in the free energy expression depend on the physical and geometrical

---

Nanostructures in Biological Systems: Theory and Applications
Aleš Iglič, Veronika Kralj-Iglič, and Damjana Drobne
Copyright © 2015 Pan Stanford Publishing Pte. Ltd.
ISBN 978-981-4267-20-5 (Hardcover), 978-981-4303-43-9 (eBook)
www.panstanford.com

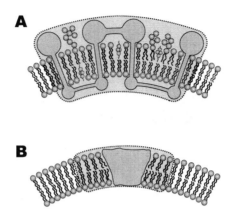

Figure 8.1 Schematic illustration of flexible membrane nanodomains (shaded area): a flexible membrane nanodomain including a chain-like protein (A), and a flexible membrane nanodomain induced by a membrane-embedded rigid protein (B).

properties of the molecules that constitute the membrane. Special consideration is devoted to membrane nanodomains induced by rigid membrane-embedded proteins. The cases of constrained and unconstrained local shape perturbations of the membrane around a rigid membrane inclusion are discussed. The total free energy of the membrane bilayer with membrane nanodomains is derived.

8.1 Phenomenological Expression for the Energy of a Flexible Membrane Nanodomain

The thin surface of the membrane is in general anisotropic with respect to the curvature of the normal cuts (Helfrich and Prost, 1988; Iglič et al., 2005a; Oda et al., 1999) and can attain various equilibrium shapes that are not flat or spherical (Iglič et al., 2005a,b).

The local shape of the membrane surface is described by two principal curvatures C_1 and C_2 (Fig. 5.1). The flexible membrane nanodomain can be treated as a small two-dimensional flexible plate with area a_0. The nanodomain is in general anisotropic, therefore its intrinsic shape can be described by the two intrinsic principal

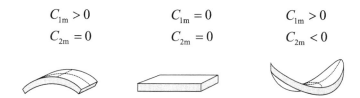

Figure 8.2 Schematic illustration of the most favourable shapes (cylindrical, flat, and a saddle-like) of a flexible membrane nanodomain having different values of the intrinsic (spontaneous) mean curvatures C_{1m} and C_{2m}.

curvatures C_{1m} and C_{2m} (Fig. 8.2) and by the in-plane orientation of the nanodomain in the membrane.

Accordingly, we define the elastic energy of a small plate-like membrane nanodomain (see Fig. 8.1) with area a_0 as the energy of the mismatch between the actual local curvature of the membrane and the intrinsic (spontaneous) curvature of the nanodomain. Therefore, we define the tensor $\underline{M} = \underline{R}\,\underline{C}_m\underline{R}^{-1} - \underline{C}$ (Iglič et al., 2005a), where the tensor $\underline{C}$ describes the actual local curvature, the tensor $\underline{C}_m$ describes the intrinsic curvature of the nanodomain (see Fig. 8.2), and

$$\underline{R} = \begin{bmatrix} \cos\omega & -\sin\omega \\ \sin\omega & \cos\omega \end{bmatrix} \tag{8.1}$$

is the rotation matrix (see also Fig. 8.3). In the respective principal systems the matrices that represent curvature tensors include only the diagonal elements:

$$\underline{C} = \begin{bmatrix} C_1 & 0 \\ 0 & C_2 \end{bmatrix}, \quad \underline{C}_m = \begin{bmatrix} C_{1m} & 0 \\ 0 & C_{2m} \end{bmatrix}. \tag{8.2}$$

The principal systems of these two tensors are in general rotated in the tangential plane of the membrane surface by an angle ω with respect to each other (Fig. 8.3).

The elastic energy of the nanodomain per unit area (w) should be scalar quantity. Therefore each term in the expression for w must also be scalar (Landau and Lifshitz, 1997), that is, invariant with respect to all transformations of the local coordinate system. In this work, the elastic energy density w is approximated by an expansion in powers of all independent invariants of the tensor $\underline{M}$ up to the

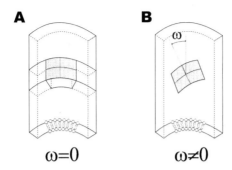

Figure 8.3 Schematic illustration of different orientations of a flexible membrane nanodomain with intrinsic principal curvatures $C_{1m} > 0$ and $C_{2m} = 0$ (see also Fig. 8.2). The shape of the membrane is cylindrical ($C_1 > 0$ and $C_2 = 0$). Reprinted from *Blood Cells, Molecules and Diseases*, 39(1), Aleš Iglič, Maruša Lokar, Blaž Babnik, Tomaž Slivnik, Peter Veranič, Henry Hgerstrand, and Veronika Kralj-Iglič, Possible role of flexible red blood cell membrane nanodomains in the growth and stability of membrane nanotubes, pp. 14–23, Copyright 2007, with permission from Elsevier.

second order in the components of $\underline{M}$. The trace and the determinant of the tensor are taken as the set of invariants (Iglič et al., 2005a, 2007c):

$$w = \mu_0 + \frac{K_1}{2}(\mathrm{Tr}\underline{M})^2 + K_2 \mathrm{Det}\underline{M}, \tag{8.3}$$

where μ_0 is the minimal possible value of w, while K_1 and K_2 are constants. For the sake of simplicity $\mu_0 \equiv 0$. Taking into account the definition of the tensor $\underline{M}$ it follows from Eqs. 8.2–8.3 that the elastic energy of the flexible membrane nanodomain can be written as:

$$E = a_0(2K_1 + K_2)(H - H_m)^2 - a_0 K_2(D^2 - 2DD_m \cos 2\omega + D_m^2), \tag{8.4}$$

where

$$H = \frac{1}{2}(C_1 + C_2) \tag{8.5}$$

is the membrane mean curvature and,

$$D = \frac{1}{2}|C_1 - C_2| \tag{8.6}$$

is the membrane curvature deviator, $H_m = (C_{1m} + C_{2m})/2$ is the intrinsic (spontaneous) mean curvature and $D_m = |C_{1m} - C_{2m}|/2$ is the intrinsic (spontaneous) curvature deviator.

It can be seen from Eq. 8.4 that the geometrical and material properties of an anisotropic flexible membrane nanodomain can be expressed in a simple way by only two intrinsic curvatures C_{1m} and C_{2m} and constants K_1 and K_2. Figure 8.2 shows a sketch of cylindrical, flat, and saddle-like intrinsic (spontaneous) shapes of flexible membrane nanodomains.

The values of the membrane mean curvature $H = (C_1 + C_2)/2$, the curvature deviator $D = |C_1 - C_2|/2$ and the orientation angle of the nanodomain ω that correspond to the minimum of the function E for given values of $H_m = (C_{1m} + C_{2m})/2$ and $D_m = |C_{1m} - C_{2m}|/2$ can be calculated from the necessary conditions for the extreme of the function E (Iglič et al., 2007c):

$$\frac{\partial E}{\partial H} = 2a_0(2K_1 + K_2)(H - H_m) = 0, \tag{8.7}$$

$$\frac{\partial E}{\partial D} = -K_2 a_0 (2D - 2D_m \cos 2\omega) = 0, \tag{8.8}$$

$$\frac{\partial E}{\partial \omega} = -4a_0 K_2 D D_m \sin 2\omega = 0, \tag{8.9}$$

and the sufficient conditions for the minimum of E (Widder, 1947):

$$\frac{\partial^2 E}{\partial H^2} = 2a_0(2K_1 + K_2) > 0, \tag{8.10}$$

$$\left(\frac{\partial^2 E}{\partial H^2}\right)\left(\frac{\partial^2 E}{\partial D^2}\right) - \left(\frac{\partial^2 E}{\partial H \partial D}\right)^2 = -4K_2 a_0^2 (2K_1 + K_2) > 0, \tag{8.11}$$

$$\frac{\partial^2 E}{\partial H^2}\left[\left(\frac{\partial^2 E}{\partial D^2}\right)\left(\frac{\partial^2 E}{\partial \omega^2}\right) - \left(\frac{\partial^2 E}{\partial D \partial \omega}\right)^2\right]$$
$$= 16K_2^2 a_0^3 \frac{\partial^2 E}{\partial H^2} \left(D D_m \cos 2\omega - D_m^2 \sin^2 2\omega\right) > 0, \tag{8.12}$$

where it was taken into account that $\partial^2 E / \partial H \partial D = 0$ and $\partial^2 E / \partial H \partial \omega = 0$. Considering only positive values of ω, it follows from Eqs. 8.7–8.9 and 8.12 that at the minima of E:

$$H = H_m, \ D = D_m, \ \omega = 0, \pi, \tag{8.13}$$

and (Iglič et al., 2007c)

$$K_1 > -K_2/2, \ K_2 < 0. \tag{8.14}$$

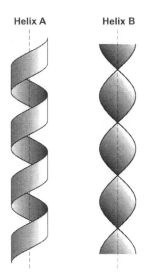

Figure 8.4 Schematic representation of helical configurations A and B.

If flexible membrane nanodomains have $C_{1m} > 0$ and $C_{2m} = 0$ (see Fig. 8.2), the energetically favourable membrane shapes would be tubular or collapsed tubular (in the form of a twisted strip – helix A, see Fig. 8.4). For $C_{1m} > 0$ and $C_{2m} < 0$ (Fig. 8.2), the favourable membrane shape would be saddle-like (constituting the neck connecting a daughter vesicle and the parent cell), or collapsed tubular, twisted in the form of helix B strip (see Fig. 8.4 and Iglič et al., 2005a).

The flexible membrane nanodomain adapts its shape in order to fit its curvature to the actual membrane curvature (which is also influenced by the nanodomains). Since all orientations of the single flexible nanodomain do not have the same energy (see Eq. 8.4), the partition function of a single nanodomain can be written in the form:

$$Q = \frac{1}{\omega_0} \int_0^{2\pi} \exp\left(-\frac{E(\omega)}{kT}\right) d\omega, \qquad (8.15)$$

with ω_0 as an arbitrary angle quantum. The free energy of the flexible membrane nanodomain is then obtained by the expression $f_i = -kT \ln Q$. Combining Eqs. 8.4 and 8.15 allows us to write the free energy of a single flexible membrane inclusion up to the constant as

$$f_i = (2K_1 + K_2)(H - H_m)^2 a_0$$
$$- K_2(D^2 + D_m^2)a_0 - kT \ln\left(I_0\left(\frac{2K_2 D D_m a_0}{kT}\right)\right). \quad (8.16)$$

By knowing the equilibrium density distribution of the membrane nanodomains (inclusions) over the membrane (see Kralj-Iglič et al., 1996), the contribution of the nanodomains to the overall membrane free energy can be attained by integration of Eq. 12.12 over the whole membrane surface. This possibility makes the above described approach an efficient theoretical tool to study equilibrium (closed) shapes of membranes with anisotropic membrane nanodomains (inclusions) (Fosnarič et al., 2005; Iglič et al., 2007b; Kralj-Iglič et al., 1999, 2005).

8.2 Membrane Nanodomains Induced by Rigid Proteins

8.2.1 Perturbation of Lipid Molecules around Rigid Membrane Embedded Proteins

A rigid protein, intercalated in the lipid bilayer, perturbs the structure of the surrounding lipids. Therefore we can define a membrane nanodomain (inclusion) as an embedded rigid protein and the surrounding lipids that are significantly distorted due to the presence of the embedded rigid protein (Kralj-Iglič et al., 1999). The energy of such a membrane nanodomain induced by the embedded rigid protein is therefore mainly attributed to the change in energy of the surrounding lipids. The energy of a lipid molecule depends on the particular sequence of *trans*, *gauche*$^+$ and *gauche*$^-$ orientations along the lipid chain, van der Waals interactions of the lipid chain with its neighbours, steric repulsion between the hard cores of each atom of neighbouring lipid chains and ionic interactions between polar lipid headgroups (Marčelja, 1974, 1976). The change in the ordering of lipids that surround the rigid protein leads to an indirect lipid mediated interaction between two rigid proteins when they approach each other (Marčelja, 1976). If the two proteins are close enough, the total lipid perturbation decreases, which may result in a net attractive force between the membrane-embedded rigid proteins and therefore in their aggregation (Marčelja, 1976).

Cone-like rigid proteins (Gruler, 1975) are characterized by a cone angle (Dan and Safran, 1998) to which the membrane shape has to adapt. The mesoscopic-level description of the membrane identifies the rigid protein's cone-shape with a local discontinuity in the membrane curvature field. On a more microscopic level, another degree of freedom of the membrane becomes significant, namely the *tilt* of the lipid molecules (Fournier, 1999; Helfrich, 1973). Helfrich and Prost (Helfrich and Prost, 1988) have shown that a symmetric lipid bilayer may exhibit an intrinsic bending force if the lipid molecules are collectively tilted.

However, membrane perturbations that involve lipid tilt are often short-ranged, with a characteristic length extending over a few lipids. Lipid tilt may be thus important for processes where the local membrane geometry changes over short distances such as for non-bilayer lipid phases (May and Ben-Shaul, 1999; Perutková et al., 2009; Rappolt et al., 2003), or for the periodic "ripple" phase (Fournier, 1998; Lubensky and MacKintosh, 1993; Seifert et al., 1996).

In the different works cited above, the membrane-embedded rigid proteins exhibit cylindrical symmetry about their axis normal to the membrane, that is, they are *isotropic*. More generally, if cylindrical symmetry of the rigid membrane protein is absent (Fig. 8.6), the membrane nanodomain (inclusion) free energy depends on the protein's in-plane orientation within the membrane. The intrinsic shape of the rigid protein is then characterized by two intrinsic principal curvatures C_{1m} and C_{2m}. The lateral organization of *anisotropic* proteins can be quite complex, ranging from a chain-like assembly (Dommersnes and Fournier, 1999), saddle-like membrane regions (Kralj-Iglič et al., 1999) to periodic pattern formation (Dommersnes and Fournier, 2002).

Within the standard theory of elasticity of the lipid bilayer, its elastic energy is decomposed into contributions due to area stretching, tilt of the lipid molecules, local bending, and non-local bending (Evans and Skalak, 1980; Helfrich, 1973, 1974). On a mesoscopic scale level, the local and non-local bending energies can be described in terms of its two local principal membrane curvatures

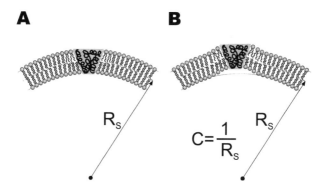

Figure 8.5 Schematic illustration of a lipid bilayer of prescribed spherical curvature ($C = C_1 = C_2 = H = 1/R_s$) defined at the mesoscopic scale level. The intercalated rigid protein has a conical shape. In case A, the local membrane shape does not differ from the mesoscopic spherical curvature of the membrane (C), while in the case B the local microscopic (nanoscale) membrane shape perturbation of the spherical surface with curvature C is also induced due to the presence of the rigid protein. In the case B, the lipids accommodate to the intrinsic shape of the intercalated rigid protein through curvature deformation and via changes in lipid tilt, while in case A lipids accommodate to the protein intrinsic shape via changes in lipid tilt only. Figure reprinted with permission from Fošnarič, M., Iglič, A., and May, S. Influence of rigid inclusions on the bending elasticity of a lipid membrane. *Phys. Rev. E*, 174, pp. 051503. Copyright 2006 by the American Physical Society.

C_1 and C_2 (Evans and Skalak, 1980; Helfrich, 1974). The question arises how the elastic behaviour of a membrane bilayer is affected by membrane-embedded rigid proteins, if the local microscopic membrane shape perturbation (at the nanoscale level) due to each individual protein is taken into account (Fig. 8.5). In general, the theoretical description of local microscopic perturbations of lipid molecules around the intercalated rigid protein falls between two limiting cases.

In the first case the membrane-intercalated rigid proteins are distributed over the whole membrane surface or at least over a large portion of it (Hägerstrand et al., 2006). Therefore, possible local microscopic perturbations of the membrane shape around each of the rigid proteins (as schematically shown in Fig. 8.5B) would greatly increase the non-local bending energy of the bilayer membrane (see Eq. 7.68). This energy contribution, also called the relative stretching energy (since it originates from the different stretching of the two monolayers during bending of the bilayer at constant average membrane area (Evans and Skalak, 1980; Helfrich, 1974; Hwang and Waugh, 1997), can be written as (Eq. 7.70)

$$W_n = 2k_r A(\langle H \rangle - H_0)^2 \qquad (8.17)$$

where $\langle H \rangle = \frac{1}{A} \int H \, dA$ is the average mean curvature, $H = (C_1 + C_2)/2$, H_0 is the spontaneous mean curvature (Kralj-Iglič et al., 2005), k_r is the non-local bending constant (Evans and Skalak, 1980; Hwang and Waugh, 1997), A is the membrane area and dA is the membrane area element. For a closed, nearly flat bilayer membrane (where $\langle H \rangle \approx 0$, $H_0 \approx 0$), with N homogeneously distributed intercalated rigid proteins, the membrane's non-local bending energy W_n can be approximately written as (Fošnarič et al., 2006)

$$W_n \cong 2k_r A(N\langle H \rangle_p - NH_{0p})^2 \propto N^2, \qquad (8.18)$$

where H_{0p} and $\langle H \rangle_p$ refer to the disturbed membrane patch around a single membrane-intercalated rigid protein (Fig. 8.5B). Since the energy favour W_n increases quadratically with the total number of membrane-embedded rigid proteins, the local microscopic perturbation of the membrane shape around each of the intercalated rigid proteins (Fig. 8.5B) would be energetically less favourable for large enough N than the locally unperturbed membrane shape where the lipids accommodate to the intrinsic shape of the rigid protein predominantly via changes in the lipid tilt (Fig. 8.5A).

In the opposite limit, the membrane region with intercalated rigid proteins is spatially confined (i.e., small) and in contact with a reservoir of relaxed lipid bilayers. Therefore, the lipids surrounding the intercalated rigid protein are also free to adjust their conformation by perturbation of the local membrane shape, as schematically shown in Fig. 8.5B.

In biological membranes the majority of membrane proteins are laterally distributed over the whole membrane area. In addition, the number of membrane proteins (N) is very large. Therefore the first scenario, that is, the case of constrained microscopic deviations of the membrane shape around the intercalated rigid inclusions (Fig. 8.5A), seems to be more relevant.

8.2.2 Energy of a Membrane Nanodomain Induced by a Single Rigid Membrane Protein

Coupling between a non-homogeneous lateral distribution of membrane-embedded rigid proteins and membrane shapes may be a general mechanism of generation and stabilization of highly curved membrane structures (spherical buds, membrane necks, thin tubular membrane protrusions) (Allain and Ben Amar, 2004; Kralj-Iglič et al., 1999, 2005; Laradji and Kumar, 2004; Markin, 1981; Seifert, 1997).

On the phenomenological level, membrane bending may be coupled energetically to the local density of membrane-embedded rigid proteins by introducing a composition-dependent local bending constant and the spontaneous curvature. The underlying model (including direct interactions between rigid proteins and the configurational entropy of rigid proteins) was suggested by Markin (Markin, 1981) and used in subsequent applications (Seifert, 1993). Leibler (1986) proposed a similar thermodynamic model.

Another theoretical approach starts from a phenomenological expression for the energy of a *single* membrane nanodomain induced by intercalation of the rigid protein (Kralj-Iglič et al., 1996, 1999) where the term nanodomain (inclusion) is used for an entity consisting of the embedded rigid protein and lipids that are significantly distorted due to the presence of the embedded rigid protein (Kralj-Iglič et al., 1999) (see also Fig. 8.1).

It is proposed that the energy of such a nanodomain derives from the mismatch between the local shape of the membrane and the intrinsic shape of the membrane-embedded rigid protein. The local curvature of the membrane is represented by the curvatures of all possible normal cuts of the surface through the site of the inserted rigid protein. The energy of a single nanodomain assumed to be induced by intercalation of a single rigid protein is then given by a phenomenological expression consisting of two terms (Kralj-Iglič et al., 1999),

$$E = \frac{\xi}{4\pi} \int_0^{2\pi} (C - C_m)^2 d\psi + \frac{\xi^*}{16\pi} \int_0^{2\pi} \left(\frac{d}{d\psi}(C - C_m)\right)^2 d\psi, \tag{8.19}$$

where ξ and ξ^* are positive interaction constants, $C = 1/R$ is the curvature of the membrane normal cut (Eq. 5.15) that is rotated by an angle ψ in the principal axes system of the membrane surface, and C_m is the curvature of the normal cut corresponding to the protein intrinsic shape. The first contribution takes into account the differences in curvatures of the normal cuts of the two systems, while the second contribution takes into account the coupling between the neighbouring curvatures of the normal cuts of the two systems.

The orientation of the membrane embedded rigid protein is described by considering that the principal directions of the membrane surface are in general different from the principal directions of the protein intrinsic shape. The mutual orientation of the two systems is determined by the angle ω. We consider the Euler equations for the curvatures of the respective normal cuts of the continuum

$$C = C_1 \cos^2 \psi + C_2 \sin^2 \psi \qquad (8.20)$$

and

$$C_m = C_{1m} \cos^2(\psi + \omega) + C_{2m} \sin^2(\psi + \omega), \qquad (8.21)$$

where C_1 and C_2 are the principal curvatures describing the local shape of the surface (Fig. 5.2), and C_{1m} and C_{2m} are the principal curvatures describing the intrinsic shape of the membrane-embedded rigid protein. By performing integrations in Eq. 8.19, we get

$$E = \mu_m + \frac{\xi}{2}(H - H_m)^2 + \frac{\xi + \xi^*}{4}(D^2 - 2DD_m \cos 2\omega + D_m^2), \qquad (8.22)$$

where μ_m is the constant, $H = (C_1 + C_2)/2$ is the mean curvature, $D = |C_1 - C_2|/2$ is the curvature deviator, while $H_m = (C_{1m} + C_{2m})/2$ and $D_m = |C_{1m} - C_{2m}|/2$ are the intrinsic mean and deviatoric curvatures that reflect the preferred local macroscopic membrane curvature of the membrane-embedded rigid protein. The membrane-inserted protein is called isotropic if $C_{1m} = C_{2m}$, while it is called anisotropic if $C_{1m} \neq C_{2m}$. Figure 8.6 gives a schematic representation of different intrinsic shapes of inserted rigid proteins.

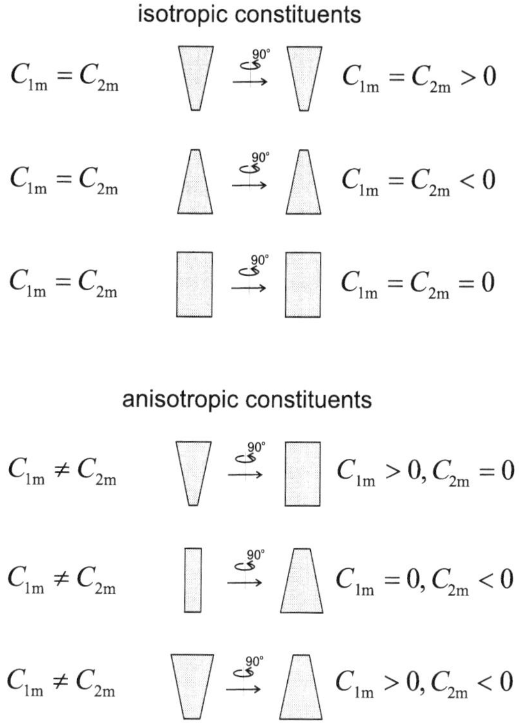

isotropic constituents

$C_{1m} = C_{2m}$ ⬙ $\xrightarrow{90°}$ ⬙ $C_{1m} = C_{2m} > 0$

$C_{1m} = C_{2m}$ △ $\xrightarrow{90°}$ △ $C_{1m} = C_{2m} < 0$

$C_{1m} = C_{2m}$ ▯ $\xrightarrow{90°}$ ▯ $C_{1m} = C_{2m} = 0$

anisotropic constituents

$C_{1m} \neq C_{2m}$ ⬙ $\xrightarrow{90°}$ ▯ $C_{1m} > 0, C_{2m} = 0$

$C_{1m} \neq C_{2m}$ ▯ $\xrightarrow{90°}$ △ $C_{1m} = 0, C_{2m} < 0$

$C_{1m} \neq C_{2m}$ ⬙ $\xrightarrow{90°}$ △ $C_{1m} > 0, C_{2m} < 0$

Figure 8.6 Schematic illustration of different isotropic and anisotropic shapes of membrane-embedded constituents (rigid proteins). The intrinsic shape of the rigid protein is characterized by two intrinsic principal curvatures C_{1m} and C_{2m}. Front and side views are shown. Upper: isotropic inclusion ($C_{1m} = C_{2m}$), lower: examples of anisotropic inclusions ($C_{1m} \neq C_{2m}$).

At this point, let us stress that the energy of a single membrane inclusion induced by a membrane-embedded rigid protein (Eq. 8.22) is mathematically equivalent to the energy of a single flexible membrane inclusion (Eq. 8.4). Combining Eqs. 8.4 and 8.22 yields relations between the interaction constants, $\xi = 2a_0(2K_1 + K_2)$ and $\xi^* = -2a_0(2K_1 + 3K_2)$. However, the origin of the interaction constants can be different in each case. Namely, in the case of a membrane nanodomain induced by membrane-embedded rigid protein (Fig. 8.1B), the interaction constant originates in the deformation of the lipids surrounding the rigid protein only, while in the case of a flexible membrane protein chain-like biopolymer(s), the biopolymer(s) itself is (are) also deformed (Fig. 8.1A).

The maximum and the minimum of $E_i(\omega)$ occur for the protein orientation angle $\omega = 0$ and $\omega = \pi/2$, respectively. The single nanodomain energy (Eq. 8.22) comprises the intrinsic energy of the intercalated rigid protein, as well as the contribution due to deformation of the lipids that surround the intercalated protein (Fig. 8.5) (Fournier, 1996; Kralj-Iglič et al., 1996, 1999).

Possible microscopic (nanoscale) perturbations of the membrane shape around the intercalated rigid protein (Fig. 8.5B) are not explicitly taken into account in Eq. 8.22, but rather hidden in the phenomenological constants $\mu_m, \xi, \xi^*, C_{1m}$ and C_{2m} (or H_m and D_m) (Fig. 8.6), where it is assumed that the distorted regions of lipids of the neighbouring proteins do not overlap.

The concept of the single-nanodomain energy was taken as the basis for a self-consistent description of the equilibrium shapes of a closed bilayer vesicle and the related lateral distribution of intercalated proteins (Božič et al., 2006; Kralj-Iglič et al., 1996, 1999). In accordance with previous results (Markin, 1981), clustering and lateral phase separation of the nanodomains has been predicted (Hägerstrand et al., 2006).

Within the above described phenomenological (mean-field) approach, the influence of membrane-embedded rigid proteins on the elastic properties of the lipid bilayer can be calculated in terms of the properties of the host membrane and the properties (geometry) of the intercalated rigid proteins. The non-homogeneous lateral distribution of the isotropic rigid proteins are an internal degree of freedom that lowers the equilibrium free energy of the membrane and in this way contributes to the decrease in the local bending modulus (Božič et al., 2006; Kralj-Iglič et al., 1996; Leibler, 1986). The change in membrane elasticity depends linearly on the density of the membrane-embedded rigid proteins. In the case of anisotropic rigid proteins, their rotational ordering is another internal degree of freedom, which additionally decreases the membrane local bending constant (Fournier, 1996; Kralj-Iglič et al., 1999).

8.3 Estimation of Model Parameters

8.3.1 Basic Model

In the previous section we derived an expression for the energy of the membrane nanodomain induced by the membrane-embedded rigid protein (Eq. 8.22). In this section, the phenomenological parameters describing the single inclusion energy H_m, D_m and ξ (Eq. 8.22) are estimated using a simple theoretical model of the elasticity of the lipid bilayer (Fosnarič et al., 2005).

In this analysis we assume that the local microscopic shape deformations of the membrane around the membrane-embedded rigid protein are constrained (Fig. 8.5A) and the lipids accommodate to the intrinsic shape of the rigid protein only via changes in lipid tilt. This corresponds to the biologically relevant case of membrane proteins that are distributed all over the cell membrane.

Let us consider a single cone-like rigid protein. To render the protein anisotropic, we introduce the dependence of the cone angle $\theta = \theta(\omega)$ on the azimuthal angle ω (Fig. 8.7). For small variations of θ we can write

$$\theta(\omega) = \bar{\theta} + \Delta\theta \cos(2\omega), \qquad (8.23)$$

where $\bar{\theta}$ is the average conicalness of the protein and $\Delta\theta$ is the corresponding deviator.

The rigid protein is embedded in a lipid bilayer of mean and deviatoric curvatures H and D, respectively. Hence, according to the lemma of Euler, the curvature of the normal cut measured in the radial direction of the inclusion at azimuthal angle ω is

$$C(\omega) = H + D\cos(2\omega). \qquad (8.24)$$

Formally, the protein-induced perturbation free energy of the lipid bilayer can be expressed as the integral of the free energy density $\tilde{E}(\omega)$ per unit length of the circumference of the inclusion's core, $L = 2\pi r_0$, where r_0 is the radius of the inclusion's core (i.e., rigid protein): $E = \int_L \tilde{E} dL = (L/2\pi) \int \tilde{E}(\omega) d\omega$ (see Fig. 8.7). For sufficiently large radius r_0 we expect that $\tilde{E} = \tilde{E}[C(\omega), \theta(\omega)]$ depends only on ω, namely via the relations $C(\omega)$ and $\theta(\omega)$. More generally, $\tilde{E}$ should also depend on the derivatives of $C(\omega)$ and $\theta(\omega)$ with respect to ω. This additional dependence should become

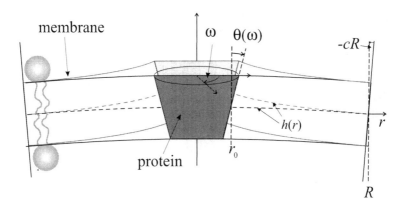

Figure 8.7 Schematic illustration of a membrane-embedded protein in the membrane constrained local shape perturbation (dark grey, in front) (see Fig. 8.5A), and an unconstrained local shape perturbations (light grey, at back) (see Fig. 8.5B). For anisotropic inclusions the cone angle θ depends on the azimuthal angle ω.

relevant if the radius r_0 is smaller than the characteristic decay length ζ of the membrane perturbations. Using membrane elasticity theory, the characteristic decay length ζ has recently been calculated (May, 2002) for a planar ($C = 0$) lipid layer in contact with a wall tilted by an angle θ; it depends on the thickness of the lipid bilayer, the lateral stretching modulus, and the tilt modulus (κ_t). Typical values of ζ for a lipid monolayer (Fosnarič et al., 2005) are about 0.9 nm. Hence, assuming that $r_0 \geq \zeta$, we can write

$$\frac{E}{L} = \frac{1}{2\pi} \int_0^{2\pi} \tilde{E}[C(\omega), \theta(\omega)] d\omega. \qquad (8.25)$$

In this case, $\tilde{E}$ can be calculated using a one-dimensional model for the elastic interaction of a lipid layer with an infinitely extensive, rigid wall. Such a model has frequently been suggested in previous works (Dan and Safran, 1998; May, 2002) and can be generalized to a bent lipid layer of curvature C (Fosnarič et al., 2005),

$$\tilde{f}(C, \theta) = \frac{\kappa_0}{2\zeta}(\theta - Cr_0)^2 + (C_0 - C)(\theta - Cr_0), \qquad (8.26)$$

where κ_0 is the bending stiffness of the lipid monolayer and C_0 is the spontaneous curvature.

After substituting $\theta(\omega)$ from Eq. 8.23 and $C(\omega)$ from Eq. 8.24 into Eq. 8.26, comparison of the expression obtained with Eq. 8.22 yields (Fosnarič et al., 2005):

$$H_{m,1} = \frac{\bar{\theta}}{r_0}\left(\frac{r_0+\zeta}{r_0+2\zeta}\right) + \frac{\zeta C_0}{r_0+2\zeta}, \quad D_{m,1} = \frac{\Delta\theta}{r_0}\left(\frac{r_0+\zeta}{r_0+2\zeta}\right),$$

$$\xi = 2\pi r_0^2 \kappa_0 \left(\frac{r_0}{\zeta}+2\right), \quad \xi^* = 0. \tag{8.27}$$

This confirms the expectation that the shape of the nanodomain's core (i.e., the shape of the membrane-embedded rigid protein) is incorporated in the expressions for the nanodomain spontaneous mean curvature and the spontaneous curvature deviator so that $H_{m,1} = \bar{\theta}/r_0$ and $D_{m,1} = \Delta\theta/r_0$, respectively. Note the strong dependence of the interaction constant $\xi \sim r_0^3$ on the protein radius (for $r_0 \gg \zeta$); this is a consequence of both the rigidity of the membrane-embedded protein (contributing $\sim r_0^2$) and the linear increase of the circumference with r_0. The dependence of ξ on the protein radius (r_0) is plotted in Fig. 8.10 for the characteristic decay length $\zeta = 0.9$ nm.

Note also that the last relation in Eqs. 8.27, that is, $\xi^* = 0$, follows from our assumption that the rigid protein has a sufficiently large radius and that $\tilde{E}$ does not depend on the derivatives of $C(\omega)$ and $\theta(\omega)$ with respect to ω.

8.3.2 Advanced model

In this section we introduce a more advanced theoretical model in order to estimate the constants H_m and ξ, where now the tilt deformation is explicitly taken into account (Fošnarič et al., 2006). In the model of Section 8.3.1, the tilt degree of freedom enters the model only through the characteristic decay length ζ.

In the advanced model (Fošnarič et al., 2006), we consider a lipid membrane consisting of two opposed monolayers, an external (E) and an internal (I) one. Both monolayers are described by a height profile, h_E and h_I, and by their local directors (unit vectors), $\mathbf{t}_E$ and $\mathbf{t}_I$, that describe the average orientation of the lipid chains; see Fig. 8.8.

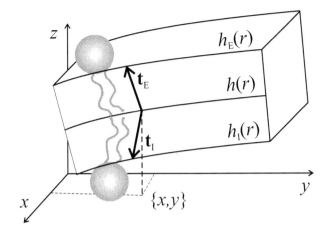

Figure 8.8 Illustration of a perturbed lipid bilayer showing local directors t_E and t_I and height profiles h_E and h_I of the external and internal leaflet, respectively. The average height of the bilayer is $h = (h_E + h_I)/2$. Two lipid molecules are shown schematically. Figure reprinted with permission from Fošnarič, M., Iglič, A., and May, S. Influence of rigid inclusions on the bending elasticity of a lipid membrane. *Phys. Rev. E*, 174, pp. 051503. Copyright 2006 by the American Physical Society.

The elastic free energy per unit area, $\hat{f}_E$, of the external monolayer can be written up to quadratic order in h_E and t_E as (Fošnarič et al., 2006):

$$\hat{f}_E = \frac{\kappa_s}{2}(\nabla \cdot \mathbf{t}_E)^2 + \frac{\kappa_t}{2}(\mathbf{t}_E - \nabla h_E)^2 + \frac{B}{2}(h_E - h)^2$$
$$+ \frac{\kappa_h}{2}(\Delta h_E)^2 + \frac{K}{2}(\nabla \times \mathbf{t}_E)^2 + \bar{\kappa} \det h_{E,ij} \qquad (8.28)$$

The first term in Eq. 8.28 characterizes the splay energy of the lipid chains with κ_s being the corresponding splay modulus. The second term accounts for the energy cost of tilting the director $\mathbf{t}_E$ away from its orientation normal to the surface h_E; the prefactor κ_t is the tilt modulus (Helfrich, 1973). Thickness changes of the monolayer are accounted for by the third term where B is the compression modulus and h is a reference surface with respect to which the compression or expansion of the monolayer is measured. It is reasonable to assume that for a given membrane thickness $h_E - h_I$ the thickness of each monolayer is allowed to relax; this specifies $h = (h_E + h_I)/2$ to be the average height profile of the bilayer. The fourth term in Eq. 8.28 expresses the bare bending energy of the external monolayer with corresponding modulus κ_h. Note that this term is distinct from the splay energy; only for $\kappa_t \to \infty$ do splay and bare bending refer to the same deformation. While the splay energy mainly accounts for the splay deformation of the lipid chains, the bending term originates predominantly in the headgroup region of the monolayer. For example, the electrostatic contribution to the bending modulus is solely responsible for κ_h. One might therefore refer to the modulus κ_h as the head group contribution to the bending stiffness. The last two terms in Eq. 8.28 describe the energetic contribution of the twist deformation of the chains (with corresponding modulus K) and of the saddle deformation of h_E (with the modulus $\bar{\kappa}$).

Starting from $\hat{f}_E$, we can obtain the elastic free energy of the internal leaflet, $\hat{f}_I$, by replacing $h_E \to h_I$ and $\mathbf{t}_E \to -\mathbf{t}_I$ (the minus sign in the latter reflecting the opposite orientation of the two opposed monolayers). Hence,

$$\hat{f}_I = \frac{\kappa_s}{2}(\nabla \cdot \mathbf{t}_I)^2 + \frac{\kappa_t}{2}(\mathbf{t}_I + \nabla h_I)^2 + \frac{B}{2}(h_I - h)^2$$
$$+ \frac{\kappa_h}{2}(\Delta h_I)^2 + \frac{K}{2}(\nabla \times \mathbf{t}_I)^2 + \bar{\kappa} \det h_{I,ij}. \qquad (8.29)$$

The elastic free energy of the lipid bilayer per unit area $\hat{f}_{bl}$ is then

$$\hat{f}_{bl} = \hat{f}_E + \hat{f}_I. \qquad (8.30)$$

At this point it is convenient to switch to a new set of variables, namely to the average shape h and thickness dilation u, defined through $h_E = h + u$ and $h_I = h - u$ (see also Fig. 8.8). Similarly, we define the average director $\mathbf{t}$ and the difference director $\mathbf{d}$ via the relations $\mathbf{t}_E = \mathbf{t} + \mathbf{d}$ and $\mathbf{t}_I = \mathbf{t} - \mathbf{d}$. This allows us to express $\hat{f}_{bl} = \hat{f}_{tu} + \hat{f}_{dh}$ as the sum of the two independent contributions (Fournier, 1999)

$$\hat{f}_{tu} = \kappa_s(\nabla \cdot \mathbf{t})^2 + \kappa_t(\mathbf{t} - \nabla u)^2 + B u^2$$
$$+ \kappa_h(\Delta u)^2 + K(\nabla \times \mathbf{t})^2 + 2\bar{\kappa} \det u_{ij} \qquad (8.31)$$

and

$$\hat{f}_{dh} = \kappa_s(\nabla \cdot \mathbf{d})^2 + \kappa_t(\mathbf{d} - \nabla h)^2$$
$$+ \kappa_h(\Delta h)^2 + K(\nabla \times \mathbf{d})^2 + 2\bar{\kappa} \det h_{ij} \qquad (8.32)$$

The two contributions can be treated separately. The first one (Eq. 8.31) depends on the tilt difference **t** and thickness dilation u which is relevant for proteins with up–down symmetry, including the case of a hydrophobic mismatch. The corresponding rigid protein-induced deformation is short-ranged and has been studied intensively in the past (Dan et al., 1994, 1993; Nielsen et al., 1998). In the present chapter we focus entirely on the second contribution (namely Eq. 8.32). In other words, we consider membrane deformations due to isotropic, cone-like rigid proteins with no hydrophobic mismatch (implying $\hat{f}_{tu} = 0$). We thus seek to minimize the overall elastic free energy $F_{dh} = \int \hat{f}_{dh}\, da$ where $da = dxdy\, [1 + (\nabla h)^2]^{1/2}$ denotes the area element of the lipid bilayer. The corresponding Euler–Lagrange equations pertaining to F_{dh} are (Fošnarič et al., 2006) :

$$\kappa_t(\mathbf{d} - \nabla h) - \kappa_s \nabla(\nabla \cdot \mathbf{d}) + K \nabla \times (\nabla \times \mathbf{d}) = 0$$
$$\kappa_h \nabla^4 h + \kappa_t(\nabla \cdot \mathbf{d} - \triangle h) = 0 \qquad (8.33)$$

We assume cylindrical symmetry around a rigid protein, since we are interested only in inclusions (i.e., membrane nanodomains) induced by isotropic membrane-embedded rigid proteins. Also, we adopt a cell model, that is, we assume that the proteins are homogeneously distributed over a membrane segment of prescribed spherical curvature ($C_1 = C_2 = C$), defined at the mesoscopic level. The cell model starts from a hexagonal arrangement of spatially fixed cone-like proteins of (average) radius r_0 (see Fošnarič et al., 2006 and Fig. 8.9). The radius R of the unit cell (Fig. 8.7) then defines the (uniform) area fraction $m = r_0^2/R^2$ of rigid proteins in the membrane segment. Our aim is to characterize—at the mesoscopic scale—the bending stiffness of a rigid protein-containing membrane patch with prescribed sphere-like membrane curvature. Hence, the membrane curvatures at the boundaries of each unit cell are fixed to be $C_1 = C_2 = C$, where C is the sphere-like (mesoscopic level) membrane curvature. The fact that the curvatures at the cell boundaries are all equal is a consequence of both the symmetry of the deformation and the isotropy of the protein. The local, microscopic, membrane shape perturbation within the unit cell is allowed to minimize the membrane free energy (see also Fig. 8.9).

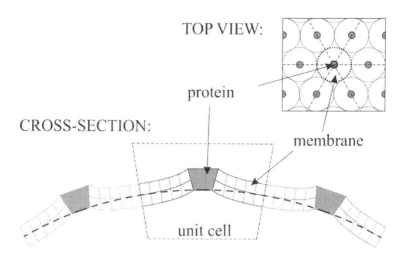

Figure 8.9 Top view: Schematic illustration of a hexagonal array of laterally fixed isotropic cone-like membrane-embedded rigid proteins (shaded circles). The unit cell around each protein is approximated by a circle. The membrane shape is also given in cross-section. The shaded cones represent cross-sections through the inclusions. Figure reprinted with permission from Fošnarič, M., Iglič, A., and May, S. Influence of rigid inclusions on the bending elasticity of a lipid membrane. *Phys. Rev. E*, 174, pp. 051503. Copyright 2006 by the American Physical Society.

Equations 8.33 can be solved analytically for cylindrical symmetry and the corresponding free energy F_{dh} can be calculated. This derivation is explained in detail elsewhere (Fošnarič et al., 2006); here we discuss only the dependences of the constants H_m and ξ (Eq. 8.22) on the parameters of the microscopic model.

In the model presented in Section 8.2.2, the single inclusion energy (Eq. 8.22) induced by an isotropic rigid protein ($D_m = 0$) in a spherical membrane curvature field ($H = C = $ const. and $D = 0$) simplifies to:

$$E = \mu_m + \frac{\xi}{2}(H - H_m)^2, \tag{8.34}$$

where curvature C is defined at the mesoscopic level. In other words, the possible local microscopic curvature deformation around the rigid protein (Fig. 8.5B) is not shown directly in C, instead, it is hidden in the phenomenological parameters ξ and H_m.

By comparing Eq. 8.34 with the free energy F_{dh} from the model described in this section, we can obtain the relations (Fošnarič et al., 2006)

$$H_m \simeq \frac{(1+\kappa_{rel})}{\kappa_{rel}} C_0, \qquad (8.35)$$

$$\xi \simeq \pi R^2 \kappa_0 \kappa_{rel}. \qquad (8.36)$$

Here κ_0 is the (local) bending stiffness of the (rigid protein-free) lipid bilayer, R the radius of the cylindrically symmetric unit cell (Fig. 8.9), c_0 is the spontaneous curvature of the rigid protein-containing membrane and κ_{rel} the relative change of the bending stiffness κ due to the presence of rigid proteins in the membrane bilayer; namely $\kappa_{rel} = \kappa/\kappa_0 - 1$. The expressions for C_0 and κ_{rel} can be derived analytically (Fošnarič et al., 2006). In compact form they can be written in terms of the relative cell size $\rho = (R/r_0)^2 - 1$ and the quantities

$$\eta^2 = \kappa_h/\kappa_s, \qquad (8.37)$$

$$\tilde{\eta} = (1+\eta^2)/\eta^2 = (\kappa_s/\kappa_h) + 1, \qquad (8.38)$$

$$\tilde{\alpha} = \bar{\kappa}/[2(\kappa_s + \kappa_h)], \qquad (8.39)$$

$$\tilde{\zeta} = (\kappa_t/\kappa_s + \kappa_t/\kappa_h)^{-1/2}, \qquad (8.40)$$

and

$$P = \frac{2\tilde{\zeta}}{r_0} \frac{I_1(R/\tilde{\zeta})K_1(r_0/\tilde{\zeta}) - I_1(r_0/\tilde{\zeta})K_1(R/\tilde{\zeta})}{I_1(R/\tilde{\zeta})K_0(r_0/\tilde{\zeta}) + I_0(r_0/\tilde{\zeta})K_1(R/\tilde{\zeta})} \qquad (8.41)$$

where I_n and K_n give the modified Bessel functions of the first and second kind, respectively. We find that

$$\frac{R^2 C_0}{\theta r_0} = \frac{-(1-P\tilde{\alpha}\tilde{\eta})(1+\rho)}{1+\rho(1+\tilde{\alpha})+P\tilde{\alpha}\eta^2\{1-\tilde{\eta}^2[1+\rho(1+\tilde{\alpha})]\}} \qquad (8.42)$$

and

$$\kappa_{rel} = \frac{1}{1+\tilde{\alpha}} \frac{1 - P\eta^2(1+\tilde{\alpha}\tilde{\eta}^2)}{\rho + P\eta^2(1-\tilde{\alpha}\tilde{\eta}^2\rho)} \qquad (8.43)$$

The local stability condition implies $\kappa_0 > -\bar{\kappa}/2 > 0$ (Ben-Shaul, 1995; Kralj-Iglič et al., 2005) (where κ_0 and $\bar{\kappa}$ are the local bending (splay) modulus and saddle-splay (Gaussian) modulus, respectively), therefore $-0.5 < \bar{\alpha} < 0$. The estimated values of κ_t (Helfrich, 1973; May et al., 2004) yield $\tilde{\zeta} \sim 0.2$ nm.

The above equations express contain the microscopic membrane shape perturbations around a rigid protein through curvature deformation and through changes in lipid tilt (Fig. 8.5B). However, the model described in this section can also be used for the biologically important case of restricted local shape perturbations (see Fig. 8.5A). Relations for H_m and ξ (Eqs. 8.35 and 8.36) remain the same, but the expression for the relative bending stiffness becomes

$$\kappa_{rel} = \frac{1}{1+\rho} \left[\frac{1}{P(1+\eta^2)(1+\bar{\alpha})} - 1 \right], \tag{8.44}$$

where the function P is the same as in Eq. 8.41, with $\tilde{\zeta}$ now being replaced by $\tilde{\zeta}_c = \tilde{\zeta}(\kappa_h \to \infty)$:

$$\tilde{\zeta}_c = (\kappa_t/\kappa_s)^{-1/2}. \tag{8.45}$$

The relations in Eqs. 8.22, 8.35 and 8.36 are valid only as long as local deformations around the membrane-embedded neighbouring rigid proteins do not overlap. Otherwise the interaction constant ξ (Eq. 8.22) would depend on the area fraction of proteins ($m = r_0^2/R^2$) in the membrane patch considered. It can be seen from the above relations that for the case of unconstrained local shape perturbations around the rigid proteins (Fig. 8.5B) is valid up to a certain value of the area fraction of the proteins. For most of the relevant cases the actual area fraction of rigid proteins (m) is well below this value.

In the case of restricted local (microscopic) shape perturbations around the rigid protein (see Fig. 8.5A), the decay of the lipid (tilt) deformation around the protein is exponential (i.e., short-ranged). Therefore, overlapping of the short-ranged lipid deformations around neighbouring proteins becomes important only if the proteins are very close. Consequently the interaction constants (ξ, ξ^*, H_m and D_m) depend on the local density of the inclusions only for very large m.

For small values of m, we can expand the expression for ξ. For unconstrained local membrane shape relaxations we get

$$\xi = \frac{\pi r_0^2 \kappa_0}{1-\bar{\alpha}} \left[1 - \frac{2\eta^2 \tilde{\zeta}(1+\bar{\alpha}\tilde{\eta}^2)}{r_0} \frac{K_1(r_0/\tilde{\zeta})}{K_0(r_0/\tilde{\zeta})} \right], \tag{8.46}$$

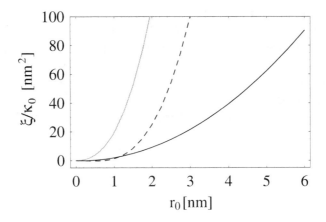

Figure 8.10 Interaction constant ξ (Eq. 8.22) as a function of the average radius of the rigid protein (r_0) in the model of constrained local membrane microscopic shape perturbations (Fig. 8.5A) calculated from Eq. 8.27 for $\zeta = 0.9$ nm (grey full curve) and from Eq. 8.47 (dashed curve) for $\eta^2 = 1$, $\tilde{\alpha} = -0.2$ and $\tilde{\zeta}_c = 0.2$ nm. The figure also shows the dependence of ξ on r_0 for unconstrained local membrane microscopic shape perturbations (Fig. 8.5B), as calculated from Eqs. 8.46 for $\tilde{\zeta} = 0.2$ nm and same values of η^2 and $\tilde{\alpha}$ (black solid curve).

whereas the case of constrained local membrane shape relaxation yields

$$\xi = \pi r_0^2 \kappa_0 \left[\frac{r_0}{2\tilde{\zeta}_c(1+\eta^2)(1+\tilde{\alpha})} \frac{K_0(r_0/\tilde{\zeta}_c)}{K_1(r_0/\tilde{\zeta}_c)} - 1 \right]. \quad (8.47)$$

It can be seen in Eqs. 8.46 and 8.47 that the interaction constant ξ adopts negative values for $r_0 < 2\tilde{\zeta}\eta^2(1+\tilde{\alpha}\tilde{\eta}^2)K_1(r_0/\tilde{\zeta})/K_0(r_0/\tilde{\zeta})$ (unconstrained case) and $r_0 < 2\tilde{\zeta}_c(1+\eta^2)(1+\tilde{\alpha})K_1(r_0/\tilde{\zeta}_c)/K_0(r_0/\tilde{\zeta}_c)$ (constrained case). Therefore, for large enough $\tilde{\alpha}$ and $\tilde{\zeta}$ (or $\tilde{\zeta}_c$), and for a small enough radius of the protein, rigid inclusions could locally soften the membrane (Fošnarič et al., 2006). This could not be predicted within the theory presented in Section 8.3.1, where the tilt degree of freedom is not explicitly taken into account and enters the model only through the characteristic decay length ζ.

In Figure 8.10, the dependence of ξ on the average radius of the membrane-embedded rigid protein r_0 is shown for the different models presented. The case of constrained local membrane shape perturbations (Fig. 8.5A) is shown in the grey curve for the model from Section 8.3.1, and in the dashed curve for the above described model (Eq. 8.47). The case of unconstrained local shape perturbations (Fig. 8.5A) is shown in the black solid curve (see Eq. 8.46).

Chapter 9

Tubular Budding of Biological Membranes

The formation of tubular membrane bilayer structures (nanotubes) is a common phenomenon in both artificial membranes (see Iglič et al., 2003; Karlsson et al., 2001; Kralj-Iglič et al., 2001a; Kralj-Iglič, 2002; Mathivet et al., 1996, and Section 6.4) and cellular systems (Chinnery et al., 2008; Davis and Sowinski, 2008; Galkina et al., 2005; Gerdes et al., 2007; Gerdes and Carvalho, 2008; Gimsa et al., 2007; Hurtig et al., 2010; Iglič et al., 2007b; Koyanagi et al., 2005; Önfelt et al., 2004; Rustom et al., 2004; Sun et al., 2005; Veranič et al., 2008; Vidulescu et al., 2004; Watkins and Salter, 2005).

Sometimes vesicles which seem to be freely diffusing in solution, are attached to the parent cell by nanotubes. This was found to be the case for erythrocytes that moved synchronously with some small released vesicles nearby (Kralj-Iglič et al., 2001b). Once pulled out from the liposome membrane (see, e.g., Roux et al., 2002), the nanotubular membrane protrusions in liposomes or the nanotubular connections between two liposomes can be mechanically stable, even without any permanent external (pulling) stabilization force. This was theoretically explained by the weak average orientational ordering and direct interactions between

---

Nanostructures in Biological Systems: Theory and Applications
Aleš Iglič, Veronika Kralj-Iglič, and Damjana Drobne
Copyright © 2015 Pan Stanford Publishing Pte. Ltd.
ISBN 978-981-4267-20-5 (Hardcover), 978-981-4303-43-9 (eBook)
www.panstanford.com

lipids in highly curved tubular membrane regions (see Section 7.7). Recently, thin membranous bridging tubes have been discovered in several cell lines (for a review see Gerdes et al., 2007; Hurtig et al., 2010; Schara et al., 2009), among which the so-called tunnelling nanotubes (TNTs) are the most interesting (Hurtig et al., 2010; Önfelt et al., 2004; Rustom et al., 2004; Veranič et al., 2008).

In this chapter, we present a possible mechanism that may explain experimentally observed detergent-induced tubular budding of the erythrocyte membrane. The proposed mechanism is based on the energetically favourable self-assembly of anisotropic membrane nanodomains (raft elements) into larger membrane domains forming nanotubular membrane protrusions (Iglič et al., 2007b; Kralj-Iglič et al., 2005). This mechanism of the growth and stability of erythrocyte membrane tubular membrane protrusions may also be relevant for stabilization of tubular membrane protrusions in other cellular systems (Iglič et al., 2006, 2007b; Janich and Corbeil, 2007) and for the stability of tunnelling nanotubes that connect cells, and could be important in intracellular and intercellular transport and communication (Chinnery et al., 2008; Veranič et al., 2008). Since TNTs are difficult to visualize and are also very fragile, they have been overlooked in the past, but it could be expected that in the future they will receive more attention due to their vital importance.

9.1 Bilayer Membrane with Nanodomains

As already pointed out, much experimental and theoretical evidence indicates the existence of membrane micro- and nanodomains (see (Corbeil et al., 2001; Huttner and Zimmerberg, 2001; Iglič et al., 2006; Janich and Corbeil, 2007; Salzer and Prohaska, 2003) and references therein). Considering the biological membrane simply as a mixture of different types of individual molecules with different intrinsic shapes, without explicitly taking into account the possibility of their self-assembly into mixed energetically favourable membrane micro and/or nonanodomains (which are composed of molecules of different shapes), would overestimate the role of the individual molecular intrinsic shape in the mechanics of biological

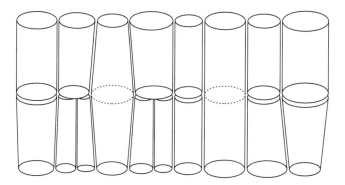

Figure 9.1 The average intrinsic shape of the membrane nanodomain may be different from the intrinsic shapes of the molecules (lipids and proteins) which constitute the domain. Reprinted from *Blood Cells, Molecules and Diseases*, 39(1), Aleš Iglič, Maruša Lokar, Blaž Babnik, Tomaž Slivnik, Peter Veranič, Henry Hägerstrand, and Veronika Kralj-Iglič, Possible role of flexible red blood cell membrane nanodomains in the growth and stability of membrane nanotubes, pp. 14–23, Copyright 2007, with permission from Elsevier.

membranes and neglect the role of direct interactions between the molecules that compose the membrane. For example, membrane lipids, which comprise an impressively large number of molecular species with different intrinsic shapes (see Figs. 7.1 and 7.5, and also Israelachvili, 1997; Kralj-Iglič et al., 2006; Roelofsen et al., 1989), may self-assemble into various micro- and nanodomains with an average intrinsic shape (spontaneous curvature) of the domain which can be different from the intrinsic shapes of the lipids constituting it (see Iglič et al., 2007b; Kuypers et al., 1984, and Fig. 9.1). A proper theoretical description of the mechanics of biological membranes should therefore also take into account the possibility that membrane molecules may form small flexible micro and nanodomains with different intrinsic shapes (see Chapter 8).

As described in Chapter 8, the expression for the energy of a membrane nanodomain induced by a single rigid membrane protein (Fig. 8.1B) can be written as (see Eq. 8.22):

$$E(\omega) = \frac{\xi}{2}(H - H_m)^2 + \frac{\xi + \xi^*}{4}(D^2 - 2DD_m \cos 2\omega + D_m^2), \quad (9.1)$$

which is mathematically equivalent to the expression for the energy of a flexible membrane nanodomain including chain-like proteins and lipids (Fig. 8.1A), where (see Section 8.2.2)

$$\xi = 2a_0(2K_1 + K_2) , \quad \xi^* = -2a_0(2K_1 + 3K_2). \quad (9.2)$$

Therefore in this section, only Eq. 9.1 is used to describe the energy of membrane nanodomains of different types (see Fig. 8.1).

The membrane nanodomain adapts its shape in order to fit its curvature to the actual membrane curvature which is also influenced by the nanodomains. Since all orientations of the nanodomain do not have the same energy (see Eq. 9.1 and Fig. 8.3), the partition function of a single nanodomain can be written in the form:

$$Q_i = \frac{1}{\omega_0} \int_0^{2\pi} \exp\left(-\frac{E(\omega)}{kT}\right) d\omega, \quad (9.3)$$

with ω_0 as an arbitrary angle quantum (Eq. 8.15). The free energy of the membrane nanodomain is then obtained by the expression

$$f_{in} = -kT \ln Q_i. \quad (9.4)$$

Combining Eqs. 9.1, 9.3 and 9.4 allows us to write the free energy of the single flexible membrane nanodomain (up to the constant terms) as:

$$f_{in} = \frac{\xi}{2}(H-H_m)^2 + \frac{\xi+\xi^*}{4}(D^2+D_m^2) - kT \ln\left(I_0\left(\frac{(\xi+\xi^*)D_m D}{2kT}\right)\right), \quad (9.5)$$

where I_0 is a modified Bessel function.

In the following, we derive the free energy of a bilayer membrane with membrane-embedded nanodomains. The excluded volume principle, that is, the finite volume of the membrane nanodomains (inclusions), is taken into account within the lattice statistics (see Section 1.2.2.5) (Hill, 1986). Therefore, the membrane is divided into small patches (Fig. 1.8), which still contain a large number of molecules so that the methods of statistical mechanics can be used. The membrane curvature is taken to be constant over the patch. A lattice is postulated with M sites in one patch, each having area a_0. In the chosen patch, there are N nanodomains. The area of a single nanodomain is a_0.

The direct interactions between nanodomains are taken into account using the Bragg–Williams approximation (Hill, 1986). We assume that direct interactions are possible only between nanodomains, while there are no direct interactions between nanodomains and the rest of the membrane:

$$W_{ii} = \bar{N}_{ii} w, \qquad (9.6)$$

where w is the interaction energy of nanodomain–nanodomain pair (for $w < 0$ the interaction between nanodomains is attractive) and $\bar{N}_{ii}$ is the average number of nearest neighbour nanodomains,

$$\bar{N}_{ii} = \frac{1}{2} N c \frac{N}{M}, \qquad (9.7)$$

where N is the number of nanodomains in the patch, M is the number of (lattice) sites in the patch and c is the number of nearest neighbours around one nanodomain. For a two-dimensional square net $c = 4$ (see Fig. 1.8). The factor $1/2$ was introduced in order to avoid counting each nanodomain–nanodomain pair twice.

Within the lattice statistics approach (Section 1.2.2.5), the canonical partition function of the nanodomains in one patch is:

$$Q^P = Q_i^N \exp\left(-cN^2 w/2MkT\right) \frac{M!}{N!\,(M-N)!}, \qquad (9.8)$$

where Q_i is the single nanodomain partition function. The Helmholz free energy of the patch is $F^P = -kT \ln Q^P$:

$$F^P = -NkT \ln Q_i + \frac{cwN^2}{2M} + kT N \ln \frac{N}{M} + kT(M-N)\ln\left(1 - \frac{N}{M}\right), \qquad (9.9)$$

where we applied the Stirling approximation $\ln x! \cong x \ln x - x$. The free energy of all nanodomains in the membrane is obtained by summing the contributions of all patches:

$$F_i = \int_A n f_{in} m_0 \, dA + \int_A \frac{cwm_0}{2} n^2 dA$$
$$+ kT m_0 \int_A (n \ln n + (1-n)\ln(1-n)) \, dA, \qquad (9.10)$$

where $n = N/M$ is the local membrane area fraction occupied by the membrane nanodomains, dA is the membrane area element (area of a patch), $m_0 = M/dA = 1/a_0$, a_0 is the area of a single nanodomain and the free energy of the single nanodomain f_{in} is defined in Eq. 9.5. The constant term proportional to $\ln Q_i$ was neglected.

The free energy of the membrane bilayer (F) should also include the bending energy of the membrane regions without nanodomains.

The normalized (reduced) membrane free energy ($f = F/(m_0 A)$) can be therefore, written in the form (Hägerstrand et al., 2006; Iglič et al., 2006):

$$f = \int_A (1-n)\tilde{w}_b \, da + \int_A n f_{in} \, da$$
$$+ \int \frac{cw}{2} n^2 da + kT \int_A (n \ln n + (1-n)\ln(1-n)) \, da, \quad (9.11)$$

where $da = dA/A$ is the relative membrane area element, $\tilde{w}_b$ is the local isotropic bending energy of the membrane regions without nanodomains (see Eq. 7.57):

$$\tilde{w}_b = \frac{a_0 k_c}{2} (2H)^2 + a_0 k_G K \quad (9.12)$$

and k_c is the corresponding (local) bending constant.

Due to their lateral mobility and specific intrinsic shapes, the membrane nanodomains may accumulate in regions of favourable curvature, while they are depleted from regions of unfavourable curvature (Hägerstrand et al., 2006; Holopainen et al., 2000; Iglič et al., 2006; Kralj-Iglič et al., 1999; Markin, 1981). The influence of the intrinsic shape of membrane nanodomains on the equilibrium configuration of the membrane and the corresponding lateral distribution of the membrane nanodomains is determined by minimizing the membrane free energy

$$\delta f = 0 \quad (9.13)$$

under relevant geometrical constraints. We require that there is a fixed number of nanodomains in the membrane

$$\int n \, da = \bar{n}, \quad (9.14)$$

where $\bar{n}$ is the average value of n.

In the following the variational problem is solved rigorously with respect to the lateral distribution of nanodomains n only. Accordingly, a functional $G = \int \mathcal{L} dl$ is constructed, where

$$\mathcal{L} = \frac{(1-n)\tilde{w}_b}{kT} + \frac{n f_{in}}{kT} + \frac{cw}{2kT} n^2 + (n \ln n + (1-n)\ln(1-n)) + \lambda n$$

and λ is the global Lagrange multiplier. The relevant Lagrange–Euler differential equation

$$\frac{\partial \mathcal{L}}{\partial n} = 0 \quad (9.15)$$

yields

$$\ln\left[\frac{n}{1-n} \cdot \exp\frac{c\,w\,n}{kT}\right] = -\lambda - \frac{f_{\text{in}}}{kT} + \frac{\tilde{w}_{\text{b}}}{kT}. \quad (9.16)$$

For simplicity the term $\exp(c\,w\,n/kT)$ in Eq. 9.16 is replaced by the term $(1 + c\,w\,n/kT)$:

$$\ln\left[\frac{n}{1-n}\left(1+\frac{c\,w\,n}{kT}\right)\right] = -\lambda - \frac{f_{\text{in}}}{kT} + \frac{\tilde{w}_{\text{b}}}{kT}. \quad (9.17)$$

After rearrangement, Eq. 9.17 is solved to obtain

$$n = -\frac{(1+e^{-(\lambda+\beta)})kT}{8w} + \frac{(1+e^{-(\lambda+\beta)})kT}{8w}\sqrt{1 + \frac{\frac{16w}{kT}e^{-(\lambda+\beta)}}{(1+e^{-(\lambda+\beta)})^2}}. \quad (9.18)$$

where

$$\beta = f_{\text{in}}/kT - \tilde{w}_{\text{b}}/kT \quad (9.19)$$

and $c = 4$. In the limit of weak interaction (small w) Eq. 9.18 transforms into (Hägerstrand et al., 2006; Iglič et al., 2006):

$$n \cong \frac{\vartheta\,\exp(-\beta)}{(1+\vartheta\,\exp(-\beta))}\left[1 - \frac{4w}{kT}\frac{\vartheta\,\exp(-\beta)}{(1+\vartheta\,\exp(-\beta))^2}\right], \quad (9.20)$$

where $\vartheta = \exp(-\lambda)$ and $w < 0$ for attractive interactions. The parameter ϑ is determined from the constraint (Eq. 9.14). For $w = 0$, the above equation (Eq. 9.20) simplifies to:

$$n \cong \frac{\vartheta\,\exp(-\beta)}{(1+\vartheta\,\exp(-\beta))}. \quad (9.21)$$

9.2 Accumulation of Anisotropic Nanodomains and the Stability of Tubular Membrane Protrusions

In the following, the above described model of a bilayer membrane with nanodomains (Section 9.1) is used to elucidate the possible physical mechanism which may explain the curvature-induced accumulation of small anisotropic prominin–lipid complexes (i.e., prominin nanodomains) on highly curved tubular membrane protrusions (Corbeil et al., 2001; Iglič et al., 2006, 2007b; Janich and Corbeil, 2007). It was suggested that prominin rafts play an important role in the stabilization of plasma membrane protrusions

(Huttner and Zimmerberg, 2001). Since prominin does not directly interact with the actin-based cytoskeleton (Huttner and Zimmerberg, 2001), the predominant localization of prominin nanodomains in tubular membrane protrusions may be explained by the specific anisotropic intrinsic shape of the prominin nanodomains which may represent the main driving force of nanotube formation (Hurtig et al., 2010; Iglič et al., 2006; Janich and Corbeil, 2007; Veranič et al., 2008). The redistribution of prominin nanodomains after mild cholesterol depletion from the protrusions indicates the importance of cholesterol (Röper et al., 2000) and other lipids as partners (Huttner and Zimmerberg, 2001) in the formation of small prominin nanodomains.

Recently, the inhomogeneous lateral distribution of flotillins and their accumulation during cytokinesis was also observed (Rajendran et al., 2003), while ganglioside GM1 was enriched in membrane exvaginations induced by cytosolic calcium and amphiphiles (Hägerstrand and Mrowczynska, 2008; Hägerstrand et al., 2006). Based on these and other experimental results and on theoretical considerations, it was suggested that membrane skeleton-detached, laterally mobile nanodomains may preferentially accumulate in the curved or flat membrane regions depending on their intrinsic shape and/or the direct interactions between them (Hägerstrand and Mrowczynska, 2008; Hägerstrand et al., 2006; Hurtig et al., 2010; Iglič et al., 2006; Veranič et al., 2008).

In order to estimate the importance of the curvature-induced accumulation of small anisotropic prominin–lipid nanodomains on highly curved tubular membrane protrusions in the model, the membrane can be divided into two parts: firstly, the flat part with relative area a_f and the fraction of the area covered by prominin nanodomains n_f, and secondly, the highly curved tubular part of the membrane with mean curvature $H = D = 1/2r$ (where r is the radius of a tubular protrusion), relative area a_t and the fraction of the area covered by inclusions (nanodomains) equal to n_t. The parameter ϑ may be determined numerically from the condition

$$n_f a_f + n_t a_t = \bar{n}, \qquad (9.22)$$

where $a_f + a_t = 1$ and n_f and n_t are given by Eq. 9.20.

Figure 9.2 shows the fraction of the area of the tubular membrane protrusions covered by anisotropic nanodomains (n_t) as a function

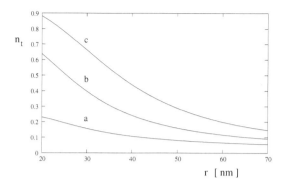

Figure 9.2 Fraction of the area of membrane tubular protrusions covered by anisotropic nanodomains (n_2) as a function of the curvature radius of the tube (r) for three values of the intrinsic curvature deviator of the nanodomains (inclusions) (D_m): 0.03 nm^{-1} (a), 0.04 nm^{-1} (b) and 0.05 nm^{-1} (c). The values of the other model parameters are: $\bar{n} = 0.02$, $a_2 = 0.02$, $H_m = D_m$, $w/kT = 0.125$ and $\xi = 5000$ kT nm^2. Reprinted from *Journal of Theoretical Biology*, 240(3), Aleš Iglič, Henry Hägerstrand, Peter Veranič, Ana Plemenitaš, and Veronika Kralj-Iglič, Curvature-induced accumulation of anisotropic membrane components and raft formation in cylindrical membrane protrusions, pp. 368–373, Copyright 2006, with permission from Elsevier.

of the radius (r) of the tubular protrusion for three values of the intrinsic curvature deviator of the nanodomains (D_m).

It can be seen that for small r and large D_m, the fraction of the membrane tubular area occupied by nanodomains (n_t) is much larger than $\bar{n}$, while n_f is smaller than $\bar{n}$. This indicates the possibility of curvature-induced accumulation of prominin nanodomains in highly curved tubular membrane regions. Due to the high concentration of nanodomains in the tubular protrusion the nanodomains in protrusions may then coalesce into larger prominin domains (rafts) as observed in experiments (Corbeil et al., 2001; Huttner and Zimmerberg, 2001; Janich and Corbeil, 2007). It can also be seen in Fig. 9.2 that for high enough values of the intrinsic curvature deviator of the nanodomains D_m, the value of n_t approaches unity, indicating the possibility of lateral phase separation of nanodomains for high values of D_m and small values of r (see also Fig. 9.3).

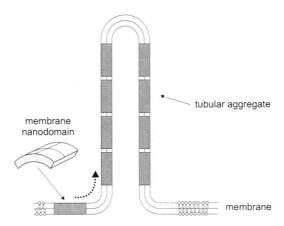

Figure 9.3 Schematic figure of an energetically favourable self-assembly of anisotropic prominin nanodomains (characterized by $C_{1m} > 0$ and $C_{2m} = 0$) into larger membrane domains forming cylindrical aggregates. Reprinted from *Blood Cells, Molecules and Diseases*, 39(1), Aleš Iglič, Maruša Lokar, Blaž Babnik, Tomaž Slivnik, Peter Veranič, Henry Hägerstrand, and Veronika Kralj-Iglič, Possible role of flexible red blood cell membrane nanodomains in the growth and stability of membrane nanotubes, pp. 14–23, Copyright 2007, with permission from Elsevier. (See also Hurtig et al., 2010; Veranič et al., 2008).

In the theoretical consideration presented (Fig. 9.2), the value applied for the interaction constant ξ is considerably larger than the corresponding value for the isotropic lipid bilayer membrane (Kralj-Iglič, 2002). This means that the isotropic bending energy of the isotropic lipid bilayer is insufficient to stabilize the tubular membrane protrusion and also may not significantly contribute to sorting of lipids between tubular membrane protrusions and the parent membrane due to the excessive decrease in configurational (mixing) entropy (Iglič et al., 2006; Tian and Baumgart, 2009). As shown in the Section 7.7, the very thin nanotubular protrusion of one component liposomes can be stabilized by the average orientational ordering of anisotropic lipids in nanotubes (Kralj-Iglič, 2002), while in more complex bilayer membrane systems (as shown also in this chapter), the lipid–lipid and lipid–protein direct interactions may result in the formation of small membrane (in general anisotropic) nanodomains (clusters, inclusions) which can stabilize tubular membrane protrusion and also significantly contribute to lipid sorting (Iglič et al., 2006; Kralj-Iglič et al., 2005; Tian and Baumgart, 2009). As shown in Fig. 9.2, such nanodomains may coalesce into larger domains (rafts) by their curvature induced clustering in membrane protrusions, as observed in (Holthius et al., 2003; Hurtig et al., 2010; Huttner and Zimmerberg, 2001). To conclude, within the standard isotropic Helfric–Evans membrane elasticity model (Eq. 7.68), the stability of tubular membrane protrusions cannot be explained without an inner supporting rod-like structure or mechanical pulling force (Derényi et al., 2002; Miao et al., 1991, 1994). However, thin tubular membrane protrusions can be stabilized by anisotropic membrane nanodomains (components) (Iglič et al., 2006, 2007b; Kralj-Iglič et al., 2005), as also shown in Fig. 9.4.

Our theoretical model may thus provide an explanation for the observed curvature-induced enrichment of prominin raft markers in tubular membrane protrusions. Accumulation of anisotropic nanodomains in tubular membrane protrusions and their average orientational ordering lowers the membrane free energy and therefore, stabilizes the tubular structure. It is therefore expected that the tubular shape of the protrusion is stable even without an inner rod-like structure (Hurtig et al., 2010; Iglič et al., 2006; Kralj-Iglič et al., 2005). This was confirmed in an experiment where the inner rod-like structures of tubular protrusions of the cell membrane were disintegrated. The membrane of the protrusions retained its tubular shape as described below.

Cytochalasin B is a substance that disintegrates the actin filaments of the cell cytoskeleton. Consequently, microtubules segregate into rod-like structures that exert an impact on the cell membrane. Fibroblasts treated with cytochalasin B for 30 minutes exhibit long flattened protrusions on a globular cell body which are attached to the support (Fig. 9.5-1A). Inside such a protrusion, a parallel array of microtubules can be seen in Fig. 9.5-1B.

In cytochalasin B-treated cells with a reduced content of cholesterol in the membrane (as a result of growth in a medium without cholesterol for 24 hours), the protrusions are much thinner (Fig. 9.5-2A), while no rod-like structures of microtubules could be found within the protrusions (Fig. 9.5-2B). Further, no microspikes

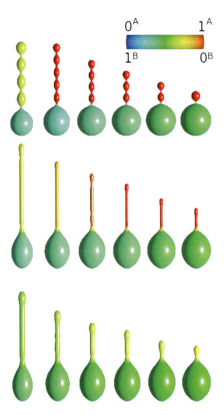

Figure 9.4 Comparison of calculated closed shapes of vesicles having a two component membrane. The shape are presented for different relative (reduced) volume v. The values of the reduced volume are (from left to right) $v = 0.54,\ 0.67,\ 0.75,\ 0.80,\ 0.85,\ 0.90$. The first two rows show the shapes of the vesicles when the entropy contribution (see the last term in Eq. 9.10) is neglected. In the first row, the shapes of the vesicles are calculated within the *isotropic* model of the two component membrane with *isotropic* flexible nanodomains. In the second and third row, the shapes of the vesicles are calculated within the anisotropic model of a two component membrane with *anisotropic* flexible nanodomains. The colour of the surface represents the fraction of the area covered by nanodomains. The fully red colour corresponds to a membrane composed of nanodomains only (isotropic in the first row and anisotropic in the second and third rows). Reprinted from *Journal of Biomechanics*, 45(2), Doron Kabaso, Nataliya Bobrovska, Wojciech Góźdź, Nir Gov, Veronika Kralj-Iglič, Peter Veranič, and Aleš Iglič, On the role of membrane anisotrophy and BAR proteins in the stability of tubular membrane structures, pp. 231–238, Copyright 2012, with permission from Elsevier.

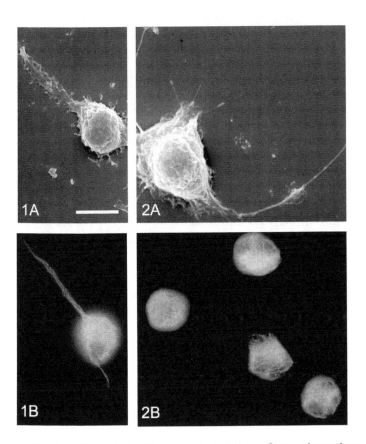

Figure 9.5 In cells treated with cytochalasin B, long- flattened membrane protrusions on globular cell bodies were found attached to the support (1A). Immunofluorescence labelling of tubulin showed a parallel rod-like organization of the microtubules in these membrane protrusions (1B). Cytochalasin treatment of cells causing mild cholesterol depletion resulted in thinner and smoother tubular membrane protrusions (2A) where the rod-like microtubular structure completely disappeared (2B). Bar = 10 µm. Reprinted from *Journal of Theoretical Biology*, 240(3), Aleš Iglič, Henry Hägerstrand, Peter Veranič, Ana Plemenitaš, and Veronika Kralj-Iglič, Curvature-induced accumulation of anisotropic membrane components and raft formation in cylindrical membrane protrusions, pp. 368–373, Copyright 2006, with permission from Elsevier..

could be found on the protrusions (Fig. 9.5-2A) in contrast to the case shown in Fig. 9.5-1A. In cholesterol-depleted cells microtubules are concentrated only in the globular bodies of the cells close to the nuclei (Fig. 9.5-2B). These experiments present evidence for membrane tubular shapes which are also stable without inner rod-like structures (Iglič et al., 2006, 2007b). Although rod-like protrusions were formed due to the impact of the inner rod-like structure, the tubular shape was stable after disintegration of the inner structure, in agreement with the theoretical predictions presented.

We therefore suggest that the observed stability of thin tubular membrane protrusions without an inner supporting rod-like cytoskeleton (Fig. 9.5-2B) may be a consequence of the accumulation of anisotropic membrane nanodomains in the bilayer membrane of these protrusions.

Lubrol rafts are considered to be a special type of membrane raft (microdomain) found in tubular-shaped membrane regions and are distinct from the cholesterol–sphingolipid (Triton resistent) rafts that were found in the planar parts of the membrane (Röper et al., 2000). In the present theoretical consideration the value of the interaction constant ξ was chosen to describe a small protein–lipid complex (Fosnarič et al., 2005; Iglič et al., 2006, 2007b) and could therefore, well describe the prominin–lipid complex (nanodomain). Small anisotropic protein–lipid complexes (i.e., anisotropic membrane inclusions) may associate into larger two-dimensional aggregates (Lubrol rafts) following their curvature-induced accumulation in tubular protrusions as previously observed (Holthius et al., 2003; Hurtig et al., 2010; Huttner and Zimmerberg, 2001; Iglič et al., 2006). The theoretical model described in this chapter may therefore, provide an explanation for the observed curvature-induced enrichment of Lubrol raft markers in tubular membrane protrusions.

The predicted and observed stability of thin tubular membrane protrusions without an inner supporting rod-like skeleton (see Figs. 9.5 and 9.8) is in line with the assumption that prominin nanodomains and other strongly anisotropic membrane nanodomains play an important role in the generation and stabilization of plasma membrane protrusions (Huttner and Zimmerberg, 2001; Kabaso et al., 2012b; Kralj-Iglič et al., 2005). However, also in cases where there is a rod-like structure inside the tubular protrusion (Boulbitch, 1998; Derényi et al., 2002), the described accumulation of anisotropic membrane nanodomains in tubular membrane protrusions represents a complementary physical mechanism for stabilization of tubular membrane protrusions (Iglič et al., 2006, 2007b; Kralj-Iglič et al., 2000, 2005; Yamashita et al., 2002).

9.3 Tubular Budding of the Erythrocyte Membrane

It was also observed that addition of amphiphilic molecules (detergents, peptides) to a suspension of erythrocytes causes changes in their shape. When the detergent molecules intercalate into the membrane, undulations of the membrane appear. Outward bending of the membrane leads to formation of an echinocyte (spiculated) shape, while inward bending of the membrane leads to formation of cup shaped erythrocytes (stomatocytes) and further (in both cases), to microvesiculation of the membrane. Echinocytosis or stomatocytosis is determined by the species of detergent molecules intercalated. For example, dodecaylmaltoside, dodecylzwittergent, and dioctyl-di-QAS induce echinocytosis and exovesiculation, while chlorpromazine and ethyleneglycolethers induce stomatocytosis and endovesiculation (Hägerstrand and Isomaa, 1992; Kralj-Iglič et al., 2000, 2005). The spherical/tubular/torocytic shape of the released vesicles is connected to the intrinsic shape of the nanodomains generated by the intercalated detergent molecules.

According to the bilayer couple hypothesis, transformation of the echinocyte shape is driven by binding of the exogeneously added molecules preferentially to the outer membrane layer (Fig. 9.6). When red blood cells approach the type III echinocytic shape, budding, and nanoexovesicle release (spherical or tubular) from the membrane surface starts (Fig. 9.6).

It has been shown theoretically that the stability of the echinocyte shape is primarily determined by competition between the membrane bilayer Helfrich–Evans bending energy (Eq. 7.70) and the membrane skeleton shear energy (Iglič, 1997). A constitutive

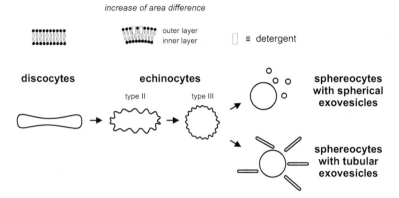

Figure 9.6 Schematic figure of erythrocyte shape transformations due to preferential intercalation of detergents into the outer membrane layer. At low detergent concentrations echinocytes of type I and II (see Bessis, 1973) appear in the erythrocyte suspension, while at higher molecular concentrations echinocytes of type III are the most frequent. At still higher molecular concentrations, that is, at sublytic molecular concentrations, the budding (exovesiculation) and release of spherical or tubular vesicles start (see Hägerstrand and Isomaa, 1992; Iglič et al., 1998, 2007b; Kralj-Iglič et al., 2005, and references therein). As a result the erythrocytes are transformed into spherocytes. Reprinted from *Blood Cells, Molecules and Diseases*, 39(1), Aleš Iglič, Maruša Lokar, Blaž Babnik, Tomaž Slivnik, Peter Veranič, Henry Hägerstrand, and Veronika Kralj-Iglič, Possible role of flexible red blood cell membrane nanodomains in the growth and stability of membrane nanotubes, pp. 14–23, Copyright 2007, with permission from Elsevier.

model for membrane skeleton behaviour takes into account the fact that the membrane skeleton is locally compressible (Discher and Mohandas, 1996; Discher et al., 1994; Mohandas and Evans, 1994). However, for reasons of simplicity the membrane skeleton shear energy is usually calculated using an approximate expression (Evans and Skalak, 1980; Iglič, 1997):

$$W_{\text{shear}} = \frac{\mu}{2} \int (\lambda_m^2 + \lambda_m^{-2} - 2)\, dA, \qquad (9.23)$$

where the membrane skeleton is considered laterally incompressible (Waugh, 1996), μ is the membrane skeleton area shear modulus, λ_m is the principal extension ratio along the meridional direction (Evans and Skalak, 1980; Iglič, 1997) and dA is the membrane area element. The Helfrich–Evans membrane bending energy F_b (Eq. 7.70) is the sum of a local and a non-local term (Evans and Skalak, 1980; Helfrich, 1974; Miao et al., 1994; Stokke et al., 1986):

$$F_b = \frac{k_c}{2} \int (2H)^2 \, dA + 2k_r A(\langle H \rangle - H_0)^2, \qquad (9.24)$$

where the Gaussian local bending term is omitted since according to the Gauss–Bonnet theorem it is constant for the closed surfaces. For thin and not too strongly curved membrane bilayers the average mean curvature $\langle H \rangle$ is proportional to the difference between the two membrane monolayer areas (ΔA) (see Eq. 7.66):

$$\langle H \rangle = \Delta A / 2 A \delta. \qquad (9.25)$$

The normalized average mean curvature $\langle h \rangle = R_0 \langle H \rangle$ is equal to the normalized area difference $\Delta a = \Delta A / 8\pi \delta R_0$, where R_0 is defined by $R_0 = \sqrt{A/4\pi}$ (see also Sections 7.7 and 7.8).

The normalized effective spontaneous mean curvature $h_0 = R_0 H_0$ is equal to the normalized optimal area difference Δa_0:

$$h_0 = \Delta a_0 = \Delta A_0 / 8\pi \delta R_0. \qquad (9.26)$$

The optimal area difference ΔA_0 is determined by the difference in the number of molecules, differences in the area per molecule and the difference in the intrinsic molecular shapes in the outer and the inner monolayer (see also Helfrich, 1974; Miao et al., 1994; Mukhopadhyay et al., 2002, and references therein). The normalized optimal area difference Δa_0 (or normalized spontaneous mean curvature h_0) therefore, depends on the number of excess detergent molecules bound in the outer layer (N), determined with respect to the number of detergent molecules in the inner layer of the membrane bilayer:

$$\Delta a_0 = \Delta a_{0,ref} + N S_a / 8\pi \delta R_0, \qquad (9.27)$$

where S_a is the average area per detergent molecule and $\Delta a_{0,ref}$ is the value of Δa_0 before intercalation of the detergent starts. As may be seen from Eq. 9.27, the value of Δa_0 increases linearly with the number of excess detergent molecules bound to the outer layer of the membrane bilayer.

Figure 9.7 shows the erythrocyte shapes calculated by minimization of the membrane elastic energy (bending and shear) for

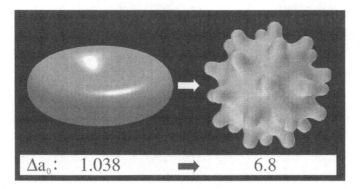

Figure 9.7 Calculated erythrocyte shapes determined by minimization of the membrane elastic energy (bending and shear) for two different values of Δa_0: 1.038 and 6.8 and for $k_r/k_c = 4$ (Hwang and Waugh, 1997), $\mu/k_c = 10^{13} m^{-2}$ (Evans and Skalak, 1980) and a relative cell volume of 0.6. The cell shapes are calculated as described in Božič et al. 2006 for the left shape and Iglič et al. 1998 for the right shape. The calculated equilibrium difference between the two cell membrane monolayer areas Δa is 1.038 for shape a and 2.06 for shape b. Reprinted from *Blood Cells, Molecules and Diseases*, 39(1), Aleš Iglič, Maruša Lokar, Blaž Babnik, Tomaž Slivnik, Peter Veranič, Henry Hägerstrand, and Veronika Kralj-Iglič, Possible role of flexible red blood cell membrane nanodomains in the growth and stability of membrane nanotubes, pp. 14–23, Copyright 2007, with permission from Elsevier.

two different values of the relative optimal area difference Δa_0. In addition to bending and shear energy the echinocyte shape is also modulated by stretching of the membrane skeleton (Mohandas and Evans, 1994; Mukhopadhyay et al., 2002) and by membrane embedded proteins (Hägerstrand et al., 2000).

The spherical erythrocyte shape (spherocyte) at sublytic concentrations of echinocytogenic detergents arises due to reduction of the size of the echinocyte spicules. The spicules become smaller mainly due to the release of daughter exovesicles from the cell surface (Fig. 9.6), predominantly from the echinocyte spicules (Fig. 9.8A). It was believed that progressive narrowing of echinocyte spicules due to the release of daughter exovesicles might lead to formation of thin tubular membrane spicules (protrusions) which are finally released from the cell surface as a whole in the form of long tubular exovesicles (Wagner et al., 1986). However, based on the results

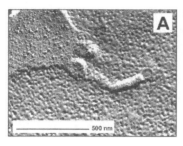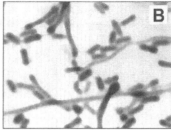

Figure 9.8 TEM micrograph of freeze fracture replicas showing a tubular bud on top of an echinocyte spicule (A) (adapted from Kralj-Iglič et al., 2005) and a TEM micrograph of a dried sample showing free tubular nanoexovesicles released from the membrane (B). The radius of the tubular nanovesicles is about 40 nm. The budding or vesiculation was induced by adding 40 μM dodecyl D-maltoside to an erythrocyte suspension. The molecule of dodecyl D-maltoside has a dimeric headgroup, therefore it is strongly anisotropic (see also Fig. 7.1). Reprinted from *Blood Cells, Molecules and Diseases*, 39(1), Aleš Iglič, Maruša Lokar, Blaž Babnik, Tomaž Slivnik, Peter Veranič, Henry Hägerstrand, and Veronika Kralj-Iglič, Possible role of flexible red blood cell membrane nanodomains in the growth and stability of membrane nanotubes, pp. 14–23, Copyright 2007, with permission from Elsevier.

presented in Fig. 9.8, it can be concluded that tubular budding at the echinocyte spicules is the principal source of the tubular exovesicles released from the erythrocyte membrane (Kralj-Iglič et al., 2005).

Most of the echinocytogenic detergents studied hitherto induce spherical budding and nanoexovesicles, while strongly anisotropic detergent molecules (e.g., dimeric detergents or detergents with a dimeric headgroup (Kralj-Iglič et al., 2000, 2005)) were found to induce mainly tubular buds and tubular nanoexovesicles (Fig. 9.8). The observed tubular budding does not need any additional driving (pulling) force.

Since the spherical and tubular daughter nanovesicles released from the erythrocyte membrane are highly depleted in the membrane skeleton (Hägerstrand et al., 1999; Knowles et al., 1997), the shape of the buds or vesicles is determined by the properties of the membrane bilayer only. It is of interest to understand the mechanisms which determine the observed detergent-induced tubular budding of the bilayer membrane (Fig. 9.8). It is generally accepted (Derényi et al., 2002; Kralj-Iglič et al., 2005; Miao et al., 1991; Tsafrir et al., 2003) that the standard theory of isotropic membrane elasticity (Sackmann, 1994) which is based on a description of the membrane as a bilayer composed of two compressible isotropic monolayers (Eq. 9.24), does not provide an explanation for tubular budding (as observed in this work) if no pulling force is applied (Derényi et al., 2002; Kralj-Iglič et al., 2005; Miao et al., 1991; Tsafrir et al., 2003). Therefore, the above described accumulation of anisotropic membrane nanodomains in tubular parts of the membrane (Fig. 9.4) was suggested as a possible mechanism that might explain the detergent-induced tubular budding of the erythrocyte membrane *with no pulling force* (see Figs. 9.3 and 9.4) required for the formation of these structures (Kralj-Iglič et al., 2005).

The predominant binding of anisotropic detergent molecules in the outer membrane monolayer also increases the optimal difference between the two membrane monolayer areas (Δa_0) (Eq. 9.27) and in this way starts the process of formation of tubular membrane protrusions corresponding to a high difference between the two cell membrane monolayer areas ΔA (Kralj-Iglič et al., 2000, 2005).

To conclude, strongly anisotropic detergent molecules such as dimeric detergents or detergents with a dimeric headgroup (like dodecyl D-maltoside) (Kralj-Iglič et al., 2000, 2005) induce mainly tubular buds and tubular nanoexovesicles (Fig. 9.8). We therefore propose that anisotropic detergents may induce formation of anisotropic nanodomains in the erythrocyte membrane and/or increase the lateral mobility of such (already existing) nanodomains. The increased lateral mobility of the nanodomains may be enabled due to detergent-induced changes in the skeleton–bilayer interactions, or due the changed physical properties of the nanodomains influenced by the incorporated detergent molecules.

9.4 Possible Limiting Shapes of Released Vesicles

The released erythrocyte tubular vesicles induced by anisotropic detergents keep a tubular shape even after their detachment from the parent cell (Fig. 9.8B). The tubular shape represents one of the possible limiting shapes of prolate vesicles (Fig. 9.9). An other limiting shape of prolate vesicles is the necklace structure shown in Fig. 9.9. In the following it is shown that both kinds of limiting shapes (tubular and necklace-like) correspond to extreme average invariants of the curvature tensor (Kralj-Iglič et al., 2000). The shapes of the extreme average invariants of the curvature tensor (Eq. 5.32) correspond to the extreme of the average mean curvature (see also Eq. 5.33):

$$\langle H \rangle = \frac{1}{A} \int H \, dA \qquad (9.28)$$

and to the extreme of the average curvature deviator (see also Eq. 5.35:

$$\langle D \rangle = \frac{1}{A} \int D \, dA \qquad (9.29)$$

at a given area of the membrane surface A and a given volume enclosed by the membrane V.

The corresponding variational problems are stated by constructing the respective functionals (Iglič et al., 1999; Kralj-Iglič et al., 2000):

$$\mathcal{G}_H = \langle H \rangle - \lambda_A \cdot \left(\int dA - A \right) + \lambda_V \cdot \left(\int dV - V \right), \qquad (9.30)$$

$$\mathcal{G}_D = \langle D \rangle + \lambda_A \cdot \left(\int dA - A \right) - \lambda_V \cdot \left(\int dV - V \right), \qquad (9.31)$$

where λ_A and λ_V are the Lagrange multipliers. The analysis is restricted to axisymmetric shapes. The shape is given by rotation of the function $y(x)$ around the x axis. In this case the principal curvatures are expressed by $y(x)$ and its derivatives with respect to x as $C_1 = \mp y''/(1+y'^2)^{3/2}$ (Eq. 5.30) and $C_2 = \pm 1/y(1+y'^2)^{1/2}$ (Eq. 5.31), where $(y' = \partial y/\partial x$ and $y'' = \partial^2 y/\partial x^2)$. The area element is $dA = 2\pi \sqrt{1+y'^2}\, y\, dx$, and the volume element is $dV = \pm \pi y^2 \, dx$. The $\pm$ sign takes into account that the function $y(x)$ may be multiple valued. The sign may change at the points where $y' \to \infty$. The variations

$$\delta \mathcal{G}_H = \delta \int g_H(x, y, y', y'') \, dx = 0 \qquad (9.32)$$

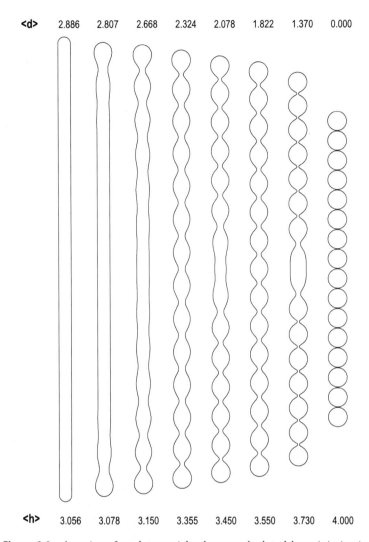

Figure 9.9 A series of prolate vesicle shapes calculated by minimization of the local membrane bending energy (Eq. 7.30) as described in (Iglič et al., 1999). The relative volume $v = 1/\sqrt{16}$ (see also Section 7.8). The corresponding values of $\langle h \rangle = R \langle H \rangle$ and $\langle d \rangle = R \langle D \rangle$ are also given. Here $R = \sqrt{A/4\pi}$. Reprinted from *Journal of Biomechanics*, 43(8), Šarká Perutková, Veronika Kralj-Iglič, Mojka Frank, and Aleš Iglič, Membrane stability of membrane nanotubular protrusions influenced by attachment of flexible rod-like proteins, pp. 1612–1617, Copyright 2010, with permission from Elsevier.

and

$$\delta \mathcal{G}_D = \delta \int g_D(x, y, y', y'') \, dx = 0 \qquad (9.33)$$

are performed by solving the corresponding Euler–Lagrange equations

$$\frac{\partial g_i}{\partial y} - \frac{d}{dx}\left(\frac{\partial g_i}{\partial y'}\right) + \frac{d^2}{dx^2}\left(\frac{\partial g_i}{\partial y''}\right) = 0, \quad i = H, D. \qquad (9.34)$$

By substituting g_H and g_D into Eq. 9.34 we can express both variational problems by a Poisson–Euler equation of single form. After performing the necessary differentiations, this Poisson–Euler equation is (Iglič et al., 1999; Kralj-Iglič et al., 2000)

$$\delta_1 \frac{2y''}{(1+y'^2)^2} + \lambda_A \left(\frac{1}{\sqrt{1+y'^2}} - \frac{yy''}{(\sqrt{1+y'^2})^3} \right) - \delta_2 y \lambda_V = 0, \qquad (9.35)$$

where δ_1 and δ_2 may be + or −, depending on the actual situation. It follows from the above that the solutions for the extremes of average invariants of the curvature tensor are equal. The nature of the extreme obtained may, however, be different. As can be seen in Fig. 9.9, it is possible that some solution corresponds to the maximal average mean curvature and the minimal average curvature deviator (necklace shape in Fig. 9.9). Some other solution may correspond to the minimal average mean curvature and the maximal average curvature deviator (tubular shape in Fig. 9.9).

Some simple analytic solutions of Eq. 9.35 were found: the cylinder $y = $ constant and the circle of radius r_{cir}, $y = y_0 \pm \sqrt{r_{cir}^2 - (x - x_0)^2}$, where (x_0, y_0) is the centre of the circle (Kralj-Iglič et al., 2000). If $x_0 \neq 0$ and $y_0 = 0$, the ansatz fulfils Eq. 9.35 for two different radii (Iglič et al., 1999), representing spheres with two different radii. If $x_0 = 0$ and $y_0 \neq 0$, the circle is the solution of Eq. 9.35 only when the Lagrange multipliers are interdependent; for $r_{cir} < y_0$, the solution represents a torus and a torocyte (Iglič et al., 2000).

As the sum of the solutions of the differential equation within each of the above categories is also a solution of the same equation at the chosen constraints, different combinations of shapes within the corresponding category are possible, provided that the combined shape fulfils the constraints (Elsgolc, 1961). In these cases, the

Lagrange multipliers may be interdependent (Iglič et al., 1999, 2000; Kralj-Iglič et al., 2000). For example, by combining different solutions it can be shown that a cylinder closed by two hemispheres fulfils the conditions for the extremes of the average invariants of the curvature tensor (left tubular shape in Fig. 9.9).

9.5 Theoretical Description of Self-Assembly of Anisotropic Nanodomains into Tubular Membrane Protrusions

In this section, we use the theory of self-assembly to describe the accumulation of nanodomains into cylindrical membrane protrusions. The nanodomains (of total number N) are initially distributed in the (nearly) flat membrane. We assume that the nanodomains protrude through both layers (see also Figs. 8.1 and 9.3) and are laterally mobile over the membrane surface. For a cylindrical protrusion of equal radius $H = D = 1/2r$ (where r is the radius of the protrusion) everywhere on the membrane except on the tip and at the base of the protrusion, while in the flat regions $H = D = 0$.

For the sake of simplicity we assume $\xi \approx \xi^*$, therefore the free energy of a single nanodomain (Eq. 9.5) can be written in the form:

$$f_{in} = \frac{\xi}{2}(H - H_m)^2 + \frac{\xi}{2}(D^2 + D_m^2) - kT \ln\left(I_0\left(\frac{\xi D_m D}{kT}\right)\right). \quad (9.36)$$

Nanodomains in aggregates interact with neighbouring nanodomains. We denote the corresponding interaction energy per nanodomain (monomer) in an aggregate composed of i nanodomains as $\chi(i)$ where we assume that the energy $\chi(i)$ depends on the size of the aggregate i. Hence, the mean free energy per nanodomain in a cylindrical aggregate (where $H = D = 1/2r$) composed of i nanodomains can be written as:

$$\mu_i = f_c - \chi(i), \quad (9.37)$$

where $f_c = f_{in}(H = D = 1/2r)$ and $\chi(i) > 0$. We assume that in the planar regions of the membrane (having $H = D = 0$) the concentration of nanodomains is always below the critical aggregation concentration and therefore the nanodomain cannot form two-dimensional flat aggregates. The mean energy per nanodomain in the flat membrane regions is therefore $\tilde{\mu}_1 = f_p$, where $f_p = f_{in}(H = D = 0)$.

The number density of nanodomains in the flat membrane regions is

$$\tilde{x}_1 = \frac{\tilde{N}_1}{M}, \qquad (9.38)$$

where $\tilde{N}_1$ is the number of monomeric nanodomains in flat regions and M is the number of (lattice) sites in the whole system. The size distribution of cylindrical aggregates on the scale of number density is expressed as

$$x_i = \frac{i N_i}{M}, \qquad (9.39)$$

where N_i denotes the number of cylindrical aggregates with aggregation number i, that is, the number of tubular membrane protrusions (N_i) consisting of i nanodomains each. The number densities $\tilde{x}_1$ and x_i should fulfil the conservation conditions for the total number of nanodomains in the membrane

$$\tilde{x}_1 + \sum_{i=1}^{\infty} x_i = N/M. \qquad (9.40)$$

The free energy (F) of all nanodomains in the membrane can thus be written as

$$F = M \left[\tilde{x}_1 \tilde{\mu}_1 + kT \tilde{x}_1 (\ln \tilde{x}_1 - 1) \right]$$
$$+ M \sum_{i=1}^{\infty} \left[x_i \mu_i + kT \frac{x_i}{i} \left(\ln \frac{x_i}{i} - 1 \right) \right] - \mu M \left(\tilde{x}_1 + \sum_{i=1}^{\infty} x_i \right), \qquad (9.41)$$

where μ is the Lagrange parameter. The above expression for the free energy also involves also the contributions of configurational (mixing) entropy (see Eq. 1.107). Minimization of F with respect to $\tilde{x}_1$ and x_i:

$$\frac{\partial F}{\partial \tilde{x}_i} = 0, \frac{\partial F}{\partial x_i} = 0, i = 1, 2, 3, \ldots, \qquad (9.42)$$

leads to equilibrium distributions

$$\tilde{x}_1 = \exp\left(-\frac{f_p - \mu}{kT}\right), \qquad (9.43)$$

$$x_i = i \exp\left(-\frac{i}{kT}[f_c - \chi - \mu]\right), \qquad (9.44)$$

where we assumed for simplicity that $\chi(i)$ is a constant. The quantity μ can be expressed from Eq. 9.43 and substituted in Eq. 9.44 to get

$$x_i = i\left[\tilde{x}_1 \cdot \exp\left(\frac{f_p + \chi - f_c}{kT}\right)\right]^i. \qquad (9.45)$$

Since x_i can never exceed unity, it follows from Eq. 9.45 that when $\tilde{x}_1$ approaches $\exp\left[f_c - f_p - \chi\right]/kT]$ it cannot increase further. The maximal possible value of the number density of monomeric nanodomains in flat parts of the membrane $\tilde{x}_1$ is therefore (Gimsa et al., 2007; Iglič et al., 2007b):

$$\tilde{x}_c \approx \exp\left(\frac{\Delta f - \chi}{kT}\right), \qquad (9.46)$$

where $\Delta f = f_c - f_p$ is the difference between the energy of a single nanodomain on the cylindrical protrusion and the energy of the nanodomain in the flat membrane region. The number density $\tilde{x}_c$ is the critical aggregation number density (concentration) (Israelachvili, 1997). In the case of cylindrical aggregates where $H = D = 1/2r$, the value of Δf is:

$$\Delta f = \xi H(H - H_m) - kT \ln\left[I_0(\xi D_m D/kT)\right]. \qquad (9.47)$$

For $1/2r < H_m$ the value of Δf is always negative. If $\tilde{x}_1$ is above $\tilde{x}_c$, the formation of a very long cylindrical protrusion(s) composed of anisotropic membrane nanodomains is energetically favourable. It can be seen from Eq. 9.46 that longitudinal growth of the cylindrical membrane protrusion is promoted by the energy difference Δf, as well as by the strength of the direct interaction between the nanodomains χ. The critical concentration $\tilde{x}_c$ strongly decreases with increasing D_m (Fig. 9.10).

The theoretically predicted stability of thin tubular membrane protrusions without an inner supporting rod-like skeleton is in line with the assumption that prominin nanodomains (and other strongly anisotropic membrane nanodomains) have an important role in the generation and stabilization of plasma membrane protrusions (Hurtig et al., 2010; Veranič et al., 2008). However,

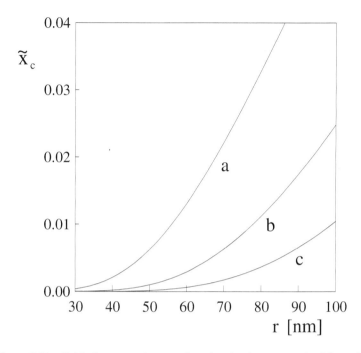

Figure 9.10 Critical aggregation number density (concentration) for self-assembly of anisotropic membrane nanodomains into larger membrane domains forming cylindrical aggregates calculated as a function of the radius of cylindrical aggregates (r). The intrinsic shape of the single nanodomains are characterized by $H_m = D_m$ of 0.06 nm^{-1} (a), 0.08 nm^{-1} (b) and 0.1 nm^{-1} (c). The values of other model parameters are: $\chi = 1\ kT$ and $\xi = 5000\ kT\ nm^2$. Reprinted from *Blood Cells, Molecules and Diseases*, 39(1), Aleš Iglič, Maruša Lokar, Blaž Babnik, Tomaž Slivnik, Peter Veranič, Henry Hägerstrand, and Veronika Kralj-Iglič, Possible role of flexible red blood cell membrane nanodomains in the growth and stability of membrane nanotubes, pp. 14–23, Copyright 2007, with permission from Elsevier.

also in cases where there is a rod-like structure inside the tubular protrusion, the described accumulation of anisotropic membrane nanodomains in tubular membrane protrusions represents a complementary physical mechanism for stabilization of tubular membrane protrusions.

Chapter 10

Spherical Budding of Biological Membranes

The proposed mechanism of stabilization of membrane nanotubes by coupling of the local membrane shape and the lateral density of the membrane constituents (nanodomains) is also one of the mechanisms relevant for the formation and stabilization of highly curved spherical membrane buds. Figures 10.1 and 10.2 (Hägerstrand et al., 2006; Iglič et al., 2007b; Laradji and Kumar, 2004; McMahon and Gallop, 2005; Sens and Turner, 2004, 2006; Staneva et al., 2005; Thiele et al., 1999) show the accumulation of isotropic membrane nanodomains (having $C_{1m} = C_{2m}$), which favour high isotropic curvature, on a small bud. The fraction of the area covered by nanodomains increases towards the tip of the bud. As the neck becomes narrower, the distribution approaches a step function, while the free energy of the nanodomains lowers the free energy of the membrane.

In the limit of an infinitesimally thin neck, the shape of the vesicle approaches a spherical shape as shown in Fig. 10.2. It can be seen that the limiting shape corresponding to the minimal average mean curvature consists of a section of a sphere while the limiting shape corresponding to the maximal average mean curvature consists of a segment of a flat surface and a spherical vesicle (Iglič and Hägerstrand, 1999).

Nanostructures in Biological Systems: Theory and Applications
Aleš Iglič, Veronika Kralj-Iglič, and Damjana Drobne
Copyright © 2015 Pan Stanford Publishing Pte. Ltd.
ISBN 978-981-4267-20-5 (Hardcover), 978-981-4303-43-9 (eBook)
www.panstanford.com

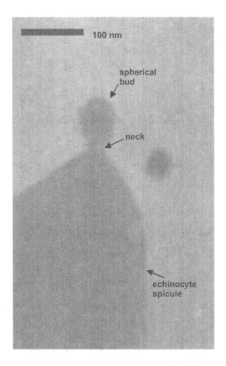

Figure 10.1 Transmission electron microscope (TEM) image of a spherical bud at the top of an echinocyte spicule induced by adding the detergent dodecylzwittergent to an erythrocyte suspension. Figure reprinted with permission from Kralj-Iglič, V., Iglič, A., Hägerstrand, H., and Peterlin, P. Stable tubular microexovesicles of the erythrocyte membrane induced by dimeric amphiphiles. *Phys. Rev. E*, 61, pp. 4230–4234. Copyright 2000 by the American Physical Society.

The influence of the anisotropy of the membrane constituents or nanodomains (see Fig. 8.2) on the stability and configuration of the neck-shaped membrane regions can be studied theoretically in a system of undulating tubular shapes (Fig. 10.3). In the model the membrane is composed of anisotropic membrane constituents or nanodomains and components of the isotropic phospholipid moiety. The anisotropic nanodomains with $H_m = 0$ and $D_m \neq 0$ (see also Fig. 8.2) favour a saddle-like shape. Figure 10.3 shows a part of the calculated membrane shape for two values of the intrinsic curvature deviator D_m of the anisotropic nanodomains.

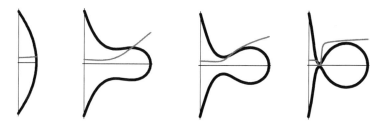

Figure 10.2 The accumulation of isotropic membrane constituents (nanodomains) in the budding region. The line represents the relative number density of membrane nanodomains characterized by positive intrinsic curvatures ($C_{1m} = C_{2m} > 0$) (see also Fig. 8.2) and attractive direct interactions during the budding of the membrane. Hägerstrand, H., Mrowczynska, L., Salzer, U., Prohaska, R., Michelsen, K. A., Kralj-Iglič, V., and Iglič, A. Curvature dependent lateral distribution of raft markers in the human erythrocyte membrane. *Mol. Membr. Biol.*, 23, pp. 277–288, copyright © 2006, Informa Healthcare. Reproduced with permission of Informa Healthcare.

For small values of the intrinsic curvature deviator D_m the tubular shape is energetically favourable. However, with increasing D_m, a certain critical value of D_m is reached where the tubular shape is changed discontinuously to an undulating shape with a narrow neck (Fig. 10.3). With increasing values of D_m the neck becomes thinner. As can be seen in Fig. 10.3, the saddle-preferring anisotropic membrane constituents/nanodomains accumulate in the energetically favourable saddle-like neck regions.

The results presented in Figs. 10.2 and 10.3 indicate that two complementary mechanisms may take place in the budding of heterogeneous membranes containing isotropic and anisotropic membrane constituents or nanodomains: accumulation of saddle-preferring membrane constituents or nanodomains in the neck connecting the bud to the parent membrane, and accumulation of spherically curved membrane-preferring constituents or nanodomains in the spherical region of the bud (i.e., daughter vesicle).

As an example of the experimental evidence for the accumulation of membrane components in the spherical region of the bud, Fig. 10.4 shows an increased fluorescence signal of choleratoxin-labelled rafts on buds of the membrane of the human urothelial

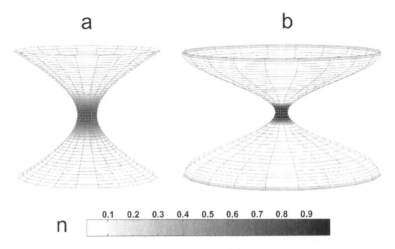

Figure 10.3 The neck region of a membrane with anisotropic nanodomains or constituents and the corresponding fraction of the membrane covered by nanodomains (shaded) for two values of the intrinsic curvature deviator of anisotropic nanodomains: $D_m = 0.4\,\text{nm}^{-1}$ (a) and $0.7\,\text{nm}^{-1}$ (b). Both values of D_m are above its critical value. The membrane free energy was minimized with respect to the shape and lateral and orientational distributions of anisotropic membrane constituents or nanodomains, as described in detail in Iglič et al. (2007a).

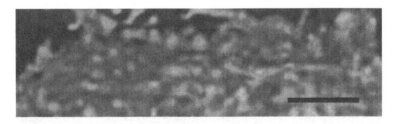

Figure 10.4 A fluorescence microscope image of the budding membrane of human urothelial line RT4 cells. Differences in the intensity of the fluorescence signal indicate that cholera toxin–labelled rafts accumulate on the buds. Bar = 200 nm (Kralj-Iglič and Veranič, 2007).

line (RT4) cell. Clustering of rafts and membrane proteins in highly curved membrane regions (invaginations) and vesicles has also been observed previously (Hägerstrand et al., 2006; Harder and Simons, 1997).

To conclude, the membrane configuration of a budding vesicle connected to the parent cell by a very thin neck (right hand shape in Fig. 10.2) may be stabilized by the accumulation and average orientational ordering of anisotropic membrane components or nanodomains in the neck. As the suggested mechanism of stabilization of the neck connecting the budding vesicle and the parent membrane is nonspecific, and as there is no *a priori* reason for the membrane constituents or nanodomains to be in general isotropic, it could be expected to take place in any cell type (Jorgačevski et al., 2010). For example, in was shown recently that the orientational and lateral redistribution of membrane constituents or nanodomains may explain the transient energetically stable narrow fusion necks (pores) connecting fused vesicles to the target membrane which were observed in resting lactotrophs (Jorgačevski et al., 2010).

The stability of the narrow neck connecting the budding vesicle to the parent membrane has also been addressed previously within the area-difference-elasticity (ADE) model (see Fig. 7.18A). A minimum of free energy corresponding to a narrow neck was obtained; however, the values of the model constants in the ADE model (Eq. 7.70 had to be taken outside the range estimated by experiments (see, e.g., the discussion in Miao et al., 1994; Seifert, 1997).

At first glance the stabilizing effect of the saddle-preferring anisotropic membrane constituents or nanodomains (Fig. 10.3) may completely prevent fission of the daughter vesicle, so the question arises as to what might be the possible mechanism of vesicle fission if the highly curved neck geometry is strongly stabilized by accumulation of saddle-preferring membrane constituents possessing average orientational ordering. As suggested recently, beside biologically active mechanisms, the creation of localized topologically defects in average orientational order in the membrane neck might play an important role in membrane fission processes (Jesenek et al., 2012, 2013). Namely, topological defects of the average orientational ordering of the membrane components in the region of a very thin neck (Fig. 10.5) may induce strong fluctuations of the membrane neck. Consequently, interactions among neighbouring membrane constituents in the neck are weakened. The resulting softer structure could enable

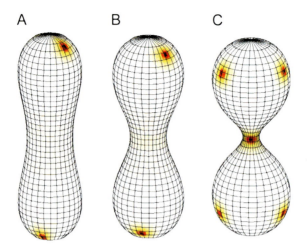

Figure 10.5 Change in the number and position of topological defects or anti-defects in the average in-plane membrane ordering during formation of the membrane neck. For large enough values of the curvature deviator $D = |C_1 - C_2|/2$ (i.e., strongly negative $C_1 C_2 < 0$) (see Eqs. 5.34 and 5.35) in the neck, defect–antidefect pairs are created as shown in Figure C, where two antidefects are formed at the neck. Republished with permission of DOVE Medical Press, from biological membrane driven by curvature. induced frustrations in membrane orientational ordering, Jesenek, D., Perutková, Š, Gozdzd, W., Kralj-Iglič, V., Iglič, A. and Kralj, S., *Int. J. Nanomed*, 8, copyright 2013; permission conveyed through Copyright Clearance Center, Inc.

molecular reorganization in the neck, and the consequent breaking of the neck, that is, fission (Jesenek et al., 2012, 2013).

If separation of the budding vesicle from the mother membrane is prevented, the neck can grow into a nanotube, pushing the vesicle at its tip. Such a situation can frequently be seen with a scanning electron microscope (Fig. 10.6). The growth of the nanotube by elongation of the neck can be supported by actin filaments or can be independent of the cytoskeleton. However, it is also possible that the vesicles at the tip of the nanotube are attached to the membrane surface of the neighbouring cell and afterwards detached (torn apart) from the nanotube so that finally one end of the nanotube becomes free as shown in Fig. 10.6. The possibility that the tip vesicles are attached to the substrate cannot be excluded either.

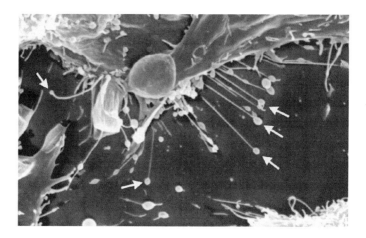

Figure 10.6 Scanning electron micrograph of membrane nanotubes of RT4 urothelial cancer cells. Some of the nanotubes have spherical vesicles at their free tips, as indicated by the arrows. Bar = 10 μm. Figure adapted from Schara et al. (2009).

The spherical vesicle at the tip of the nanotube is assumed to be stabilized by isotropic nanodomains characterized by positive $C_{1m} = C_{2m} > 0$, while the nanotube is assumed to be formed from anisotropic cylindrical curvature-preferring membrane constituents or nanodomains ($C_{1m} > 0, C_{2m} = 0$) (Fig. 8.2) connecting the vesicle and the parent cell membrane (Schara et al., 2009).

In accordance with the assumption that the composition of the membrane of the nanotubes is different from the composition of the membrane of the vesicles at the tip of the nanotube (see Schara et al., 2009, and Fig. 10.7), the brightness (originating from the ganglioside GM1-bound fluorescent label choleratoxin B-FITC) of the vesicles at the tips of the nanotubes that are not attached to neighbouring cells is more intense than the brightness of non-exvaginated regions of the cell membrane. This result supports the hypothesis that the vesicles at the tips of the nanotubes (having one free end) tend to accumulate ganglioside GM1 (Fig. 10.7), one of the characteristic components of lipid rafts, that is, membrane domains that accumulate several types of membrane proteins, such as growth factor receptors and enzymes (Brown and London, 1998a; Simons and Ikonen, 1997). The appearance of lipid rafts in vesicular

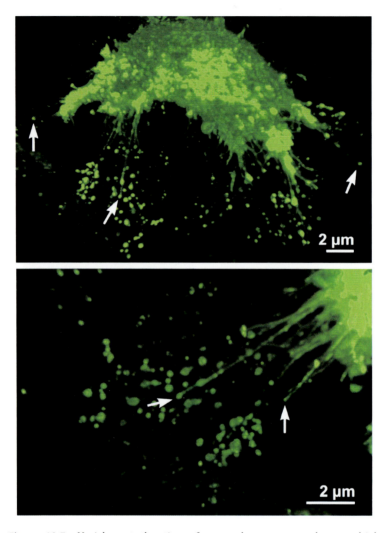

Figure 10.7 Vesicles at the tips of nanotubes seem to have a high concentration of the ganglioside GM1, labelled with choleratoxin B-FITC (seen as brighter labelling; arrows show examples) in the urothelial cell line T24. Bar = 2 μm. Figure adapted from Schara et al. (2009).

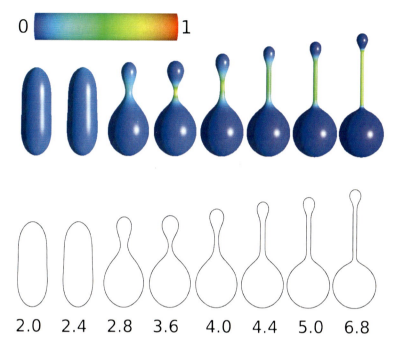

Figure 10.8 Calculated cell shapes having a two component membrane composed of isotropic and anisotropic flexible nanodomains. The values of the intrinsic mean curvature of isotropic membrane component ($H_{m,iso}$) are 2.0, 2.4, 2.8, 3.6, 4.0, 4.4, 5.0 and 6.8. The anisotropic membrane component having $D_{m,aniso} = H_{m,aniso} = 8$ prefers a cylindrical membrane curvature (see also Fig. 8.2). The relative volume $v = 0.8$. The colour of the surface represents the fraction of the area covered by isotropic nanodomains. The fully blue colour corresponds to a membrane composed of isotropic nanodomains only. The shift towards green and red colours indicates increased lateral density of the anisotropic nanodomains. Figure adapted from Bobrowska et al. (2013).

protrusions at the tips of the nanotubes might be crucial for the attachment of the nanotube to the target cell, because N-cadherins were found among the proteins comprising the lipid raft domains (Causeret et al., 2005). These cadherins are responsible for making intercellular connections between mesenchymal cells and are also found in urothelial T24 cells (Laidler et al., 2000) where nanotubes are frequently seen (Veranič et al., 2008). Differences in membrane composition between the tip vesicles and the nanotubes have also

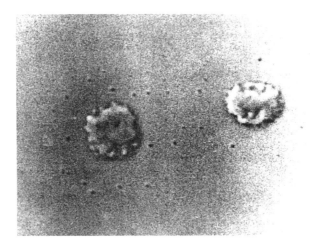

Figure 10.9 Vesiculation of human erythrocytes at high pH with exogeneously added dibucaine. The vesicles around the parent cell move synchronously with the parent cell, indicating that they are connected to the parent cell by thin membrane nanotubes. Reprinted from Kralj-Iglič, V., Gomišček, G., Majhenc, J., Arrigler, V., and Svetina, S. (2001a). Myelin-like protrusions of giant phospholipid vesicles prepared by electroformation. *Colloids. Surf. A*, 181, pp. 315–318, Copyright 2001, with permission from Elsevier.

been suggested by other authors (Huttner and Schmidt, 2002). Accordingly Fig. 10.8 shows that cylindrical curvature-preferring membrane constituents or nanodomains favour elongation of the neck in a thin tube and a long tube, similarly as observed in Fig. 10.7. The daughter vesicles observed to be connected to the parent red blood cells by thin membrane nanotubes (Fig. 10.9) indicate that membrane nanotubular protrusions with vesicles at their tips can be indeed stabilized by the membrane itself, that is, without cytoskeleton structures which are completely absent in red blood cells.

Chapter 11

Fusion of Vesicles with a Target Plasma Membrane

Membrane fusion (Fig. 11.1) is an essential event in many biological processes of eukaryotic cells (Jahn et al., 2003), such as for instance, in the vesicular release of hormones. Membrane fusion is thought to begin with the formation of a hemifusion stalk, an intermediate structure connecting the outer leaflets of fusing membranes (for a review see Chernomordik and Kozlov, 2008). The hemifusion stalk then develops into a fusion neck (pore), the membrane bilayer channel connecting a spherical vesicle and a plasma membrane, through which cargo molecules may diffuse from the vesicle lumen into the cell exterior (Jorgačevski et al., 2010). After formation, the fusion neck either closes and allows the vesicle to be reused in another round of (transient) exocytosis (Ceccarelli et al., 1973), or it fully opens, leading to full fusion exocytosis, that is, complete merging of the vesicle membrane with the target plasma membrane (see Heuser and Reese, 1973, and Fig. 11.1). The mechanisms by which the initial fusion neck between the vesicle and the plasma attains stability are still poorly understood (Jorgačevski et al., 2010). Formation of the fusion neck at first glance may be considered to be energetically

---

Nanostructures in Biological Systems: Theory and Applications
Aleš Iglič, Veronika Kralj-Iglič, and Damjana Drobne
Copyright © 2015 Pan Stanford Publishing Pte. Ltd.
ISBN 978-981-4267-20-5 (Hardcover), 978-981-4303-43-9 (eBook)
www.panstanford.com

unfavourable by the argument that the repulsive electrostatic forces between two closely opposed phospholipid bilayers need to be overcome in order to reach metastable transition states leading to fusion neck formation (Kozlov and Markin, 1983). However, in cellular systems the repulsive electrostatic force between like-charged membrane surfaces can be reduced or even changed into an attractive force, for example, by protein-mediated interactions between like-charged membrane surfaces, where the proteins (or some other biological nanoparticles, such as lipoproteins) should have a distinctive internal charge distribution (see Chapter 14 and Kim et al., 2008; May et al., 2008; Urbanija et al., 2007, 2008a,b). Another example of possible mediators that may reduce the energy barrier between the vesicles and the target plasma membrane in regulated exocytosis is soluble N-ethylmaleimide-sensitive factor attachment protein (SNARE) receptor (Duman and Forte, 2003; Jahn and Scheller, 2006; Martens et al., 2007).

It was suggested that without stabilizing factors the fusion necks would spontaneously close or widen swiftly and irreversibly after their formation (Jackson and Chapman, 2008) (see also Fig. 11.1). On the other hand, in the absence of stimulation, repetitive transient fusion events of the same vesicle were also observed, indicating the possibility of formation of a stable thin membrane neck connecting the vesicle and the plasma membrane (Jorgačevski et al., 2010; Stenovec et al., 2004; Vardjan et al., 2007). In addition to some proteins, negatively charged lipid molecules have also been shown to strongly affect the probability of exocytosis (Churchward et al., 2008). To understand how lipid molecules may affect fusion neck dynamics, we need to have an appropriate theoretical model which in the first place could describe the stability of the initially formed fusion neck (Fig. 11.1), and then predict how interacting molecules (proteins and/or lipids) mediate changes in neck stability (Jorgačevski et al., 2010).

Such a model should take into account the high curvature in the region of the fusion neck, as well as the specific shape of interacting molecules, which in general may be anisotropic (see Figs. 7.1, 8.6 and Kralj-Iglič et al., 1999; Mareš et al., 2008). In Chapter 10, a theory was presented which may explain the stability of narrow necks connecting daughter vesicles with the

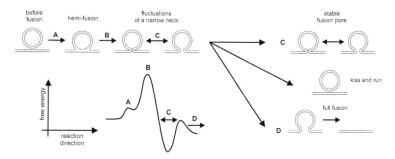

Figure 11.1 Fusion of a vesicle and a plasma membrane is thought to begin with the formation of a hemifusion stalk (transition A), an intermediate structure connecting the outer leaflets of the fusing membranes (reviewed in Chernomordik and Kozlov, 2008). The hemifusion stalk then develops into a fusion neck (transition B). The fusion neck (pore) exhibits stability (see Fig. 11.2) and can therefore reversibly vary its diameter around an "equilibrium" value (transitions C). In state C the fusion neck (pore) diameter may be too narrow to permit transport of luminal cargo molecules and therefore this state could be considered release incompetent (see Stenovec et al., 2004; Vardjan et al., 2007) vesicles in state C may transform into a state with a wider fusion neck diameter and further into a state of full fusion. The fusion pore can also be disrupted (kiss and run scenario) (reviewed in Masedunskas et al., 2012), or remain stable for a longer time in state C. Figure adapted from Jorgačevski et al. (2010) and Jesenek et al. (2012).

parent membrane (Fig. 10.3) (Bobrowska et al., 2013; Kralj-Iglič et al., 1999; Urbanija et al., 2008a). It was shown that in the thin neck that connects the vesicle with the plasma membrane the difference between the two principal membrane curvatures C_1 and C_2 (see also Fig. 5.2) is very high, reaching a regime where the anisotropic intrinsic shape of the membrane constituents becomes locally and globally important (Fig. 10.3) because of the average membrane in-plane orientational ordering of anisotropic membrane components (Fournier and Galatola, 1998; Iglič et al., 2007b; Kralj-Iglič et al., 2000, 2006). As shown in Chapter 10, in multicomponent membranes strong lateral redistribution of membrane components takes place in thin membrane necks, representing a degree of freedom of the system which contributes with decrease in the membrane free energy (Bobrowska et al., 2013; Hägerstrand et al.,

2006; Iglič et al., 2006, 2007a; Kralj-Iglič et al., 1999; Markin, 1981; Sorre et al., 2009; Staneva et al., 2005; Tian and Baumgart, 2009).

It should be pointed out that considering the average orientational ordering of anisotropic membrane components, which may be single molecules (Fig. 7.1) or small membrane nanodomains (see Fig. 8.1 and Iglič et al., 2007b), does not assume lattice-like packing of these components with fixed orientation and fixed position of membrane constituents, but merely takes into account the possibility with decrease in the membrane free energy due to the average orientation (see Fig. 7.2) and position of laterally mobile rotating anisotropic membrane constituents (lipids, proteins, or nanodomains).

Recently, repetitive fusion neck events in resting lactotrophs were observed experimentally using cell-attached patch–clamp capacitance and fusion neck conductance measurements (Jorgačevski et al., 2010). The results revealed a bell-shaped distribution of the fusion neck conductance. The observed stability of the fusion neck (Jorgačevski et al., 2010) was explained within the theoretical model of multicomponent membrane described in Chapter 10. In this model the membrane is considered as a pair of coupled monolayers composed of different constituent species (molecules or nanodomains) (Jorgačevski et al., 2010). In calculating the energy (Fig. 11.2) however, the two membrane monolayers are considered separately, the outer layer having a larger area than the inner layer. The sign of the principal curvatures of the outer membrane layer is equal to the sign of the curvature of the membrane surface, while the sign of the curvatures of the inner surface is opposite to the sign of the curvature of the membrane surface. As the curvature radii in the neck connecting the vesicle and plasma membrane approach the membrane thickness (Fig. 11.2), the membrane thickness should be taken into account when calculating the principal curvatures of the outer and inner membrane lipid layers (Jorgačevski et al., 2010).

In the model, each of the membrane layers were assumed to contain isotropic constituents (type 1) and anisotropic constituents (type 2) which are free to redistribute laterally over a lattice with equal lattice sites. We can describe this degree of freedom by the local relative area densities of the species in the outer and inner membrane layer. Direct interactions between constituents can

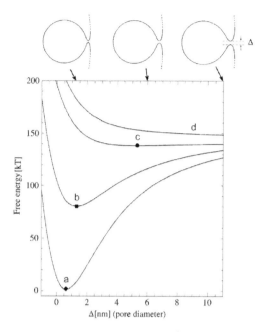

Figure 11.2 Configuration of a vesicle fused a the two-component bilayer membrane and the corresponding free energy as a function of the fusion neck diameter (Δ) calculated for different values of the intrinsic mean curvature of the anisotropic membrane component $H_m = -D_m = -|C_{1m} - C_{2m}|/2 = -1/5.75$ nm^{-1} (A), $-1/6$ nm^{-1} (B), $-1/6.2$ nm^{-1} (C), $-1/6.5$ nm^{-1} (D). A deeper energy minimum corresponds to stronger accumulation of anisotropic membrane components in the region of the fusion neck (see also Fig. 10.3). Jorgačevski, J., M. Fošnarič, N. V., Stenovec, M., Potokar, M., Kreft, M., Kralj-Iglič, V., Iglič, A., and Zorec, R. Fusion Pore Stability of Peptidergic Vesicles. *Mol. Membr. Biol.*, 27, pp. 65–80, copyright © 2010, Informa Healthcare. Reproduced with permission of Informa Healthcare.

be taken into account within the Bragg–Williams approximation (see Section 9.1). The free energy of each membrane layer thus contains the contributions of membrane constituents of both types, their configurational entropy and the contribution of the direct interactions between anisotropic constituents (Jorgačevski et al., 2010). The free energy of the system, considering the effects of the positional and orientational distribution of membrane constituents in both membrane layers, was minimized within the sequence of calculated closed shapes with an endovesicle simulating narrowing of the neck connecting the vesicle and the cell membrane (Fig. 11.2). The shape corresponding to the configuration with minimal free energy was considered to be the equilibrium shape attained by the model system. The diameters of the neck, corresponding to the minimum of free energy (Fig. 11.2), are in agreement with the respective experimental results (Fig. 11.4) (Jorgačevski et al., 2010). It can be seen in Fig. 11.2 that the energy curves express minima at certain neck diameters only in the cases of sufficiently high anisotropy of type 2 membrane constituents, where the anisotropy is described by the intrinsic curvature deviator $D_m = |C_{1m} - C_{2m}|/2$. This is consistent with the experimental results indicating that fusion necks may exhibit an energetically favourable state (Fig. 11.4) (Jorgačevski et al., 2010). If the anisotropy is small enough no minimum is observed (curve d in Fig. 11.2). Moreover, one can also observe in Fig. 11.2 that the higher is the anisotropy, the smaller is the stable fusion neck diameter. Within the model parameters used, a high enough anisotropy of the membrane constituents is therefore required to describe a stable narrow fusion neck (Jorgačevski et al., 2010). It should be stressed that the average orientation (see Fig. 7.2) of the anisotropic membrane constituents is not equal in the two membrane layers of the fusion neck, the difference being about 90 degrees for sufficiently large curvature of the neck (Jorgačevski et al., 2010). Isotropic (axisymmetric) inverted conical constituents (with $C_{1m} = C_{2m} < 0$ as defined in Figs. 7.1 and 8.2) only weakly accumulate in the inner and outer membrane layer in the vicinity of the saddle-like fusion neck (not shown), while anisotropic membrane constituents (with $C_{2m} < 0$ at $C_{1m} \approx 0$) (Fig. 7.1) strongly accumulate in both membrane layers of the fusion neck (Jorgačevski et al., 2010).

This phenomenon may be explained as follows. While the effect of isotropic inverted conical constituents in the two membrane layers partly cancel each other due to the opposing signs of the principal curvature in the two membrane layers, the effect of the average orientational ordering of the anisotropic constituents in the two membrane layers is summed, since the average orientation of the anisotropic membrane constituents is different in the two membrane layers in the region of the fusion neck (Fig. 11.3 and

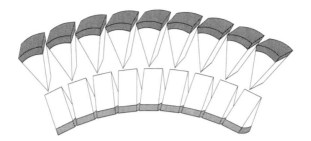

Figure 11.3 The average orientation of anisotropic membrane constituents is different in the two membrane layers if the bilayer curvature deviator is large enough. Jorgačevski, J., M. Fošnarič, N. V., Stenovec, M., Potokar, M., Kreft, M., Kralj-Iglič, V., Iglič, A., and Zorec, R. Fusion Pore Stability of Peptidergic Vesicles. *Mol. Membr. Biol.*, 27, pp. 65–80, copyright © 2010, Informa Healthcare. Reproduced with permission of Informa Healthcare.

Fournier and Galatola, 1998; Kralj-Iglič et al., 2000). This is one of the main reasons for the strong difference in the effects of anisotropic and isotropic membrane constituents on fusion neck stability (Jorgačevski et al., 2010).

Most importantly, in the case when the accumulation of isotropic inverted conical membrane constituents may stabilize the fusion neck, the equilibrium necks (corresponding to minima of the free energy) are much wider (i.e., more than 50 nm wide) than the necks stabilized by accumulation of anisotropic membrane components and do not correspond to the experimentally determined values given in Fig. 11.4.

In the calculations presented in Fig. 11.2, values of the intrinsic principal curvature of anisotropic membrane constituents C_{2m} around $-1/3$ nm^{-1} at $C_{1m} \approx 0$ (i.e., $H_m \simeq -D_m \simeq -1/6$ nm^{-1}) were considered (see also Figs. 7.1 and Fig. 7.5), since they are very close to the measured values of the negative intrinsic (spontaneous) curvatures of lipids necessary to trigger membrane fusion (Churchward et al., 2008). It can therefore, be concluded that, the same components with negative intrinsic (spontaneous) curvatures which are essential for membrane fusion can also stabilize the narrow fusion neck after its formation. The diameter of the fusion neck remains stable, as observed in experiments

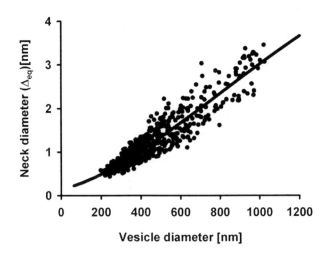

Figure 11.4 Experimentally determined relationship between vesicle diameter and fusion neck diameters. The fusion neck diameter was estimated from the fusion neck conductance. The vesicle diameter was estimated from the vesicle capacitance, by assuming a spherical shape of the vesicles (adapted from Jorgačevski et al., 2010).

(Jorgačevski et al., 2010), since the membrane shape is trapped within an energy minimum (Fig. 11.2).

Although exocytotic fusion necks were hitherto believed to be energetically unfavourable in the absence of specific stabilizing factors (Israelachvili, 1997), repetitive fusion neck events in resting lactotrophs (Stenovec et al., 2004; Vardjan et al., 2007) indicate (in agreement with the theoretical predictions given in Fig. 11.2) that an open neck may be energetically favourable and likely trapped in an energy minimum (Jorgačevski et al., 2010). Therefore, we next discuss the nature of a stable fusion neck, a highly complex curved structure in which anisotropic membrane constituents may play a stabilizing role.

In the theoretical model used to calculate the energies given in Fig. 11.2, it is assumed that the inner membrane layer of the vesicle and the neck of the vesicle (i.e., the fusion neck) both contain sugar residues (Jorgačevski et al., 2010). For this reason the inner part of the membrane is considered to be thicker than the outer part of the membrane. Both layers of sugar residues in the region of the fusion neck together exceed 2 nm in thickness and therefore are not subject to short-range attractive van der Waals and short-range attractive or oscillatory hydration forces between the opposing membranes in the fusion neck at low separation distances, as pointed out by Israelachvili and Wennerstrom (Israelachvili and Wennerström, 1996).

In conclusion, in this chapter we show that the orientational and lateral redistribution of anisotropic membrane constituents may explain transient energetically stable narrow fusion neck events, recorded in resting lactotrophs using the cell-attached patch–clamp capacitance technique (Jorgačevski et al., 2010). A theoretical description is provided by a simple but relevant model composed of a parent cell with a small endovesicle connected by a fusion neck (Bobrowska et al., 2013; Jorgačevski et al., 2010). This model requires the minimum of free energy of sufficient depth to suppress excessive fluctuations (Bobrowska et al., 2013; Jesenek et al., 2012) of the thickness of the neck connecting the endovesicle with the membrane in order for the proposed mechanism to describe the essential features of the system.

Once the vesicle is fused with the membrane, a very thin initial fusion neck, that is, the neck connecting the vesicle and the target cell, is formed. It was shown recently that in initiation of vesicle fusion (i.e., neck formation), specific lipids with high negative intrinsic (spontaneous) curvatures play a very important role (Churchward et al., 2008). These and others specific lipids also possess high intrinsic anisotropy (see Figs. 7.1 and 7.5) and can therefore stabilize the narrow diameter of the opened fusion neck, as predicted in Fig. 11.2. Comparison of the experimental results for fusion necks (Fig. 11.4) with theoretical predictions (Fig. 11.2) enabled us to estimate that for anisotropic membrane components an intrinsic curvature deviator of anisotropic membrane components $D_m \simeq 0.2\,\mathrm{nm}^{-1}$ is needed to stabilize the neck. The corresponding values of the intrinsic principal curvatures $C_{1m} \approx 0$ and $C_{2m} < 0$ are very similar to the values of spontaneous curvatures of some lipid molecules previously determined by other authors (Chen and Rand, 1997; Churchward et al., 2008; Fang et al., 2008; Kooijman et al., 2005; Wang et al., 2007; Zimmerberg and Kozlov, 2006, and references therein), although a role for proteins in the fusion neck structure cannot be ruled out completely (reviewed in Fang et al., 2008; Jackson and Chapman, 2008). As already mentioned in the above theoretical analysis of the stability of a fusion neck (Fig. 11.2), the anisotropic membrane constituents could be single molecules (lipid or protein) or small membrane nanodomains composed of lipids or lipids and proteins. It should be stressed that besides the stable anisotropic geometry of the fusion neck, the stability of other strongly anisotropic lipid structures may be better understood by taking into account the anisotropic shape of lipid molecules, such as inverted hexagonal lipid phases (see Mareš et al., 2008; Rappolt et al., 2008, and Section 7.4) or thin tubular protrusions (Bobrowska et al., 2013) of giant lipid vesicles (Section 7.7).

The predicted local minimum of free energy for the narrow fusion necks (Fig. 11.2) suggests a neck diameter with a value corresponding to the local minimum of free energy. This cannot be predicted if the membrane constituents are described as isotropic, as no set of model parameters in the relevant range was found that would give a free energy minimum of appropriate depth and appropriate fusion neck diameter consistent with experiments. Considering isotropic inclusions with certain limitations leads to renormalization of the free energy within the accepted theory of isotropic membrane elasticity (area difference elasticity model), which considers the membrane as a thin layered isotropic elastic continuum (Seifert, 1997, and references therein). The stability of the narrow neck in phospholipid vesicles has previously been addressed by the area difference elasticity model (Miao et al., 1994; Seifert, 1997). A minimum of free energy corresponding to the narrow neck was obtained, but values of the model constants had to be assumed which are outside the range estimated by experiments (see discussions in Bobrowska et al., 2013; Iglič et al., 2007b; Kralj-Iglič et al., 2005).

Indeed, the phospholipid tails are subject to van der Waals interactions, which affect their packing in the layer. As this additionally lowers the local membrane free energy (Kralj-Iglič et al., 2006), formation of transient complexes of membrane constituents such as fusion necks is favoured. The curvature-dependent average orientation of anisotropic lipids or small anisotropic lipid complexes (nanodomains) is important for their energy (Fig. 7.2). However, taking into account the average orientational ordering of anisotropic lipid molecules does not assume their lattice-like packing with fixed molecular orientation at fixed position, but just the possibility with decrease in membrane free energy due to the average orientation and position of rotating and laterally mobile anisotropic lipid molecules.

To conclude, experimental results, along with the theoretical model (Jorgačevski et al., 2010), provide an interpretation for repetitive, transient fusion neck events with energetically stable narrow neck diameters. This represents an intermediate state in the sequence of reactions between the vesicle and the plasma membrane that take place after establishment of a hemifusion stalk and formation of a fusion neck (Fig. 11.4). The nature of the anisotropic constituents is not restricted to lipids, but may also include proteins. As the fusion neck stabilization mechanism is nonspecific and as there is no *a priori* reason for the membrane constituents to be in general isotropic (Bobrowska et al., 2013), it could be expected to take place in any cell type. Regulation of vesicle cargo discharge may therefore be attained by affecting the relationship between the vesicle size and the stable fusion neck diameter.

Chapter 12

Exogenous Membrane-Attached Nanoparticles

In this chapter, we discuss the influence of the intrinsic shape of membrane-attached nanoparticles on the elastic properties of bilayer membranes. The intrinsic shape of membrane-attached proteins is described within two different models. In the first, the membrane-attached proteins are considered as one-dimensional rod-like structures. In the second model the attached proteins are considered as small two-dimensional plates. The role of the hydrophobic protrusion of the attached nanoparticles which is embedded in the outer lipid layer is also discussed.

12.1 Rod-Like Attached Nanoparticles

In this section it is shown that a nonhomogeneous lateral distribution of membrane-attached and flexible rod-like proteins (FRPs) (Fig. 12.1) may stabilize nanotubular membrane protrusions. It is also shown that curvature-induced accumulation of FRPs in the nanotubular membrane protrusion and a corresponding decrease of the membrane free energy is possible if the decrease in deviatoric

---

Nanostructures in Biological Systems: Theory and Applications
Aleš Iglič, Veronika Kralj-Iglič, and Damjana Drobne
Copyright © 2015 Pan Stanford Publishing Pte. Ltd.
ISBN 978-981-4267-20-5 (Hardcover), 978-981-4303-43-9 (eBook)
www.panstanford.com

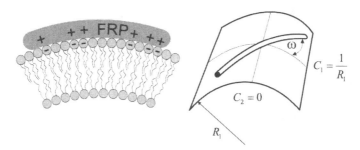

Figure 12.1 Schematic figure of a flexible rod-like protein (FRP) strongly attached to a cylindrical membrane surface having $C_1 = 1/R_1$ and $C_2 = 0$, that is, $H = D = 1/2R_1$. At a given value of the protein orientation angle ω, the protein senses the curvature $C = (C_1 + C_2)/2 + ((C_1 - C_2)/2)\cos(2\omega)$. Reprinted from *Journal of Biomechanics*, 43(8), Šarká Perutková, Veronika Kralj-Iglič, Mojka Frank, and Aleš Iglič, Membrane stability of membrane nanotubular protrusions influenced by attachment of flexible rod-like proteins, pp. 1612–1617, Copyright 2010, with permission from Elsevier.

free energy of FRPs in the nanotubular protrusions is large enough to overcome the increase in the free energy due to the decrease of configurational entropy in the process of lateral sorting of FRPs. The decrease in isotropic curvature energy of the FRPs in the region of the membrane protrusion is usually not enough for distinct protein sorting and consequent stabilization of the nanotubular protrusions of the biological (lipid bilayer) membranes.

The isotropic bending energy of lipids is not sufficient to stabilize the tubular membrane protrusion and may also not contribute significantly to the sorting of lipids between tubular membrane protrusions and the parent membrane due to the excessive decrease in configurational (mixing) entropy (Iglič et al., 2006; Tian and Baumgart, 2009) (see also Section 9.2). Very thin nanotubular protrusions of one component liposomes can be stabilized due to the average orientational ordering of lipids in nanotubes (Kralj-Iglič, 2002, and Section 7.7), while in more complex bilayer membrane systems the lipid–lipid and lipid–protein direct interactions may result in the formation of small membrane (in general anisotropic) nanodomains (clusters, inclusions) which can stabilize the tubular membrane protrusion and also significantly contribute to lipid sorting (Iglič et al., 2006; Kralj-Iglič et al., 2005; Sorre et al., 2009;

Tian and Baumgart, 2009) (see Chapter 9). The deformation of biological membranes can also be driven by proteins that are attached to the membrane surface (Iglič et al., 2007c; Powel, 2009; Tian and Baumgart, 2009). A number of proteins have been identified that directly bind to and deform biological membranes (Bouma et al., 1999; Farsad and De Camilli, 2003). The binding of proteins to the membrane surface, liposomes or lipoproteins may be driven by electrostatic forces and/or by penetration of the protein's hydrophobic protrusions into the membrane bilayer (Farsad and De Camilli, 2003; Masuda et al., 2006). The proteins attached to the membrane surface may thus influence the elastic properties of the membrane (Farsad and De Camilli, 2003; Iglič et al., 2007c; Zimmerberg and Kozlov, 2006).

Membrane-attached proteins can be more or less rigid than cellular or lipid bilayer membranes (Nossal, 2001). Some of the membrane-attached proteins may be considered to be flexible elongated curved rod-like proteins. In the limit of strong adhesion (Fig. 12.1), the elastic (curvature) energy of an FRP having similar rigidity as a membrane bilayer can be written in the form (Landau and Lifshitz, 1997):

$$E_1 = \frac{K_p L_0}{2}(C - C_p)^2, \qquad (12.1)$$

where K_p is the flexural rigidity (Iglič et al., 2007c), C_p the intrinsic (spontaneous) curvature and L_0 the length of the protein. The curvature

$$C = H + D\cos(2\omega), \qquad (12.2)$$

is the local membrane curvature seen by the FRP for a given rotation of the protein described by the angle ω between the normal plane in which the protein lies and the plane of the first principal curvature $C_1 = 1/R_1$ (Fig. 12.1), where $D = |C_1 - C_2|/2$ and $H = (C_1 + C_2)/2$ are the curvature deviator and the mean curvature, respectively. If the rigidity of the FRPs is of the same order of magnitude or not much larger than the rigidity of the membrane (see also Duwe et al., 1990; Meleard et al., 1997), the shape of the membrane is the result of interplay between the membrane and the membrane-attached proteins.

In order to take into account rotation of the FRPs (due to thermal motion), the free energy of a single FRP is calculated as:

$$f_i = -kT \ln Q, \qquad (12.3)$$

where different orientational states of the protein on the membrane surface are taken into account in the partition function Q:

$$Q = \frac{1}{\omega_0} \int_0^{2\pi} \exp\left(-\frac{E_1(\omega)}{kT}\right) d\omega = \frac{1}{\omega_0} \exp\left[-\frac{K_p L_0}{2kT}(H - C_p)^2\right] \cdot$$
$$\cdot \int_0^{2\pi} \exp\left[\frac{K_p L_0}{2kT}\left(2D(C_p - H)\cos 2\omega - D^2 \cos^2 2\omega\right)\right] d\omega, \qquad (12.4)$$

where ω_0 is an arbitrary angle quantum.

For nonzero flexural rigidity (K_p) the membrane-attached proteins have different energy on the spherical and on the tubular part of the cell membrane. For proteins which are attached to the spherical part of the cell with a constant mean curvature H and curvature deviator $D = 0$, the free energy of a single FRP is

$$f_{ps} = \frac{K_p L_0}{2}(H - C_p)^2, \qquad (12.5)$$

while for proteins attached to the tubular membrane protrusions where $H = D$, the free energy of a single FRP is (Perutková et al., 2010b)

$$f_{pt} = \frac{K_p L_0}{2}(H - C_p)^2 + \frac{K_p L_0}{4} D^2 - kT \ln\left[I_0\left(\frac{K_p L_0 D}{kT}(C_p - H)\right)\right], \qquad (12.6)$$

where I_0 is Bessel function.

The highest fraction of the protrusion area covered by FRPs corresponds to the lowest membrane free energy, also including the entropic contribution to the free energy (see Eq. 1.104) (Perutková et al., 2010b). This effect may account for stabilization of the tubular protrusions driven by accumulation of FRPs in the region of membrane tubular protrusions. It was shown (Perutková et al., 2010b) that proteins with $C_p = 1/8\,\text{nm}^{-1}$ (which corresponds to intrinsic curvature of some protein BAR domains (Peter et al., 2004)) have the highest effect on the lowering of the free energy. Moreover, for $C_p = 1/8\,\text{nm}^{-1}$ and $C_p = 1/10\,\text{nm}^{-1}$ and appropriate values of the radius of the tubular membrane protrusion (r), the area fraction occupied by FRPs on the tubular membrane protrusions may approach unity, that is, the proteins may occupy the whole tubular surface of the cell (vesicle) membrane (Perutková et al., 2010b).

It should be stressed at this point that neglecting the deviatoric term (the last term in Eq. 12.6) would considerably reduce the effect of FRPs on the stability of membrane protrusions (Perutková et al., 2010b). This indicates that the decrease of isotropic curvature energy of the FRPs (first term in Eq. 12.6) in the region of membrane protrusions for smaller C_p is not large enough for substantial protein sorting and consequent stabilization of the nanotubular membrane protrusions. In this case, with decrease in the deviatoric free energy of the attached proteins with nonzero spontaneous curvature may overcome the increase in the free energy due to decrease in the configurational entropy as a consequence of lateral sorting of FRPs and thus, stabilize the nanotubular membrane protrusion (Perutková et al., 2010b).

The deviatoric term in Eq. 12.6 originates from the expression for the elastic energy of the attached FRP given by Eqs. 12.1 and 12.2, taking into account that deformation of the protein attached to the anisotropic membrane surface (having $C_1 \neq C_2$) depends on its orientation angle ω (see Fig. 12.1). Neglecting the orientation-dependent elastic (free) energy of the single-attached FRP would omit the influence of temperature dependent rotational movement of the attached proteins from the given theoretical description. Moreover, even in the limit of infinite temperature, neglecting Eq. 12.2 and replacing the curvature C in Eq. 12.1 by the mean curvature $H = (C_1 + C_2)/2$ would lead to an incorrect expression for the elastic (free) energy of a single-attached FRP (see Eq. 12.6). Similarly, in the zero temperature limit such a simplified expression for the elastic (free) energy of a single attached FRP would not be correct for an arbitrary value of C_p.

A possible experimental example of the system described in the present work may be the membrane tethers of a giant unilamellar lipid vesicle (GUV) induced by an attached spherical bead which is moved apart from the membrane by optical tweezers. Accumulation of FRPs in the region of the GUV tubular protrusion (tether) could stabilize the tether so it may also be stable without or with only a very small external pulling force.

In cellular systems there are many examples of proteins whose attachment to the membrane surface has important physiological consequences, for instance FtsZ proteins in bacteria, which are short protofilaments constructing the Z ring incorporated in the inner layer of the cell membrane (Osawa et al., 2008). Such proteins were proposed to have an important role in the initiation of the contractile ring in cells (Shlomovitz and Gov, 2008). Other examples of membrane-attached proteins are apolipoprotein B-100 and β_2-glycoprotein I (β_2-GPI) (Gamsjaeger et al., 2005). β_2-GPI (also known as apolipoprotein H) and apolipoprotein B-100 have elongated shapes composed of distinct domains that are connected by links which allow them to change their orientation (Di Scipio, 1992; Hammel et al., 2002; Johs et al., 2006; Moore et al., 1989). The electrostatic character of the β_2-GPI attachment to the negatively charged membrane surface is attributed to the large positively charged regions of the molecule (Balasubramanian and Scroit, 1998; Bouma et al., 1999; Hamdan et al., 2007). Accordingly, it was shown that β_2-GPI strongly binds to the negatively charged outer membrane surface of apoptotic cells (Balasubramanian and Scroit, 1998). Atomic force microscopy has shown that the average height of β_2-GPI bound to supported lipid bilayers is approximately equal to the diameter of the elongated molecule. This means that bound β_2-GPI has a horizontal-like orientation on the bilayer surface (Gamsjaeger et al., 2005; Hamdan et al., 2007), as shown schematically in Fig. 12.1.

Recently, the effect of the attachment of β_2-GPI to the negatively charged membrane surface was tested experimentally in a suspension of negatively charged 1-palmitoyl-2-oleoyl-sn-glycero-3-phosphocholine (POPC)-cardiolipin-cholesterol GUVs (Fig. 12.2) prepared by a modified electroformation method (Angelova et al., 1992). It was previously indicated (Mathivet et al., 1996), but not observed, that GUVs prepared by the electroformation method are often connected by thin tubular membraneous structures. Later, it was also shown that GUV nanotubular protrusions are usually invisible under the optical microscope; however they could become visible if their diameter was sufficiently increased during

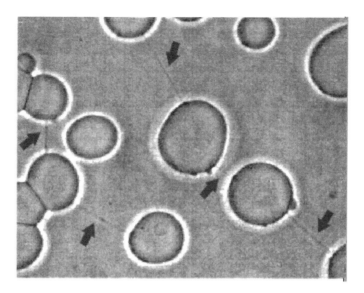

Figure 12.2 Network of thin nanotubular connections (indicated by black arrows) between negatively charged POPC-cholesterol-cardiolipin giant unilamellar vesicles (GUVs) in the presence of β_2-GPI (100 mg/L), serum IgG antibodies (75 mg/mL) and antibodies against β_2-GPI. Reprinted from *Journal of Biomechanics*, 43(8), Šarká Perutková, Veronika Kralj-Iglič, Mojka Frank, and Aleš Iglič, Membrane stability of membrane nanotubular protrusions influenced by attachment of flexible rod-like proteins, pp. 1612–1617, Copyright 2010, with permission from Elsevier.

the shape transformation of GUVs (Kralj-Iglič, 2002). Figure 12.2 shows how after addition of β_2-GPI to the suspension of GUVs (previously invisible) nanotubular connections between GUVs became visible. The effect is stronger if serum IgG (from a patient with antiphospholipid syndrome) containing antibodies against β_2-GPI (anti-β_2-GPI antibodies) are added along with β_2-GPI to the suspension of GUVs (Willems et al., 1996). These anti-β_2-GPI-IgG antibodies primarily target membrane-attached β_2-GPI, enhance β_2-GPI binding to negatively charged membranes and connect/dimerize two membrane attached β_2-GPI molecules. In accordance with theoretical predictions (Perutková et al., 2010b), it was suggested that β_2-GPI molecules accumulate on the nanotubular connections and make them visible because of the increased nanotube diameter. The enhancing effect seen after addition of IgG antibodies may be explained by the increased protein length (L_0) attained through dimerization of membrane-attached β_2-GPI by by anti-β_2-GPI IgG antibody (see also Eq. 12.6 for the role of L_0 in the single FRP free energy).

Membrane tubular protrusions can be stable after their detachment from the mother (spherical) cell (Kralj-Iglič et al., 2005) or can change to the necklace-like shape which corresponds to the maximal average mean curvature $\langle H \rangle = \frac{1}{A} \int H \, dA$ (see Section 9.4) of the detached vesicle at a given area of the membrane surface A and a given volume enclosed by the vesicle membrane V, as shown in Fig. 9.9. The initial tubular shape of the detached tubular membrane protrusion corresponds to the maximal possible average curvature deviator $\langle D \rangle = \frac{1}{A} \int D \, dA$ (see Section 9.4) and the minimal possible $\langle H \rangle$ at given A and V, as also shown in Fig. 9.9.

In the above example of protein attachment to the membrane surface the domains of the proteins are assumed to be rigid, while the flexibility of the protein is a consequence of the flexible links connecting the protein domains (units). In the limit of strong adhesion of the rigid attached proteins, the rigid domains may induce different local microscopic perturbations of the membrane shape around each of the attached rigid protein domains such as the flexible rod-like protein shown schematically in Fig. 12.1 which might increase the local bending energy around the attached protein. In addition, the nonlocal bending energy of the membrane bilayer (Evans and Skalak, 1980; Helfrich, 1974), which increases quadratically with the total number of membrane-attached FRPs, would also be increased (see also Eq. 8.18) (Iglič et al., 2007c). Consequently, the attached protein having rigid domains may induce stronger membrane rigidification than the flexible FRPs shown in Fig. 12.1.

In the case of binding (adhesion) of a positively charged FRP to a negatively charged membrane surface (Fig. 12.1), the nature of the attractive force is in large part electrostatic. To this end positively charged groups of the attached protein may induce lipid demixing (Gamsjaeger et al., 2005), that is, accumulation of negatively charged lipids (like phosphatidylserine) below the attached protein, which may in some cases facilitate protein clustering in order to reduce the line tension around the lipid domains of negatively charged proteins.

In the limit of high protein flexural rigidity K_p and strong adhesion, the membrane or part of the membrane should adapt its curvature to the spontaneous curvature of the attached proteins ($C_p > 0$). Consequently, the membrane principal curvatures C_1 and C_1 are constant in these membrane regions. The membrane surfaces with constant C_1 and C_1 can be membrane shapes composed of spheres of equal radii connected by infinitesimal necks (i.e., a string of pearls) or tubular shapes. The tubular shapes correspond to the minimal possible bending energy of the membrane within the given class of undulating shapes (Iglič et al., 1999). The nonzero principal curvature of a tubular membrane surface ($C_1 = 1/R_1$) with an attached FRP with spontaneous curvature C_p^0 is in general:

$$C_1 = C_p / \cos^2 \omega, \qquad (12.7)$$

where ω describes the rotation of the protein in the principal system of the membrane curvature tensor (see Fig. 12.1). The value $\omega = 0$ corresponds to the minimal possible value of C_1 (Fig. 12.3).

In the limit of small membrane curvatures and constant area density of the FRPs (n) we can express the contribution of attached

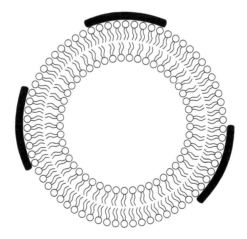

Figure 12.3 Schematic figure of the cross-section of a bilayer membrane tubular protrusion with attached FRPs having $C_p > 0$. The rotation angle $\omega = 0$.

FRPs to the total area density of the membrane local bending energy in terms of the renormalized constants k_c, k_G and $\bar{C}_0$ (see Eq. 7.68) (Iglič et al., 2007c) as:

$$\Delta k_c = \frac{3}{8} K_p L_0 n, \qquad (12.8)$$

$$\Delta k_G = -\frac{1}{4} K_p L_0 n, \qquad (12.9)$$

$$\Delta \bar{C}_0 = \frac{n K_p L_0 C_p}{2 k_c}. \qquad (12.10)$$

It can be seen in Eqs. 12.8 and 12.10 that within the adopted approximations the local bending constant of the membrane (k_c) increases with increasing area density of the attached rod-like proteins.

12.2 Plate-Like Attached Nanoparticles

Plate-like membrane-attached proteins (nanoparticles) can be treated as small two-dimensional thin semi-flexible plates with area a_0 (Iglič et al., 2007c). Here, it is assumed that the protein is in general anisotropic, therefore its intrinsic shape could be described by the two intrinsic principal curvatures C_{1m} and C_{2m} (Fig. 8.2) and by the orientation of the protein in the principal systems of the actual local membrane curvature tensor so that its energy can be expressed by Eq. 8.4. After rotational averaging of the free energy of the single plate-like membrane-attached protein, we can write the contributions of the membrane-attached proteins to the area density of membrane elastic energy $w_p = f_p n$ in the form (up to the constant terms):

$$w_p = (2 K_1 + K_2)(H - H_m)^2 n a_0 \qquad (12.11)$$
$$+ K_2 (D^2 + D_m^2) n a_0 - kT n \ln\left(I_0\left(\frac{2 K_2 D D_m a_0}{kT}\right)\right),$$

where we assumed that that lateral distribution of membrane-attached proteins is homogeneous, that is, the area density of the proteins (n) is constant. For $C_{1m} > 0$ and $C_{2m} = 0$, the attached protein-induced membrane tubulation, while for $C_{1m} > 0$ and $C_{2m} < 0$, a "saddle-like" membrane is the most favourable shape (Iglič et al., 2007c).

For small $x = 2 K_2 D D_m a_0 / kT$, the logarithm of the modified Bessel function in the last term in Eq. 12.12 can be approximated as $\ln I_0(x) \sim x^2/4$. The contribution of attached proteins to the total area density of membrane elastic energy can then be expressed in terms of the renormalized local bending constant k_c, the renormalized Gaussian saddle-splay constant k_G and the renormalized spontaneous curvature $\tilde{C}_0$ (see Eq. 7.68) as follows:

$$\Delta k_c = n (K_1 + K_2) a_0 - n D_m^2 K_2^2 a_0^2 / 2kT, \qquad (12.12)$$

$$\Delta k_G = n \left(D_m^2 K_2^2 a_0^2 / kT - K_2 a_0 \right), \qquad (12.13)$$

$$\Delta \tilde{C}_0 = H_m n (2 K_1 + K_2) a_0 / k_c, \qquad (12.14)$$

where the relation $D^2 = H^2 - C_1 C_2$ was taken into account.

Comparison of Eqs. 12.8 and 12.12 leads us to the conclusion that attachment of one-dimensional rod-like proteins to biological membranes always increases the local bending constant k_c, while the attachment of two-dimensional anisotropic (i.e., with $C_{1m} \neq C_{2m}$) proteins may reduce k_c. Also, the effect of protein attachment on the value of the Gaussian saddle-splay constant k_G could be of opposite sign in the two cases (compare Eqs. 12.9 and 12.13).

In the analysis of protein attachment to the membrane surface presented here, we did not take into account the role of the hydrophobic protrusion of the attached proteins (Bouma et al., 1999; Iglič et al., 2007c; Masuda et al., 2006) which is embedded in the outer membrane layer (Fig. 12.4). This may additionally increase the affinity of the attached proteins for highly curved membrane surfaces (Masuda et al., 2006) such as nanotubular membrane protrusions (Iglič et al., 2007c). The hydrophobic protrusion of the attached protein may also influence the elastic properties of the membrane. Typical examples of membrane-attached protein with hydrophobic protrusion(s) are banana shaped BAR domain proteins (Masuda et al., 2006) or the membrane-attached part of β_2-GPI proteins (Bouma et al., 1999).

A simple microscopic interaction model of a protein inclusion anchored in the outer lipid layer is described in Section 8.2.2

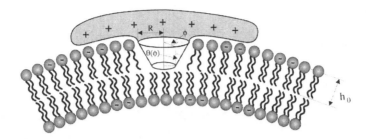

Figure 12.4 Schematic figure of a positively charged protein attached to the outer surface of a negatively charged bilayer membrane. The hydrophobic protrusion of the attached protein embedded in the outer lipid layer is also shown. The isotropic shape of the hydrophobic protrusion is characterized by a constant "cone angle" $\theta(\phi) = \bar{\theta}$ and the radius (R) at the lipid head group level. The equilibrium thickness of the monolayer is h_0.

(Fosnarič et al., 2005; Kralj-Iglič et al., 1999). The energy of the disturbed lipids surrounding the inclusion (Fig. 12.4) was estimated, where it was assumed that the protein protrusion is anchored within the lipid layer through hydrophobic interactions. In the model, the hydrocarbon core of the host lipid layer was allowed to adjust to the shape of the protein insertion (see also Fig. 12.4). The corresponding elastic lipid perturbation energy depends on the curvature of the membrane. The energy of the disturbed lipids around the isotropic protein insertion in the outer lipid layer can be approximately written in the form (see Eq. 8.22 and Fosnarič et al., 2005; Kralj-Iglič et al., 1999):

$$W_p = \mu_p + \frac{\xi}{2}(H - \bar{H}_m)^2 + \frac{\xi}{4} D^2. \qquad (12.15)$$

leading to the conclusion that Eq. 12.12 should be upgraded by an additional term (i.e., Eq. 12.15) in order to take into account the energy of the disturbed lipids due to protein insertion in the outer lipid layer.

In the most simple example, the shape of the isotropic hydrophobic protein insertion can be described by the "cone-angle" $\bar{\theta}$ and the radius R of the core of the hydrophobic protrusion at the level of the lipid head group (Fig. 12.4). The protein insertion is "cone-like" for $\bar{\theta} > 0$, cylindrical for $\bar{\theta} = 0$ and "inverted cone-like" for $\bar{\theta} < 0$. The interaction constant ξ and intrinsic curvature $\bar{H}_m$ can be expressed as (Fosnarič et al., 2005; Iglič et al., 2007c):

$$\bar{H}_m \cong \frac{\bar{\theta}}{R}\left(\frac{R+\lambda_d}{R+2\lambda_d}\right), \qquad (12.16)$$

$$\xi \cong \pi k_c R^2 \left(\frac{R}{\lambda_d}+2\right), \qquad (12.17)$$

where $\lambda_d \sim 1$ nm is the monolayer perturbation decay length. The contribution of the hydrophobic insertion of the attached proteins to the total area density of membrane elastic energy can be expressed in terms of renormalized local bending constants k_c and k_G and a renormalized spontaneous curvature C_0:

$$\Delta k_c = 3n\xi/8, \; \Delta k_G = -n\xi/4, \; \Delta C_0 = \bar{H}_m n\xi/2k_c. \qquad (12.18)$$

As can be seen from Eqs. 12.12, 12.14 and 12.18, the relative contribution of the intrinsic shape of the attached protein to the membrane elastic energy versus the corresponding contribution of its hydrophobic protrusion may vary substantially, depending on the values of the bending constants of the protein (K_1 and K_2), the intrinsic (spontaneous) curvatures of the protein (C_{1m} and C_{2m}), the shape of the hydrophobic protrusion (described by angle $\bar{\theta}$ and radius R) and the protein area a_0.

Chapter 13

Electric Double Layer Theory

13.1 Charged Biological Systems

Biopolymers, biological membranes, and other cellular components are electrically charged. Electrostatic interactions in biological systems are therefore of fundamental importance in understanding the interactions between charged molecules and membrane surfaces. Examples of electrically charged systems from biology include self-assembling dispersions such as spherical (inverse) micelles (Fig. 6.1), phospholipid vesicles (Fig. 6.6), and microemulsions (Israelachvili, 1997; Safran, 1994). Such objects are formed by aggregation of amphiphilic molecules in such a way that the hydrophilic parts of the molecules are in contact with electrolyte solutions. Microemulsions are formed in mixtures of amphiphiles, water, and oil, where domains of water (in oil) or oil (in water) are separated by surfactant monolayers.

In a biological medium (electrolyte solution), free (hydrated) ions are always present. The charges of ions and molecules are multiples of the elementary charge. Multivalent ions are commonly treated as point charges. However, real ions and particularly organic nanoparticles (such as, e.g., different proteins) often possess an internal electric charge distribution (Alvarez et al., 1983), with the

---

Nanostructures in Biological Systems: Theory and Applications
Aleš Iglič, Veronika Kralj-Iglič, and Damjana Drobne
Copyright © 2015 Pan Stanford Publishing Pte. Ltd.
ISBN 978-981-4267-20-5 (Hardcover), 978-981-4303-43-9 (eBook)
www.panstanford.com

individual charges being located at distinct, well-separated positions (Gongadze et al., 2013; May et al., 2008; Urbanija et al., 2008a,b).

The magnitude of the cell membrane charge, its spatial distribution and the spatial distribution of ions in the solution in close proximity to the inner and outer membrane surfaces determine the profile of electric potential across the biological membrane (see Heinrich et al., 1982; McLaughlin, 1989). The electrically charged molecular groups on both membrane surfaces protrude into the solution phase and therefore, the inner and outer membrane surface potentials are smaller in comparison to the situation where the charge would be distributed in the planes of both membrane surfaces (Heinrich et al., 1982; Iglič et al., 1997). Nevertheless, for the sake of simplicity the volume electric charge distribution of membrane surfaces is usually described by an effective surface charge characterized by the surface charge density σ.

The *electric double layer* (EDL) (McLaughlin, 1989) is composed of a charged surface and an electrolyte solution in contact with the charged surface. The distribution of the ions in the electrolyte solution close to the charged surface is given by competition between the electrostatic interactions and the entropy of the ions in the solution. Due to the electrostatic forces between the charged surface and the ions in solution, the counterions (ions with a charge of opposite sign to the charged surface) are accumulated close to the surface and the coions (ions with a charge of the same sign as the surface) are depleted from the surface, so that an EDL is created (Fig. 13.1). A diffuse EDL influences the overall electrostatic interaction of the charged surface with its environment, as well as the internal properties of the membrane carrying the surface charge.

The ELD has been the subject of extensive study since the pioneering work of Helmholtz, Gouy, and Chapman. Helmholtz (1879) treated the double layer mathematically as a capacitor, based on a physical model in which a layer of ions of opposite charge (counterions) with a single shell of hydration around each ion (the so-called Helmholtz layer) is adsorbed at the oppositely charged surface and neutralizes its charge. Later Gouy (1910) and Chapman (1913) also considered the thermal motion of ions and pictured a diffuse double layer composed of counterions attracted

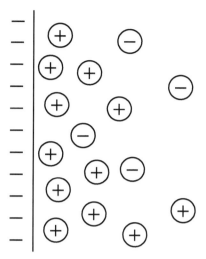

Figure 13.1 Schematic representation of a planar EDL composed of a negatively charged planar surface in contact with an electrolyte solution of positively charged counterions and negatively charged coions. The counterions accumulate near the charged surface.

to the surface and ions of the same charge (coions) repelled by it, embedded in a dielectric continuum of constant permittivity. Such a distribution of ions and the corresponding space dependence of the electric potential in the EDL can in the first approximation be theoretically described by Boltzmann distribution functions and the Poisson–Boltzmann (PB) equation (Bazant et al., 2009; Bivas and Ermakov, 2007; Chapman, 1913; Gongadze et al., 2013; Gouy, 1910; Kralj-Iglič et al., 1996; Lamperski and Outhwaite, 2002; Manciu and Ruckenstein, 2002; McLaughlin, 1989; Safran, 1994; Stern, 1924), expressing competition between the electrostatic interactions and the configurational entropy of ions in the solution. Ions within the mean-field Gouy–Chapman theory (Israelachvili, 1997; McLaughlin, 1989; Safran, 1994) are treated as dimensionless, while the electrolyte solution is accounted for by a uniform dielectric constant. The charged surfaces are considered to be uniformly charged (Heinrich et al., 1982; McLaughlin, 1989).

An improvement of the mean-field Gouy–Chapman theory can be obtained by including the direct ion–ion interactions and the finite size of ions. The fluctuation potential (Carnie et al., 1994) arising from the self-atmosphere of ions and the ion–ion exclusion volume term was taken into account in the modified PB equation (Bratko and Vlachy, 1982; Das et al., 1995, 1997; Outhwaite, 1986). Integral equation methods, such as the hypernetted chain (HNC) approximation, have also been carried out (Bacquet and Rossky, 1983, 1984; Gonzalez-Tovar et al., 1985; Lozado-Cassou and Henderson, 1983; Torrie and Valleau, 1982). A number of different attempts have been made to incorporate steric effects into the PB equation (Barbero et al., 2000; Bhuiyan and Outhwaite, 2009; Biesheuvel and van Soestbergen, 2007; Bikerman, 1942; Borukhov, 2004; Borukhov et al., 1997; Eigen and Wicke, 1954; Freise, 1952; Kralj-Iglič et al., 1996; Lamperski and Outhwaite, 2002; Lue et al., 1999; Manciu and Ruckenstein, 2002; Trizac and Raimbault, 1999). Monte Carlo simulations incorporate direct interactions between ions and interactions between ions and charged surfaces, as well as the finite size of ions (Bhuiyan et al., 1992; Bratko and Vlachy, 1982; Das et al., 1995, 1997; Hatlo and Lue, 2009; Ibarra-Armenta et al., 2009; Mills et al., 1985; Moreira and Netz, 2002; Tresset, 2008). With the Monte Carlo (MC) technique, it is possible to obtain numerically exact data and compare this data with the approximate theories. The advanced approaches (Bhuiyan et al., 1992) and the HNC integral equations (Bratko, 1990; Gonzalez-Tovar et al., 1985) lead to better agreement with MC simulations for divalent counterions.

The Gouy–Chapman theory and its PB equation as a mean-field level approach are widely used to estimate the interactions between charged surfaces in aqueous solution of counterions and coions. For a monovalent salt, its predictions are generally found to agree well with experimental results and computer simulations. However, the presence of multivalent ions can affect the nature of the interactions between charged surfaces in a way that qualitatively differs from the PB prediction. A remarkable example is the possibility of *attraction* between two identical, like-charged surfaces separated by an intermediate solution of point-like multivalent ions that the mean-field Gouy–Chapman approach is unable to predict. This attraction is currently attracting much interest (Gelbart et al., 2000) because it is observed in a number of biologically relevant processes such as condensation of DNA (Bloomfield, 1996), network formation in actin solutions (Angelini et al., 2003), virus aggregation (Butler et al., 2003) and the interactions between like-charged lipid membranes that occur during adhesion (Urbanija et al., 2007) and fusion. Various theoretical approaches ascribe this attraction to the presence of direct ion–ion correlations (Grosberg et al., 2002; Netz, 2001).

The MC simulations of Guldbrand et al. (1984) confirmed the existence of attraction between equally charged surfaces immersed in a solution composed of quadrupolar (divalent) ions in the limit of high surface charge density, which was originally predicted by Oosawa (1970). The anisotropic HNC approximation within the primitive electrolyte model for divalent ions was used (Kjellander, 1996; Kjellander and Marčelja, 1988), where the ions are described as charged hard spheres immersed in a dielectric continuum. Attractive interaction was predicted between identical like-charged surfaces in an aqueous solution composed of short divalent nanoparticles (Kim et al., 2008; May et al., 2008; Urbanija et al., 2008b).

In this chapter, we present a statistical mechanical approach to the functional density theory of the EDL using lattice statistics. First, in the mean field approximation the consistently related free energy, ion distribution function and differential equation for the electrostatic potential was obtained. We upgrade the description of the Gouy–Chapman theory by considering the effect of ion size (i.e., charged nanoparticles). The influence of ion size on the properties of the EDL is discussed. The effective thickness of the EDL is derived. Gouy–Chapman theory modified by orientational ordering of water and the excluded volume effect is also described.

13.2 Electrostatic Energy

The distribution of ions in the EDL reflects a balance between electrostatic interactions and entropy. First, we consider the electrostatic interactions. The *Poisson equation* expresses the general relation between the charge distribution and the electrostatic potential. It follows from Gauss law that

$$\nabla \cdot \mathbf{E} = \rho/\varepsilon_r \varepsilon_0, \tag{13.1}$$

in which we substitute the definition of the electrostatic potential $\mathbf{E} = -\nabla \phi$ (Jackson, 1999) (see also Section 1.1.1) so that

$$\nabla^2 \phi = -\frac{\rho}{\varepsilon_r \varepsilon_0}, \tag{13.2}$$

where ∇^2 is the Laplace operator, ∇ the nabla operator, $\mathbf{E}$ the electric field strength, ε_r the relative (dielectric) permittivity and ε_0 the permittivity of free space. From a given space charge distribution $\rho(x, y, z)$, the electrostatic potential $\phi(x, y, z)$ can be calculated provided the boundary conditions are satisfied at the geometrical boundaries.

The electrostatic energy of the system can be expressed as an integral of the square of the electric field strength over the system (Jackson, 1999):

$$F_{el} = \frac{1}{2} \int \varepsilon_r \varepsilon_0 \mathbf{E}^2 \, dV. \tag{13.3}$$

If the system possesses planar symmetry, then the electrostatic energy can be written as:

$$F_{el} = \frac{1}{2} \int \varepsilon_r \varepsilon_0 \left(\frac{d\phi}{dx}\right)^2 A \, dx, \tag{13.4}$$

where the electrostatic field varies only in the x-direction and A denotes the area of the charged surface.

13.3 Entropy

13.3.1 *Solution of Counterions*

We consider the entropy of a system composed of finite sized counterions (macro-ions) only. The lattice model (Hill, 1986) is used (see Fig. 13.2).

Following the classical, well-known approach (see Section 1.2.2.5), the system is divided into cells of equal volume ΔV. In any particular cell, there are N counterions. The excluded volume effect is taken into account in the description by considering that the counterions are distributed over M lattice sites and each lattice site cannot be occupied by more than one counterion. The number of spatial arrangements of N non-interacting counterions in a small cell with M lattice sites is

$$W = \frac{M(M-1)(M-2)\ldots(M-(N-1))}{N!}, \qquad (13.5)$$

which can be rewritten as

$$W = \frac{M!}{N!(M-N)!}. \qquad (13.6)$$

The configurational entropy of the cell S_{cell} can be computed by using the Boltzmann equation (see Section 1.2.2.5 and Hill, 1986)

$$S_{\text{cell}} = k \ln W, \qquad (13.7)$$

where k is the Boltzmann constant. Using Stirling's approximation for large N: $\ln N! \simeq N \ln N - N$, we get for $\ln W$:

$$\ln W = M \ln M - M - N \ln N + N - (M-N)\ln(M-N) + (M-N). \qquad (13.8)$$

Redistribution of the terms in Eq. 13.8 gives

$$\ln W = M \ln M - N \ln N - (M-N) \ln \left(M \left(1 - \frac{N}{M} \right) \right)$$

$$= M \ln M - N \ln N - (M-N) \ln M - (M-N) \ln \left(1 - \frac{N}{M} \right)$$

$$= -N \ln N + N \ln M - (M-N) \ln \left(1 - \frac{N}{M} \right). \qquad (13.9)$$

After summation of the first and the second terms in Eq. 13.9, we get:

$$\ln W = -N \ln \left(\frac{N}{M} \right) - (M-N) \ln \left(1 - \frac{N}{M} \right). \qquad (13.10)$$

By substituting Eq. 13.10 in Eq. 13.7, we get the expression for the entropy of a single cell:

$$S_{\text{cell}} = -k \left(N \ln \frac{N}{M} + (M-N) \ln \left(1 - \frac{N}{M} \right) \right). \qquad (13.11)$$

In the following we introduce the volume of one lattice site v_0. The volume of a cell with M lattice sites is then given by $\Delta V = M v_0$.

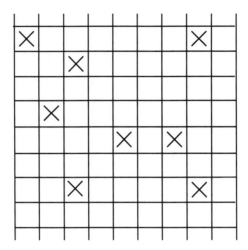

Figure 13.2 Schematic representation of the lattice model, where only counterions are included.

The entropy of the whole system can thus be obtained by integration of the entropy over all cells of the system:

$$S = \int S_{cell} \frac{dV}{\Delta V}, \qquad (13.12)$$

where S_{cell} is given by Eq. 13.11. We substitute Eq. 13.11 in Eq. 13.12 to get:

$$S = -k \int \left[n \ln(n v_0) + \frac{1}{v_0} (1 - n v_0) \ln(1 - n v_0) \right] dV, \qquad (13.13)$$

where the number density of counterions is defined by $n = N/\Delta V$ and $v_0 = \Delta V/M$. Equation 13.13 takes into account the finite size of the counterions (macro-ions). If we assume a very dilute system ($n v_0 \ll 1$ everywhere in the solution), the second term in Eq. 13.13 can be approximated by $\ln(1 - n v_0) \approx -n v_0$, where we neglected quadratic and higher order terms. In the limit of a very dilute system, the entropy (Eq. 13.13) thus becomes:

$$S = -k \int [n \ln(n v_0) - n] dV. \qquad (13.14)$$

The entropic contribution to the free energy $F_{ent} = -TS$ can therefore be expressed as (Safran, 1994)

$$F_{ent} = kT \int [n \ln(n v_0) - n] dV. \qquad (13.15)$$

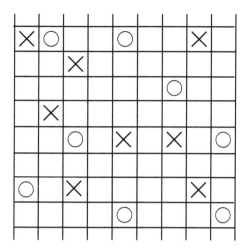

Figure 13.3 Schematic representation of the lattice model in which counterions (×) and coions (○) are included.

13.3.2 Solution of Counterions and Coions

We consider now the entropy of a solution composed of counterions and coions. The finite sizes of ions (macro-ions) are again considered within the lattice model (Fig. 13.3). The system is divided into cells of equal volume ΔV. In any particular cell chosen, there are N_+ counterions and N_- coions. The number of spatial arrangements of non-interacting counterions and coions in a small cell with M lattice sites is (Fig. 13.3):

$$W = \frac{M(M-1)(M-2)\ldots(M-(N-1))}{N_+! \, N_-!}, \quad (13.16)$$

which can be re-written as

$$W = \frac{M!}{N_+! \, N_-! \, (M-N)!}, \quad (13.17)$$

where

$$N = N_+ + N_-. \quad (13.18)$$

The translational (configurational) entropy of the mixed system of the single cell S_{cell} is then (see Section 1.2.2.5 and Hill, 1986):

$$S_{\text{cell}} = k \ln W. \quad (13.19)$$

Using Stirling's approximation for large N_i: $\ln N_i! \simeq N_i \ln N_i - N_i$, $i = \{+, -\}$, the expression for $\ln W$ transforms into:

$$\ln W = M \ln M - M - N_+ \ln N_+ + N_+ - N_- \ln N_- + N_-$$
$$- (M - N) \ln(M - N) + (M - N). \qquad (13.20)$$

Redistribution of terms in Eq. 13.20 gives

$$\ln W = -N_+ \ln\left(\frac{N_+}{M}\right) - N_- \ln\left(\frac{N_-}{M}\right) - (M - N) \ln\left(1 - \frac{N}{M}\right). \qquad (13.21)$$

To simplify the calculations, we assume that each lattice site with volume v_0 can be occupied by only one coion or counterion. The volume of the cell with M sites is given by $\Delta V = M v_0$. The number density of counterions is defined as

$$n_+ = \frac{N_+}{\Delta V}, \qquad (13.22)$$

while the number density of coions is

$$n_- = \frac{N_-}{\Delta V}. \qquad (13.23)$$

The configurational entropy of the whole system is obtained by integration over all cells of the system:

$$S = \int S_{\text{cell}} \frac{dV}{\Delta V}, \qquad (13.24)$$

where S_{cell} is given by equation (13.19). We susbstitute Eq. 13.21 into Eq. 13.19 to get from Eq. 13.24:

$$S = -k \int [n_+ \ln(n_+ v_0) + n_- \ln(n_- v_0)$$
$$+ \frac{1}{v_0} (1 - n_+ v_0 - n_- v_0) \ln(1 - n_+ v_0 - n_- v_0)] \, dV. \qquad (13.25)$$

Eq. 13.25 takes into account the finite size of the counterions.

The entropic part of the free energy $\tilde{F}_{\text{ent}} = -TS$, calculated from the Eq. 13.25, is therefore

$$\tilde{F}_{\text{ent}} = kT \int \left[\sum_{i=+,-} n_i \ln(n_i v_0) \right.$$
$$\left. + \frac{1}{v_0}\left(1 - \sum_{i=+,-} n_i v_0\right) \ln\left(1 - \sum_{i=+,-} n_i v_0\right) \right] dV. \qquad (13.26)$$

We need to subtract the reference free energy. The difference between the entropic part of the free energy $\tilde{F}_{\text{ent}}$ and the reference entropic part of the free energy F_{ref} is:

$$\tilde{F}_{\text{ent}} - F_{\text{ref}} = kT \int dV \left(\sum_{i=+,-} n_i \ln(n_i\, v_0) - 2n_0 \ln(n_0\, v_0) \right)$$

$$+ kT \int dV \frac{1}{v_0} \left(1 - \sum_{i=+,-} n_i v_0 \right) \ln \left(1 - \sum_{i=+,-} n_i v_0 \right)$$

$$- kT \int dV \frac{1}{v_0} (1 - 2n_0 v_0) \ln(1 - 2n_0 v_0). \qquad (13.27)$$

By taking into account the relation

$$\int dV \left[2n_0 - \sum_{i=+,-} n_i \right] = 0, \qquad (13.28)$$

we obtain

$$\tilde{F}_{\text{ent}} - F_{\text{ref}} = kT \int dV \Bigg\{ \sum_{i=+,-} n_i \ln(n_i\, v_0) - 2n_0 \ln(n_0\, v_0)$$

$$- \sum_{i=+,-} n_i \ln(n_0\, v_0) + 2n_0 \ln(n_0\, v_0)$$

$$+ \frac{1}{v_0} \left(1 - \sum_{i=+,-} n_i v_0 \right) \ln \left(1 - \sum_{i=+,-} n_i v_0 \right)$$

$$- \frac{1}{v_0} (1 - 2n_0 v_0) \ln(1 - 2n_0 v_0)$$

$$- \frac{1}{v_0} \left(1 - \sum_{i=+,-} n_i v_0 \right) \ln(1 - 2n_0 v_0)$$

$$+ \frac{1}{v_0} (1 - 2n_0 v_0) \ln(1 - 2n_0 v_0) \Bigg\}. \qquad (13.29)$$

By taking into account Eq. 13.29, $\ln(n_0\, v_0)$ = constant and $\ln(1 - 2n_0 v_0)$ = constant, we get the entropic part of the free energy in the form:

$$F_{\text{ent}} = \tilde{F}_{\text{ent}} - F_{\text{ref}} = +kT \int dV \sum_{i=+,-} n_i \ln\left(\frac{n_i}{n_0}\right)$$

$$+ kT \int dV \left(\frac{1}{v_0} - \sum_{i=+,-} n_i \right) \ln \left(\frac{\frac{1}{v_0} - \sum_{i=+,-} n_i}{\frac{1}{v_0} - 2n_0} \right). \qquad (13.30)$$

In our model, the number density of lattice sites is:

$$n_s = \frac{1}{v_0} = \frac{1}{a^3}, \qquad (13.31)$$

where a is the lattice constant. All lattice sites are occupied by either solvent molecules or macro-ions, therefore:

$$n_s = n_w + \sum_{j=+,-} n_j, \qquad (13.32)$$

where n_w is the number density of lattice sites occupied by solvent (water) molecules.

Different values of the lattice constant a may describe different effective sizes of macro-ions. In the following the number densities of counterions and coions are referred to as the respective concentrations. By taking into account Eq. 13.32, we may re-write Eq. 13.30 in the form:

$$F_{ent} = kT \int dV \sum_{i=+,-} n_i \ln\left(\frac{n_i}{n_0}\right)$$

$$+ kT \int dV \left(n_s - \sum_{i=+,-} n_i\right) \ln\left(\frac{n_s - \sum_{i=+,-} n_i}{n_s - 2n_0}\right). \qquad (13.33)$$

If we assume that $n_+ \ll 1, n_- \ll 1$ everywhere in the solution, as well as $n_0 \ll 1$, we can expand the third term in Eq. 13.33 up to quadratic terms to get (see, e.g., Gongadze, 2011; Kralj-Iglič et al., 1996):

$$F_{ent} = kT \int \left[n_+ \ln\left(\frac{n_+}{n_0}\right) + n_- \ln\left(\frac{n_-}{n_0}\right) - (n_+ + n_-) + 2n_0\right] dV. \qquad (13.34)$$

The expression Eq. 13.34 describes the configurational entropy of an electrolyte solution where the excluded volume is not taken into account.

13.4 Functional Density Theory of Electric Double Layer for Constant Dielectric Permittivity

Within standard Gouy–Chapman theory (Cevc, 1990), the finite size of ions is not taken into account (except by the Stern distance of closest approach), therefore the number density of counterions at the charged surface may exceed the upper value corresponding to their close packing. Different attempts have been made to incorporate steric effects into the modified PB equation in order to prevent the prediction of unrealistically high number densities of counterions close to the charged surface.

The first attempt to include the finite size of ions into Gouy–Chapman theory was made by Stern (Stern, 1924) who combined the Helmholtz (Helmholtz, 1879) and the Gouy–Chapman model (Chapman, 1913; Gouy, 1910). In its simplest version, the Stern model considers only the finite size of counterions whose centres can approach the charged surface only up to a certain distance, the so-called outer Helmholtz plane (Butt et al., 2003; Gongadze et al., 2011b, 2013).

Later, Bikerman (1942) derived a modified PB equation (the Bikerman equation) to account for the finite size of ions and solvent molecules. The Bikerman-modified PB equation and the corresponding Fermi–Dirac-like distribution of ions was later derived and justified using other different methods (Dutta and Sengupta, 1954; Eigen and Wicke, 1954; Freise, 1952; Grimley, 1950; Grimley and Mott, 1947; Kralj-Iglič et al., 1996; Lamperski and Outhwaite, 2002; Wiegel and Strating, 1993). Among these, Freise (1952) introduced the finite size of ions by a pressure-dependent potential, while Eigen and Wicke (1954) used a thermodynamic approach. More recently, Bikerman's predictions have been reformulated within the PB theory based on a lattice statistics model and density functional variation (Kralj-Iglič et al., 1996). The finite size of ions has also been described by other density functional approaches (Barbero et al., 2000; Trizac and Raimbault, 1999) and by considering the ions and solvent molecules as hard spheres (Biesheuvel and van Soestbergen, 2007; Lamperski and Outhwaite, 2002). Also, MC simulations are widely used to describe the finite-sized counterions (Biesheuvel and van Soestbergen, 2007; Ibarra-Armenta et al., 2009; Tresset, 2008; Zelko et al., 2010).

In the following section, we describe a model of the EDL in which the charged surface is assumed to carry a uniformly distributed charge with surface charge density σ. The solution in general is composed of solvent molecules and ions. The ions may be counterions or coions. Electrostatic interactions are described within the mean field approximation, while the finite size of the ions in solution is considered by means of the excluded volume effect. The latter is taken into account within the statistical mechanical description described in the previous section, where each ion in solution occupies one and only one site of a finite volume (Kralj-Iglič et al., 1996).

13.4.1 Solution of Counterions Only

13.4.1.1 Single double layer

We first consider a system composed of a charged surface and a solution of counterions only. The physical properties of the solvent (water) molecules are accounted for by a uniform relative (dielectric) constant $\varepsilon_r \sim 80$ and by the excluded volume principle. The electrostatic free energy of the system can be written as the sum of the electrostatic energy (Eq. 13.4) and the entropic contribution to the free energy (Eq. 13.13):

$$F = \frac{1}{2} \varepsilon \varepsilon_0 \int_0^\infty E^2(x)\,dx + kT \int_0^\infty \left[n(x) \ln(n(x) v_0) \right.$$
$$\left. + \frac{1}{v_0} (1 - n(x) v_0) \ln (1 - n(x) v_0) \right] dx, \quad (13.35)$$

where $E(x)$ is the electric field strength, $n(x)$ is the counterion concentration and x denotes the distance from the charged plane.

The free energy of the whole system, subject to local thermodynamic equilibrium, is

$$F = \int_0^\infty f(E(x), n(x))\,dx, \quad (13.36)$$

where the density of the free energy is given by

$$f(E(x), n(x)) = \frac{1}{2} \varepsilon_r \varepsilon_0 E^2(x) + kT \left[n(x) \ln(n(x) v_0) \right.$$
$$\left. + \frac{1}{v_0} (1 - n(x) v_0) \ln (1 - n(x) v_0) \right]. \quad (13.37)$$

The counterion number density $n(x)$ and the electric field strength are not known in advance. Thus, in the following, explicit expressions for $n(x)$ and $E(x)$ are obtained using the condition that

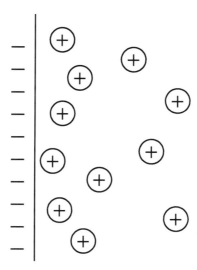

Figure 13.4 Schematic representation of a negatively charged planar surface in contact with a solution of positively charged counterions. The counterions are accumulated near the charged surface.

the free energy is at its minimum at thermodynamic equilibrium of the whole system. The condition for global equilibrium

$$\delta F = 0, \tag{13.38}$$

is subject to (Kralj-Iglič et al., 1996):

- the global constraint requiring the electro-neutrality of the whole system,

$$\int_0^\infty n(x)\,dx - \frac{\sigma A}{Z\,e_0} = 0, \tag{13.39}$$

- the local constraint requiring the validity of the differential form of Gauss's law $\varepsilon_r \varepsilon_0 \nabla \cdot \mathbf{E} = \rho(x)$, where $\rho(x) = e_0\,v\,Z\,n(r)$ is the volume charge density and

$$\varepsilon\,\varepsilon_0 \frac{\partial E(x)}{\partial x} - e_0\,Z\,n(x) = 0, \tag{13.40}$$

where Z is the valency of counterions. The method of undetermined multipliers (Bohinc et al., 2005; Elsgolc, 1961; Kralj-Iglič et al., 1996) is used to determine the extreme of the free energy (Eq. 13.36) taking into account the constraints 13.39 and 13.40. The variational problem can be expressed by the Euler–Lagrange equations

$$\frac{\partial L^*}{\partial E} - \frac{d}{dx}\left(\frac{\partial L^*}{\partial \left(\frac{\partial E}{\partial x}\right)}\right) = 0, \qquad (13.41)$$

$$\frac{\partial L^*}{\partial n} = 0, \qquad (13.42)$$

where

$$L^*\left(E(x), n(x), \frac{\partial E(x)}{\partial x}, \eta(x)\right)$$
$$= \left[f(E(x), n(x)) + \mu n(x) - \eta(x)\left(\varepsilon_r \varepsilon_0 \frac{\partial(E(x))}{\partial x} - e_0 Z n(x)\right)\right], \qquad (13.43)$$

where μ is the global Lagrange multiplier, while $\eta(x)$ is the local Lagrange multiplier. The local Lagrange multiplier $\eta(x)$ can be expressed from the Euler–Lagrange equation (see Eq. 13.41):

$$\eta(x) = \phi(x), \qquad (13.44)$$

where we took into account that $\mathbf{E} = -\nabla \phi$, while it follows from the Euler–Lagrange equation (Eq. 13.42) that

$$kT\,[\ln(n\,v_0) - \ln(1 - n\,v_0)] + \mu + e_0 Z\,\eta(x) = 0. \qquad (13.45)$$

From Eqs. 13.44 and 13.45, the Fermi–Dirac-like counterion distribution function is obtained:

$$n(r) = \frac{1}{v_0}\frac{1}{1 + e^{(\mu + e_0 Z\,\phi(x))/kT}}, \qquad (13.46)$$

where the Lagrange multiplier μ can be determined from the condition of electro-neutrality (Eq. 13.39). Gauss's law (Eq. 13.40) and the counterion distribution functions (Eq. 13.46) give the differential equation for the electrostatic potential $\phi(r)$:

$$\frac{d^2 \phi(x)}{dx^2} = -\frac{e_0 Z}{\varepsilon_r \varepsilon_0 v_0}\frac{1}{1 + e^{(\mu + e_0 Z\,\phi(x))/kT}}. \qquad (13.47)$$

In the following, the Lagrange multiplier μ is expressed from Eq. 13.46 as a function of the concentration of counterions for $\Phi = 0$ (n_0):

$$e^{\mu/kT} = \frac{1}{(n_0/n_s)} - 1, \qquad (13.48)$$

where the number density of lattice sites is $n_s = 1/v_0$ (Eq. 13.31). In the limit of a very dilute system ($n_0/n_s \ll 1$ everywhere in the system) Eq. 13.48 becomes:

$$e^{\mu/kT} \simeq \frac{1}{(n_0/n_s)}. \tag{13.49}$$

Taking into account the above approximate expression (Eq. 13.49), we can transform the distribution function (Eq. 13.46) into the form of the Boltzmann distribution function:

$$n(x) = \frac{n_s}{1 + \frac{n_s}{n_0} e^{e_0 Z \phi(x)/kT}} \simeq n_0 e^{-e_0 Z \phi(x)/kT}. \tag{13.50}$$

Accordingly, the differential Eq. 13.47 transforms into the PB equation:

$$\frac{d^2\phi(x)}{dx^2} = -\frac{e_0 Z}{\varepsilon_r \varepsilon_0} n_0 e^{-Z e_0 \phi(x)/kT}. \tag{13.51}$$

It should be stressed at this point that for higher values of the surface charge density (σ) the derived distribution function (Eq. 13.46) predicts saturation of the counterion density close to the charged surface to its close packing value. On the other hand, the usual Boltzmann distribution function (Eq. 13.50) may predict unreasonably high values beyond the close-packing value.

The condition of electro-neutrality of the whole system (Eq. 13.39) is equivalent to two boundary conditions. The first boundary condition states that the electric field is zero far from the charged surface:

$$\left.\frac{d\phi(x)}{dx}\right|_{x\to\infty} = 0, \tag{13.52}$$

while the second boundary condition (at the interface) is:

$$\left.\frac{d\phi(x)}{dx}\right|_{x=0} = \frac{-\sigma}{\varepsilon_r \varepsilon_0}. \tag{13.53}$$

13.4.2 Solution of Counterions and Coions: The Bikerman Equation

The electrostatic free energy of a system (per unit area) composed of counterions and coions is derived from Eqs. 13.4 and 13.33 (Bohinc et al., 2005; Kralj-Iglič et al., 1996):

$$F = \frac{1}{2}\varepsilon\varepsilon_0 \int_0^\infty E^2(x)\,dx$$
$$+ kT \sum_{j=+,-} \int_0^\infty n_j(x) \ln\left(\frac{n_j(x)}{n_0}\right) dx$$
$$+ kT \int_0^\infty \left(n_s - \sum_{j=+,-} n_j(x)\right) \ln\left(\frac{n_s - \sum_{j=+,-} n_j(x)}{n_s - 2n_0}\right) dx, \tag{13.54}$$

where n_+ is the concentration of counterions, n_- the concentration of coions, n_0 the bulk concentration of counterions and coions and n_s is defined by Eqs. 13.31 and 13.32.

The free energy of the whole system, subject to local thermodynamic equilibrium, is

$$F = \int_0^\infty f(E(x), n_+(x), n_-(x))\,dx, \tag{13.55}$$

where the density of the free energy is given by

$$f(E(x), n_+(x), n_-(x)) = \frac{1}{2}\varepsilon_r\varepsilon_0 E^2(x) + kT \sum_{j=+,-} n_j(x) \ln\left(\frac{n_j(x)}{n_0}\right)$$
$$+ kT \left(n_s - \sum_{j=+,-} n_j(x)\right) \ln\left(\frac{n_s - \sum_{j=+,-} n_j(x)}{n_s - 2n_0}\right).$$

The particle distribution functions $n_+(x)$ and $n_-(x)$ and the electric field strength $E(x)$ are obtained from the condition that the free energy be at its minimum at thermodynamic equilibrium of the whole system. The condition for global equilibrium:

$$\delta F = 0, \tag{13.56}$$

is subject to (Kralj-Iglič et al., 1996):

- the global constraint requiring that the total number of particles of each species per volume of the whole system, Λ_j, is constant

$$\int_0^\infty (n_j(x) - \Lambda_j)\,dx = 0; \quad j = +, -; \quad \text{and} \tag{13.57}$$

- the local constraint requiring the validity of the differential form of Gauss's law $\varepsilon_r \varepsilon_0 \nabla \cdot \mathbf{E} = \rho(x)$, where $\rho(x) = e_0 \sum_{j=+,-} Z_j n_j(x)$ is the volume charge density:

$$\varepsilon_r \varepsilon_0 \frac{\partial E(x)}{\partial x} - e_0 \sum_{j=+,-} Z_j n_j(x) = 0, \qquad (13.58)$$

where Z_j is the valency of the counterions ($j = +$) and coions ($j = -$). The method of undetermined multipliers (Bohinc et al., 2005; Elsgolc, 1961; Kralj-Iglič et al., 1996) is used to find the extrema of the free energy (see Eq. 13.55) taking into account the constraints 13.57 and 13.58. This described variational problem can be expressed by the Euler–Lagrange equations:

$$\frac{\partial L^*}{\partial E} - \frac{d}{dx}\left(\frac{\partial L^*}{\partial \left(\frac{\partial E}{\partial x}\right)} \right) = 0, \qquad (13.59)$$

$$\frac{\partial L^*}{\partial n_j} = 0, \quad j = +, -, \qquad (13.60)$$

where

$$L^*\left(E(x), n_+(x), n_-(x), \frac{\partial E(x)}{\partial x}, \eta(x) \right) = f(E(x), n_+(x), n_-(x)) \\ + \sum_{j=+,-} \lambda_j (n_j(x) - \Lambda_j) - \eta(x)\left(\varepsilon_r \varepsilon_0 \frac{\partial E(x)}{\partial x} - e_0 \sum_{j=+,-} Z_j n_j(x) \right),$$

$$(13.61)$$

λ_j, and $j = +, -$ are the global Lagrange multipliers, while $\eta(x)$ is the local Lagrange multiplier. Eqs. 13.59, 13.60 and 13.61 give

$$\eta(x) = \phi(x), \qquad (13.62)$$

$$kT \ln \frac{n_j n_{0w}}{n_0 (n_s - \sum_i n_i)} + \lambda_j + e_0 Z_j \phi(x) = 0. \qquad (13.63)$$

From Eqs. 13.62, 13.63 and 13.32, the Bikerman particle distribution functions are obtained (Bikerman, 1942; Dutta and Sengupta, 1954; Eigen and Wicke, 1954; Freise, 1952; Grimley, 1950; Grimley and Mott, 1947; Iglič and Kralj-Iglič, 1994; Kralj-Iglič et al., 1996; Wiegel and Strating, 1993):

$$n_j(r) = \frac{n_s (n_0/n_{0w}) \exp(-Z_j e_0 \phi(x)/kT)}{1 + \frac{2n_0}{n_{0w}} \cosh(Z_j e_0 \phi(x)/kT)}, \quad j = +, -, \qquad (13.64)$$

where n_{0w} is the bulk number density of lattice sites occupied by water molecules (see Eq. 13.32):

$$n_{0w} = n_s - 2n_0. \tag{13.65}$$

It can be seen from Eq. 13.64 that close to the charged plane, there may be a considerable excluded volume effect on the density profile of the counterions and on the solvent molecules. The concentration of counterions there is comparable to the concentration of solvent lattice sites, so that the concentration of the latter deviates significantly from its value far from the charged surface (Kralj-Iglič et al., 1996). Equation 13.64 also predicts a Fermi–Dirac-like distribution for counterions if the lattice constant a is large enough (see also Fig. 13.5). For higher values of surface charge density ($|\sigma|$), the counterion density saturates close to the charged surface at its close packing value, while the usual Gouy–Chapman theory predicts unreasonable high values beyond the close-packing value (Bikerman, 1942; Borukhov et al., 1997; Kralj-Iglič et al., 1996).

Gauss's law (Eq. 13.58) and the particle distribution functions (Eq. 13.64) give the Bikerman equation for the electrostatic potential $\phi(r)$ (Bikerman, 1942; Dutta and Sengupta, 1954; Eigen and Wicke, 1954; Freise, 1952; Grimley, 1950; Grimley and Mott, 1947; Kralj-Iglič et al., 1996; Wiegel and Strating, 1993):

$$\frac{d^2\phi(x)}{dx^2} = \frac{2 e_0 n_s n_0 Z}{\varepsilon_r \varepsilon_0 n_{0w}} \frac{\sinh(Z e_0 \phi(x)/kT)}{1 + \frac{2n_0}{n_{0w}} \cosh(Z e_0 \phi(x)/kT)}, \tag{13.66}$$

where $Z = |Z_+| = |Z_-|$. The first boundary condition states that the electric field is zero far away from the charged surface:

$$\left.\frac{d\phi(x)}{dx}\right|_{x \to \infty} = 0. \tag{13.67}$$

The second boundary condition at the charged surface requires the electro-neutrality of the whole system:

$$\left.\frac{d\phi(x)}{dx}\right|_{x=0} = -\frac{\sigma}{\varepsilon_r \varepsilon_0}. \tag{13.68}$$

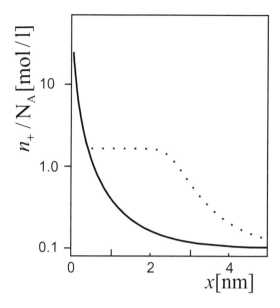

Figure 13.5 The number density of counterions as a function of distance (x) from the planar charged surface. The dashed curve presents results for finite sized ions (Bikerman model) using the lattice constant $a = 1$ nm, while the full line presents results for dimensionless ions within the Gouy–Chapman model. The model parameters are $\varepsilon_r = 78.5$, $T = 310$ K, $n_0/N_A = 0.1$ mol/l and $\sigma = -0.4$ A s/m² (Bohinc et al., 2001), where N_A is the Avogadro number.

13.5 Gouy–Chapman Model: Poisson–Boltzmann Equation

In the limit of a very dilute solution everywhere in the system:

$$\sum_{j=+,\,-} n_j(x) \ll n_w(x)$$

and by taking into account the approximation

$$n_{0w} \simeq n_s,$$

where $n_w(x)$ is the number density of lattice sites occupied by water (solvent) molecules, the second term in the denominator of Eq. 13.66 can be neglected, so that it becomes (Chapman, 1913;

Gouy, 1910; McLaughlin, 1989; Verwey and Overbeek, 1948):

$$\frac{d^2 \Psi(x)}{dx^2} = \frac{\kappa^2}{Z} \sinh(Z\,\Psi(x)), \qquad (13.69)$$

which is the well-known PB equation within the Gouy–Chapman model valid in the limit of dimensionless ions. We introduced the reduced electrostatic potential:

$$\Psi = e_0\,\phi/kT \qquad (13.70)$$

and the Debye length

$$l_D = \kappa^{-1} = \sqrt{\frac{\varepsilon_r\,\varepsilon_0\,kT}{2\,n_0\,Z^2\,e_0^2}}. \qquad (13.71)$$

Neglecting the second term in the denominator of Eq. 13.64, the particle distribution function (Eq. 13.64) transforms into the Boltzmann distribution function:

$$n_j(x) = n_0\,\exp(-Z_j\,\Psi(x)),\ j = +, -. \qquad (13.72)$$

For higher values of the surface charge density ($|\sigma|$) and close to the charged surface, the Boltzmann distribution function (Eq. 13.72) predicts unreasonably high values of the counterion number density, far beyond the corresponding close-packing value (Bikerman, 1942; Kralj-Iglič et al., 1996). For an illustration, Fig. 13.5 shows the number density n_+ as a function of the distance x from the planar charged surface. The results of the Gouy–Chapman model and the results of the functional density theory modified by the excluded volume effect (Bikerman model) with the lattice constant $a = 1$ nm are presented. Saturation of the counterions near the charged surface (i.e., a Fermi–Dirac-like shape of distribution) for ions of finite size is obtained in the Bikerman model. The effect is more pronounced for larger ions, that is, larger a.

The calculated ratio between the number density of counterions near the charged plane and the bulk counterion number density as a function of the surface charge density σ is presented in Fig. 13.6. This ratio is higher for dimensionless ions within the Gouy–Chapman model than for ions of finite size within the Bikerman model. The discrepancy between the results for dimensionless ions (Gouy–Chapman model) and for ions of finite size (Bikerman model) grows with increasing $|\sigma|$. This deviation can be attributed to the

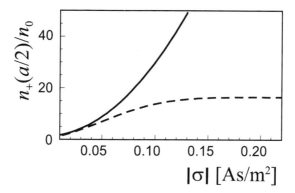

Figure 13.6 Ratio between the number density of monovalent counterions near the charged plane and the bulk counterion number density as a function of $|\sigma|$. The dashed curve represents calculation for the lattice constant, $a = 0.8$ nm. The result of the Gouy–Chapman model (for dimensionless ions) is given by the full line. The model parameters are $\varepsilon_r = 78.5$, $T = 310$ K.

steric effect of counterions and solvent molecules in the small region in the vicinity of the charged surface. The counterion number density profile shows a rapid decrease for small lattice constant and a plateau region near the charged plane for large lattice constant. For large counterions, we can therefore distinguish between two regions within the EDL: the saturated layer dominated by steric repulsion and the diffuse layer extending into the solution.

In the following we shall consider the linear regime of the PB equation for monovalent ions ($Z_+ = 1$, $Z_- = -1$), that is, we assume that the electrostatic potential energy of an ion is much smaller than its thermal energy ($\Psi \ll 1$). We linearize $\sinh(Z\Psi(x))$ in Eq. 13.69 to get the linearized PB equation:

$$\frac{d^2 \Psi(x)}{dx^2} = \kappa^2 \, \Psi(x). \tag{13.73}$$

Taking into account the boundary conditions in Eqs. 13.67 and 13.68, the solution of Eq. 13.73 is (Chapman, 1913; Gouy, 1910; Verwey and Overbeek, 1948):

$$\Psi(x) = \Psi_0 \, e^{-\kappa x}, \tag{13.74}$$

where

$$\Psi_0 = \frac{\sigma\, e_0}{\varepsilon_r\, \varepsilon_0\, \kappa\, kT} = 4\pi\, \sigma\, l_B\, l_D/e_0, \qquad (13.75)$$

is the reduced electrostatic potential near the charge surface and

$$l_B = \frac{e_0^2}{4\pi\, \varepsilon_r\, \varepsilon_0\, kT} \qquad (13.76)$$

is the Bjerrum length. Note that the electrostatic potential is proportional to the surface charge density. The electrostatic potential decreases exponentially with increase in the distance from the charged surface. The thickness of the EDL is described by the Debye length $l_D = 1/\kappa$ (see Eq. 13.71).

13.6 Langevin Poisson-Boltzmann Model

The classical Gouy–Chapman and Bikerman theories described in the previous section do not consider the solvent structure and thus, can be upgraded by hydration models, where the interplay between solvent polarization and the diffuse double layer is considered (Berkowitz et al., 2006; Gongadze, 2011; Gongadze et al., 2013; Gruen and Marčelja, 1983; Iglič et al., 2010; Manciu and Ruckenstein, 2004). Study of the orientational ordering of water dipoles at the charged surface has shown that they are on average oriented orthogonally to the charged surface (Gongadze et al., 2013; Iglič et al., 2010). Recently, Langevin dipoles were introduced into the mean-field EDL theory to study polarization of the solvent and the space dependence of the relative permittivity close to the charged membrane surface (Gongadze et al., 2010, 2011c; Velikonja et al., 2013). Spatial decay of solvent polarization with increasing distance from the charged membrane surface was predicted (Gongadze et al., 2011a,c, 2013). Most of the EDL models, for example, the Gouy–Chapman and Bikerman models, (Butt et al., 2003; Israelachvili and Wennerström, 1996; Lamperski and Outhwaite, 2002; McLaughlin, 1989; Stern, 1924) assume a constant dielectric permittivity ε_r throughout the system. But actually, close to the charged surface, the water dipoles are oriented thus, leading to a varying dielectric permittivity (Butt et al., 2003; Gongadze et al., 2013).

Therefore, in this section, first the Langevin PB mean-field model (Gongadze, 2011; Gongadze et al., 2011c, 2013) for point-like ions is derived within the functional density theory, where the orientational ordering of water molecules is taken into account. In the Langevin Poisson–Boltzmann (LPB) model described in this section, the dielectric permittivity is consistently related to the distribution of the ions involved and the electric field strength. The water molecules are considered as Langevin dipoles (Iglič et al., 2010; Outhwaite, 1976, 1983), which is a very approximate treatment of the dielectric properties of the solvent. The finite volume of ions and water molecules (Iglič et al., 2010; Lamperski and Outhwaite, 2002), that is, the excluded volume effect) is not taken into account. The volume density of water is, therefore assumed constant in the whole electrolyte solution (Gongadze et al., 2011c; Kralj-Iglič et al., 1996; Velikonja et al., 2013). The electrostatic interactions are described within the mean field approximation.

We consider a planar-charged surface in contact with a water solution of monovalent ions (counterions and coions) (Gongadze et al., 2010, 2011c, 2013). The planar charged surface bears a charge with a surface charge density σ. The Langevin dipole describes the water molecule with a non-zero dipole moment (**p**). A self-consistent statistical mechanical description of the orientational ordering of water Langevin dipoles is introduced (Gongadze et al., 2013). Using the calculus of variation, the ion number density profiles and average orientation of water dipoles corresponding to the minimum free energy are calculated (Gongadze et al., 2013). The free energy of system F is written as:

$$\frac{F}{kT} = \frac{1}{8\pi l_B} \int \left(\Psi'\right)^2 dV$$
$$+ \int \left[n_+(x) \ln \frac{n_+(x)}{n_0} - (n_+(x) - n_0) \right.$$
$$+ n_-(x) \ln \frac{n_-(x)}{n_0} - (n_-(x) - n_0) \right] dV$$
$$+ \int n_w \left\langle \mathcal{P}(x,\omega) \ln \mathcal{P}(x,\omega) \right\rangle_\omega dV$$
$$+ \int \left[\eta(x) \left(\left\langle \mathcal{P}(x,\omega) \right\rangle_\omega - 1 \right) \right] dV, \quad (13.77)$$

where averaging over all angles Ω is defined as:

$$\langle F(x) \rangle_\omega = \frac{1}{4\pi} \int F(x, \omega) d\Omega, \quad (13.78)$$

ω is the angle between the dipole moment vector **p** and the vector $\mathbf{n} = \nabla \Phi / |\nabla \Phi|$, $d\Omega = 2\pi \sin\omega \, d\omega$ is an element of a solid angle, n_w is the constant number density of the water Langevin dipoles, $n_+(x)$ and $n_-(x)$ are the number densities of counterions and coions, respectively, $\Psi(x) = e_0 \phi(x)/kT$ is the reduced electrostatic potential, $\phi(x)$ is the electrostatic potential, Ψ' is the first derivative of Ψ with respect to x, e_0 is the elementary charge, kT is the thermal energy, $dV = A \, dx$ is the volume element with thickness dx, A is the area of the charged surface and l_B is the Bjerrum length. The first term in Eq. 13.77 corresponds to the energy of the electrostatic field (Eq. 13.4). The second and third lines in Eq. 13.77 account for the mixing (configurational) free energy contribution of the positive and negative NaCl ions (see Eq. 13.34). We assumed $\Phi(x \to \infty) = 0$. The fourth line of Eq. 13.77 accounts for the orientational contribution of the Langevin dipoles to the free energy (see also Eq. 1.79). $\mathcal{P}(x, \omega)$ is the probability that the water Langevin dipole located at x is oriented at angle ω with respect to the normal to the charged surface. The last line is the local constraint for orientation of the water Langevin dipoles (valid at any position x) (Gongadze et al., 2013):

$$\langle \mathcal{P}(x, \omega) \rangle_\omega = 1, \quad (13.79)$$

where $\eta(x)$ is the local Lagrange multiplier.

The results of the variation in the above free energy (Eq. 13.77) gives (Gongadze et al., 2011c, 2013):

$$n_+(x) = n_0 \exp(-\Psi), \quad (13.80)$$

$$n_-(x) = n_0 \exp(\Psi), \quad (13.81)$$

$$\mathcal{P}(x, \omega) = \Lambda(x) \exp(-p_0|\Psi'| \cos(\omega)/e_0), \quad (13.82)$$

where $\Lambda(x)$ is constant for given x.

The charges of counterions, coions, and water molecules contribute to the average microscopic volume charge density:

$$\rho(x) = e_0 (n_+(x) - n_-(x)) - \frac{dP}{dx}. \quad (13.83)$$

Polarization P is given by

$$P(x) = n_{0w} \langle \mathbf{p}(x, \omega) \rangle_B, \quad (13.84)$$

where $\langle \mathbf{p}(x \text{ and } \omega) \rangle_B$ is its average over the angle distribution in thermal equilibrium. In our case of a negatively charged planar surface ($\sigma < 0$), the projection of the polarization vector $\mathbf{P}$ points in a direction opposite to the direction of the x-axis. Hence, $P(x)$ is considered negative. According to Eq. 13.82, the values of $\langle \mathbf{p}(x, \omega) \rangle_B$ can be calculated as (Gongadze et al., 2011c, 2013):

$$\langle \mathbf{p}(x, \omega) \rangle_B = \frac{\int_0^\pi p_0 \cos\omega\, \mathcal{P}(x, \omega)\, 2\pi \sin\omega d\omega}{\int_0^\pi \mathcal{P}(x, \omega)\, 2\pi \sin\omega d\omega} = -p_0\, \mathcal{L}\left(\frac{p_0|\Psi'|}{e_0}\right). \quad (13.85)$$

The function $\mathcal{L}(u) = (\coth(u) - 1/u)$ is the Langevin function. The Langevin function $\mathcal{L}(p_0|\Psi'|/e_0)$ determines the average magnitude of the Langevin dipole moments at given x. In our derivation, we assumed an azimuthal symmetry and a negative surface charge density σ.

Substituting the Boltzmann distribution functions of ions, Eqs. 13.80 and 13.81 and the expression for polarization, Eqs. 13.84 and 13.85 into Eq. 13.83, we get the expression for the volume charge density in an electrolyte solution (Gongadze et al., 2011c, 2013):

$$\rho(x) = -2 e_0 n_0 \sinh\Psi + n_{0w}\, p_0\, \frac{d}{dx}\left[\mathcal{L}(p_0|\Psi'|/e_0)\right]. \quad (13.86)$$

Substituting $\rho(x)$ from Eq. 13.86 into the Poisson equation (Eq. 13.2)

$$\Psi'' = -4\pi\, l_B\, \rho/e_0, \quad (13.87)$$

yields the LPB equation for point-like ions (Gongadze et al., 2010, 2011c, 2013):

$$\Psi'' = 4\pi\, l_B \left(2 n_0 \sinh\Psi - n_{0w}\, \frac{p_0}{e_0}\, \frac{d}{dx}\left[\mathcal{L}(p_0|\Psi'|/e_0)\right]\right), \quad (13.88)$$

where Ψ'' is the second derivative of Ψ with respect to x.

The LPB differential Eq. 13.88 is subject to two boundary conditions. The first boundary condition is obtained by integrating the differential equation 13.88 (Gongadze et al., 2011c, 2013):

$$\Psi'(x=0) = -\frac{4\pi l_B}{e_0} \left[\sigma + n_{0w}\, p_0\, \mathcal{L}(p_0|\Psi'|/e_0)\right]_{x=0}. \quad (13.89)$$

The condition requiring electro-neutrality of the whole system was taken into account in derivation of Eq. 13.89. The second boundary condition is:

$$\Psi'(x \to \infty) = 0. \quad (13.90)$$

Based on Eqs. 13.84 to 13.85, we can express the relative (effective) permittivity of the electrolyte solution (ε_r) in contact with the planar charged surface as (Gongadze et al., 2010, 2011c):

$$\varepsilon_r(x) = 1 + \frac{|P|}{\varepsilon_0 E} = 1 + n_{0w}\, \frac{p_0}{\varepsilon_0}\, \frac{\mathcal{L}(p_0\, E\, \beta)}{E}, \quad (13.91)$$

where $\beta = 1/kT$ and E is the magnitude of the electric field strength.

Equations 13.88 and 13.90 can be rewritten in a general and more elegant form as (Gongadze et al., 2011c):

$$\nabla \cdot [\varepsilon_0\, \varepsilon_r(x)\, \nabla \phi(x)] = -\rho_{\text{free}}(x), \quad (13.92)$$

where $\rho_{\text{free}}(x)$ is the macroscopic (net) volume charge density of coions and counterions:

$$\rho_{\text{free}}(x) = -e_0\, n_+(x) - e_0\, n_-(x) = -2\, e_0\, n_0\, \sinh(e_0\, \phi\, \beta), \quad (13.93)$$

and $\varepsilon_r(x)$ is the relative permittivity of the electrolyte solution defined by Eq. 13.91. The boundary condition at the charged surface (Eq. 13.89) is

$$\nabla \phi(x=0) = -\frac{\sigma\, \mathbf{n}}{\varepsilon_0\, \varepsilon_r(x=0)}, \quad (13.94)$$

where $\varepsilon_r(x)$ is again defined by Eq. 13.91 and $\mathbf{n}$ is the unit vector. The second boundary condition is

$$\phi(x \to \infty) = 0. \quad (13.95)$$

Equation 13.91 describes the dependence of the relative permittivity ε_r on the magnitude of the electric field strength E, calculated within the presented LPB model. This model takes into account the orientational ordering of water molecules (or water clusters) near the charged surface (Fig. 13.7) by considering them as Langevin dipoles but without considering their finite size.

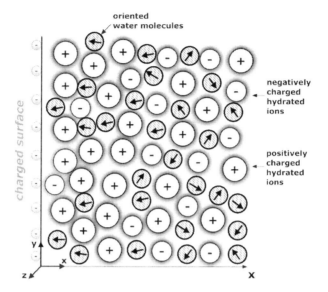

Figure 13.7 Schematic figure of the electrical double layer near a negatively charged planar surface. The water molecules in the vicinity of the charged surface are predominantly oriented towards the surface (Gongadze, 2011).

For $p_0 E/kT < 1$, we can expand the Langevin function in Eq. 13.91 into a Taylor series up to the cubic term

$$\mathcal{L}(x) \approx x/3 - x^3/45$$

to get (Gongadze et al., 2011c, 2013)

$$\varepsilon_r(x) \cong 1 + \frac{n_{0w} p_0^2 \beta}{3\,\varepsilon_0} - \frac{n_{0w} p_0^2 \beta}{45\,\varepsilon_0} (p_0 E\beta)^2 \ . \qquad (13.96)$$

It can be seen in Eq. 13.96 that $\varepsilon_r(x)$ decreases with increase in magnitude of the electric field strength E. Since the value of E increases towards the charged surface, $\varepsilon_r(x)$ decreases towards the charged surface. It can therefore be concluded that due to the preferential orientation of water dipoles in the close vicinity of the charged surface, the relative permittivity of the electrolyte $\varepsilon_r(x)$ near the charged surface is reduced relative to its bulk value, as also shown in Fig. 13.8.

To conclude, in this section the Gouy–Chapman theory for point-like ions modified by introducing the orientational ordering of water molecules is described. The corresponding LPB equation

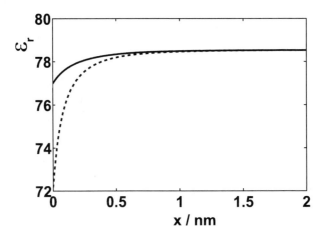

Figure 13.8 Relative dielectric permittivity ε_r as a function of the distance from the charged surface x within the presented Langevin PB theory for point-like ions. Equations 13.91–13.95 were solved numerically using the finite element method (FEM) within the program package *Comsol Multiphysics* Software as described in (Gongadze et al., 2011c). Dipole moment of water $p_0 = 4.79$ D, bulk concentration of salt $n_0/N_A = 0.15$ mol/l, bulk concentration of water $n_{0w}/N_A = 55$ mol/l, surface charge density $\sigma = -0.1$ A s/m² (full line) and $\sigma = -0.2$ A s/m² (dashed line).

is presented (Gongadze et al., 2010, 2011c). It is shown that the relative permittivity of the electrolyte solution decreases with increase in magnitude of the electric field strength (Gongadze et al., 2010; Iglič et al., 2010). Due to the increased magnitude of the electric field in the vicinity of the charged surface in contact with the electrolyte solution, the relative permittivity of the electrolyte solution in the region near the charged surface is decreased (see Gongadze et al., 2011c, 2013, and Fig. 13.8). The predicted decrease in permittivity relative to its bulk value is the consequence of the orientational ordering of the water dipoles in the vicinity of the charged surface.

In the limit of $p_0 \to 0$ the above LPB Eq. 13.92 transforms into the well-known PB equation for monovalent ions (Eq. 13.69):

$$\nabla \cdot [\varepsilon_0 \varepsilon_r \nabla \phi(x)] = -\rho_{\text{free}}(x), \quad (13.97)$$

where we made the transformation $\varepsilon_0 \to \varepsilon_r \varepsilon_0$ with $\varepsilon_r = 78.5$ and $\rho_{\text{free}}(x)$ defined by Eq. 13.93.

In the following section, a modification of the LPB model including the finite size of molecules, and the cavity and reaction fields (Gongadze and Iglič, 2012a; Gongadze et al., 2013) is presented.

13.7 Generalized Langevin–Bikerman Model

In order to develop an integral framework to clarify factors influencing the relative permittivity, recently the Langevin Poisson–Boltzman (LPB) model was generalized within the so-called generalized Langevin–Bikerman model (Gongadze and Iglič, 2012a) by taking into account the cavity field and electronic polarizability of water (Fröhlich, 1964), as well as the finite size of the molecules.

The effective dipole moment of the water molecule should be known before a satisfactory statistical mechanical study of water and aqueous solutions is possible (Adams, 1981). The dipole moment of a water molecule in liquid water differs from that of an isolated water molecule because each water molecule is further polarized (i.e., the dipole moment is further increased) and orientationally perturbed by the electric field of the surrounding water molecules (Adams, 1981). Accordingly, in the above described treatment of water ordering close to the saturation limit at high electric field within the LPB model, the effective dipole moment of water $p_0 = 4.79\,D$ is larger than the dipole moment of an isolated water molecule ($p_0 = 1.85\,D$). It is also larger than the dipole moment of a water molecule in clusters ($p_0 = 2.7\,D$) and the dipole moment of an average water molecule in the bulk ($p_0 = 2.4 - 2.6\,D$) (Dill and Bromberg, 2003) since the cavity and reaction fields, the electronic polarizability of water molecules as well as the structural correlations between water dipoles (Fröhlich, 1964; Franks, 1972), were not explicitly taken into account in the LPB model of the previous Section 13.6.

In the past treatments of the cavity and reaction fields, electronic polarizability and the correlations between water dipoles in the Onsager (1936), Kirkwood (1939) and Fröhlich (1964) models were limited to the case of small electric field strengths. Generalization of the Kirkwood–Onsager–Fröhlich theory in the saturation regime

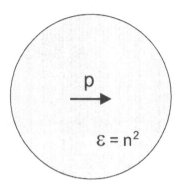

Figure 13.9 In the model, a single water molecule is considered as a sphere with permittivity n^2 and a point-like rigid (permanent) dipole with dipole moment **p** at the centre of the sphere. Here, n is the optical refractive index of water.

was performed by Booth (1951). However, Booth's model does not consider the excluded volume effect in an electrolyte solution near a charged surface. Therefore, in this section, first the LPB model (Section 13.6) is generalized to take into account the cavity and reaction fields, electronic polarizability (but not also the structural correlations between water dipoles), as well as the finite size of ions (Gongadze and Iglič, 2012a; Gongadze et al., 2013) in the saturation regime important in consideration of an electrolyte solution in contact with a highly charged surface.

In the model, the electronic polarization of water is taken into account by assuming that point-like rigid (permanent) dipole is located at the centre of a sphere which is embedded in the electrolyte solution. The volume of the sphere is equal to the average volume of a water molecule (Fig. 13.9). The permittivity of the sphere is taken to be n^2, where $n = 1.33$ is the optical refractive index of water. The relative (effective) permittivity of the electrolyte solution (ε_r) can then be expressed as:

$$\varepsilon_r(\mathbf{r}) = n^2 + \frac{|\mathbf{P}|}{\varepsilon_0 E}, \qquad (13.98)$$

where **P** is the polarization vector due to the net orientation of permanent point-like water dipoles having dipole moment **p**. The external dipole moment ($\mathbf{p}_e$) of a point-like dipole at the centre of the sphere with permittivity n^2 can then be expressed in the form

(Fröhlich, 1964):

$$\mathbf{p}_e = \frac{3}{2+n^2}\,\mathbf{p}, \qquad (13.99)$$

hence it follows:

$$\mathbf{p} = \frac{2+n^2}{3}\,\mathbf{p}_e. \qquad (13.100)$$

The short-range interactions between dipoles are neglected. The local electric field strength at the centre of the sphere at the location of the permanent (rigid) point-like dipole (Fig. 13.9) is (Fröhlich, 1964):

$$\mathbf{E}_c = \frac{3\,\varepsilon_r}{2\,\varepsilon_r + n^2}\,\mathbf{E} + g\,\mathbf{p}, \qquad (13.101)$$

where the first term represents the field inside a spherical cavity with dielectric permittivity n^2 embedded in a medium with permittivity ε_r, and the second term $g\,\mathbf{p}$ is the reaction-field acting on $\mathbf{p}$ (due to the dipole moment $\mathbf{p}$ of the point-like dipole itself). In the following, Eq. 13.101 is simplified to the form (strictly valid for $\varepsilon_r \gg n^2$ only):

$$\mathbf{E}_c = \frac{3}{2}\,\mathbf{E} + g\,\mathbf{p}. \qquad (13.102)$$

For $\varepsilon_r \gg n^2$, the value of $g \cong 1/n^2\,r_o^3$, where r_o is the effective radius of the molecule (Booth, 1951).

The energy of the point like-dipole $\mathbf{p}$ in the local field $\mathbf{E}_c$ may then be written as

$$W_i = -\mathbf{p}\cdot\mathbf{E}_c = -\mathbf{p}\cdot\left(\frac{3}{2}\mathbf{E} + g\,\mathbf{p}\right) = \gamma\,p_0\,E\cos(\omega) - g\,p_0^2, \qquad (13.103)$$

where p_0 is the magnitude of the dipole moment $\mathbf{p}_e$, ω is the angle between the dipole moment vector $\mathbf{p}$ and the vector $-\mathbf{E}$ and

$$\gamma = \frac{3}{2}\left(\frac{2+n^2}{3}\right). \qquad (13.104)$$

The polarization $P(x)$

$$P(x) = n_w(x)\left\langle \mathbf{p}(x,\omega)\right\rangle_B, \qquad (13.105)$$

is given by (Gongadze and Iglič, 2012a):

$$P(x) = n_w(x)\left(\frac{2+n^2}{3}\right) p_0 \left\langle \cos(\omega)\right\rangle_B$$

$$= -n_w(x)\left(\frac{2+n^2}{3}\right) p_0\,\mathcal{L}(\gamma\,p_0\,E\,\beta), \qquad (13.106)$$

where

$$\langle \cos\omega \rangle_B = \frac{\int_0^\pi \cos\omega \exp(-\gamma\, p_0\, E\beta\, \cos(\omega) + \beta g\, p_0^2)\, d\Omega}{\int_0^\pi \exp(-\gamma\, p_0\, E\beta\, \cos(\omega) + \beta g\, p_0^2)\, d\Omega}$$

$$= -\mathcal{L}(\gamma\, p_0\, E\, \beta)\,, \qquad (13.107)$$

and $d\Omega = 2\pi \sin\omega\, d\omega$ is an element of solid angle. Since $\sigma < 0$, the projection of polarization vector **P** on the x-axis points in the direction from the bulk to the charged surface and $P(x)$ is considered negative.

In bulk solution the number densities of water molecules (n_{0w}), counterions (n_0) and coions (n_0) are constant, therefore their number densities can be expressed in a simple way by calculating the corresponding probabilities that a single lattice site in the bulk solution is occupied by one of the three kind of particles in electrolyte solution (counterions, coions, and water molecules) (Gongadze, 2011; Gongadze et al., 2011b, 2013):

$$n_+(x \to \infty) = n_-(x \to \infty) = n_s \frac{n_0}{n_0 + n_0 + n_{0w}}, \qquad (13.108)$$

$$n_w(x \to \infty) = n_s \frac{n_{0w}}{n_0 + n_0 + n_{0w}}, \qquad (13.109)$$

where n_s is the number density of lattice sites as defined above. In the vicinity of a charged surface, the number densities of ions and water molecules are influenced by the charged surface, so the probabilities that a single lattice site is occupied by a particle of one of the three kinds should be corrected by the corresponding Boltzmann factors, leading to ion and water dipole distribution functions in the form (Gongadze and Iglič, 2012a; Gongadze et al., 2013):

$$n_+(x) = n_s \frac{n_0 e^{-e_0\phi\beta}}{n_0 e^{e_0\phi\beta} + n_0 e^{-e_0\phi\beta} + n_{0w}\left\langle e^{-\gamma\, p_0\, E\beta\, \cos(\omega)+\beta g\, p_0^2} \right\rangle_\omega},$$

$$(13.110)$$

$$n_-(x) = n_s \frac{n_0 e^{e_0\phi\beta}}{n_0 e^{e_0\phi\beta} + n_0 e^{-e_0\phi\omega} + n_{0w}\left\langle e^{-\gamma\, p_0\, E\beta\, \cos(\omega)+\beta g\, p_0^2} \right\rangle_\omega},$$

$$(13.111)$$

$$n_w(x) = n_s \frac{n_{0w}\left\langle e^{-\gamma\, p_0\, E\, \beta\, \cos(\omega)+\beta\, g\, p_0^2}\right\rangle_\omega}{n_0 e^{e_0\, \phi\, \beta} + n_0' e^{-e_0\, \phi\, \omega} + n_{0w}\left\langle e^{-\gamma\, p_0\, E\, \beta\, \cos(\omega)+\beta\, g\, p_0^2}\right\rangle_\omega}, \quad (13.112)$$

where

$$\left\langle e^{-\gamma\, p_0\, E\, \beta\, \cos(\omega)+\beta\, g\, p_0^2}\right\rangle_\omega = \frac{2\pi \int_\pi^0 d(\cos\omega)\, e^{-\gamma\, p_0\, E\, \beta\, \cos(\omega)+\beta\, g\, p_0^2}}{4\pi}$$

$$= \frac{\sinh(\gamma\, p_0\, E\, \beta)}{\gamma\, p_0\, E\, \beta}\, \exp(\beta\, g\, p_0^2). \quad (13.113)$$

is the dipole Boltzmann factor after rotational averaging over all possible angles ω. Assuming $g = 0$, Eqs. 13.111 to 13.113 can be re-written as (Gongadze and Iglič, 2012a):

$$n_+(x) = n_0\, e^{-e_0\, \phi\, \beta}\, \frac{n_s}{\mathcal{D}(\phi, E)}, \quad (13.114)$$

$$n_-(x) = n_0\, e^{e_0\, \phi\, \beta}\, \frac{n_s}{\mathcal{D}(\phi, E)}, \quad (13.115)$$

$$n_w(x) = \frac{n_{0w}\, n_s}{\mathcal{D}(\phi, E)}\, \frac{\sinh(\gamma\, p_0\, E\, \beta)}{\gamma\, p_0\, E\, \beta}. \quad (13.116)$$

where

$$\mathcal{D}(\phi, E) = 2 n_0 \cosh(e_0\, \phi\, \beta) + \frac{n_{0w}}{\gamma\, p_0\, E\, \beta}\, \sinh(\gamma\, p_0\, E\, \beta). \quad (13.117)$$

Combining Eqs. 13.106 and 13.116 gives the polarization in the form:

$$P(x) = -\left(\frac{2+n^2}{3}\right) \frac{p_0\, n_{0w}\, n_s}{\mathcal{D}(\phi, E)}\, \frac{\sinh(\gamma\, p_0\, E\, \beta)}{\gamma\, p_0\, E\, \beta}\, \mathcal{L}(\gamma\, p_0\, E\, \beta). \quad (13.118)$$

Using the definition of the function $\mathcal{F}(u)$:

$$\mathcal{F}(u) = \mathcal{L}(u)\, \frac{\sinh u}{u}, \quad (13.119)$$

Eq. 13.118 reads

$$P = -p_0\, n_{0w}\, n_s \left(\frac{2+n^2}{3}\right) \frac{\mathcal{F}(\gamma\, p_0\, E\, \beta)}{\mathcal{D}(\phi, E)}. \quad (13.120)$$

Combining Eqs. 13.98 and 13.120 yields the relative (effective) permittivity:

$$\varepsilon_r(x) = n^2 + n_{0w}\, n_s\, \frac{p_0}{\varepsilon_0} \left(\frac{2+n^2}{3}\right) \frac{\mathcal{F}(\gamma\, p_0\, E\, \beta)}{\mathcal{D}(\phi, E)\, E}. \quad (13.121)$$

Using the above expression for $\varepsilon_r(x)$, we can then write the Poisson equation (Eq. 13.2) in the form of Gongadze-Iglič (GI) equation (Gongadze and Iglič, 2012a):

$$\nabla \cdot [\varepsilon_0 \, \varepsilon_r(x) \, \nabla \phi(x)] = -\rho_{\text{free}}(x), \qquad (13.122)$$

where $\rho_{\text{free}}(x)$ is the macroscopic (net) volume charge density of coions and counterions (see Eqs. 13.114, 13.115):

$$\rho_{\text{free}}(x) = e_0 \, n_+(x) - e_0 \, n_-(x) = -2 \, e_0 \, n_s \, n_0 \, \frac{\sinh(e_0 \, \phi \, \beta)}{\mathcal{D}(\phi, E)}. \qquad (13.123)$$

The boundary conditions are (Gongadze and Iglič, 2012a; Gongadze et al., 2013):

$$\nabla \phi(x = 0) = -\frac{\sigma \, \mathbf{n}}{\varepsilon_0 \, \varepsilon_r(x = 0)}, \qquad (13.124)$$

$$\phi(x \to \infty) = 0. \qquad (13.125)$$

In the approximation of small electrostatic energy and small energy of the dipoles in the electric field compared to the thermal energy, that is, small $e_0 \, \phi \, \beta$, and small $\gamma \, p_0 \, E \, \beta$, the relative permittivity within the presented model (Eq. 13.121) can be expanded into a Taylor series (assuming $n_s \approx n_{0w}$) to get (Gongadze and Iglič, 2012a):

$$\varepsilon_r(x) \cong n^2 + \frac{3}{2} \left(\frac{2+n^2}{3} \right)^2 \frac{n_{0w} \, p_0^2 \, \beta}{3 \, \varepsilon_0} - \frac{27}{8} \left(\frac{2+n^2}{3} \right)^4 \frac{n_{0w} \, p_0^2 \, \beta}{45 \, \varepsilon_0}$$

$$(p_0 \, E \, \beta)^2 - \frac{3}{2} \left(\frac{2+n^2}{3} \right)^2 \frac{n_0 \, p_0^2 \, \beta}{3 \, \varepsilon_0} \, (e_0 \, \phi \, \beta)^2. \qquad (13.126)$$

In the limit of vanishing electric field strength ($E \to 0$) and zero potential ($\phi \to 0$), the above equations give the Onsager expression for permittivity:

$$\varepsilon_r \cong n^2 + \left(\frac{2+n^2}{3} \right)^2 \frac{n_{0w} \, p_0^2 \, \beta}{2 \, \varepsilon_0}. \qquad (13.127)$$

In the above expression derived for the relative (effective) permittivity (Eq. 13.121), the value of the dipole moment $p_0 = 3.1$ D predicts a bulk permittivity $\varepsilon_r = 78.5$. This value is considerably smaller than the corresponding value in the LPB model ($p_0 = 4.79$ D) (see Fig. 13.8), which does not take into account the cavity field.

The value $p_0 = 3.1$ D (Fig. 13.10) is also close to the experimental values of the effective dipole moment of water molecules in clusters ($p_0 = 2.7$ D) and in bulk solution ($p_0 = 2.4 - 2.6$ D) (Dill and Bromberg, 2003).

Figures 13.10 and 13.11 show the calculated spatial dependence of the relative number density of counterions (n_+/n_s), model also called water dipoles (n_w/n_s), and $\varepsilon_r(x)$ within the generalized Langevin–Bikerman also called Gongadze–Iglič (GI) model, in planar geometry for three values of the surface charge density σ.

It can be seen in Fig. 13.10 that close to the charged plane there may be a considerable excluded volume effect on the density profile of the counterions and on the solvent molecules. In the concentration of counterions, there is comparable to the concentration of solvent lattice sites, so that the concentration of solvent lattice sites deviates significantly from its value far from the charged surface (Kralj-Iglič et al., 1996).

The ratio between the concentration of counterions near the charged plane and the bulk counterion concentration as a function of the surface charge density σ is higher for dimensionless ions than for ions of finite size. The discrepancy between the results for dimensionless ions and for ions of finite size grows with increase in $|\sigma|$ (Iglič and Kralj-Iglič, 1994). The deviation can be attributed to the steric effect of counterions and solvent molecules in the small region in the vicinity of the charged surface. The counterion concentration profile shows a rapid decrease for small lattice constant and a plateau region near the charged plane for large lattice constant. For large counterions, we can therefore distinguish between two regions within the EDL: the saturated layer dominated by steric repulsion and the diffuse layer extending into the solution.

It was shown (Gongadze et al., 2013) that for high enough surface charge densities the usual trend of monotonously increasing counterion number density towards the charged surface may be completely reversed in the close vicinity of the charged surface due to competition between the counterion Boltzmann factor $n_0 e^{-e_0 \phi \beta}$ and the rotationally averaged water Boltzmann factor $n_{0w} \left\langle e^{-\gamma\, p_0 E \beta\, \cos(\omega)} \right\rangle_\omega$ in the region near the charged surface. Accordingly, the partial depletion of water molecules at the charged surface is diminished for large values of the surface charge density.

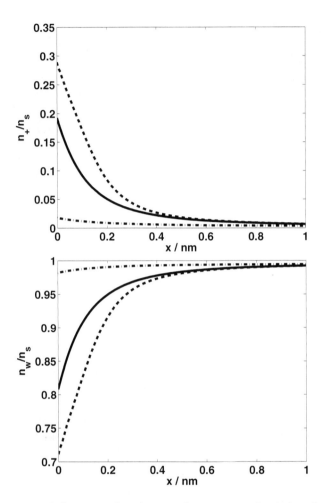

Figure 13.10 Relative number density of counterions (n_+/n_s) and water dipoles (n_w/n_s) (Eqs. 13.114 and Eq. 13.116) as a function of distance from a planar charged surface x calculated for three values of the surface charge density: $\sigma = -0.1$ A s/m² (dashed-dotted line), $\sigma = -0.2$ A s/m² (full line) and $\sigma = -0.3$ A s/m² (dashed line). Values of parameters assumed are dipole moment of water $p_0 = 3.1$ D, bulk concentration of salt $n_0/N_A = 0.15$ mol/l, optical refractive index $n = 1.33$, bulk concentration of water $n_{0w}/N_A = 55$ mol/l. Reprinted from *Bioelectrochemistry*, 87, Gongadze, E., and Iglič, A. (2012a), Decrease of permittivity of an electrolyte solution near a charged surface due to saturation and excluded volume effects, pp. 199–203, Copyright 2012, with permission from Elsevier.

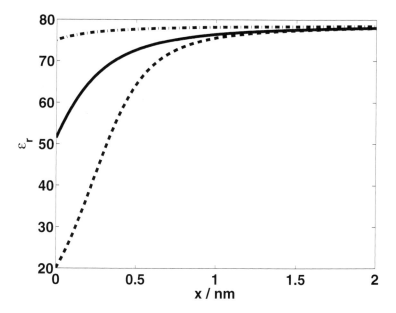

Figure 13.11 Relative permittivity ε_r (Eq. 13.121) as a function of distance from a planar charged surface x. Three values of surface charge density were considered: $\sigma = -0.1$ A s/m² (dashed-dotted line), $\sigma = -0.2$ A s/m² (full line) and $\sigma = -0.3$ A s/m² (dashed line). Values of parameters assumed were dipole moment of water $p_0 = 3.1$ D, bulk concentration of salt $n_0/N_A = 0.15$ mol/l, $n = 1.33$, $n_{0w}/N_A = 55$ mol/l. Reprinted from *Bioelectrochemistry*, 87, Gongadze, E., and Iglič, A. (2012a), Decrease of permittivity of an electrolyte solution near a charged surface due to saturation and excluded volume effects, pp. 199–203, Copyright 2012, with permission from Elsevier.

The decrease in $\varepsilon_r(x)$ towards the charged surface becomes pronounced with increase in σ (Fig. 13.11) and is a consequence of the increased depletion of water molecules near the charged surface (due to the excluded volume effect as a consequence of counterion accumulation near the charged surface) (Fig. 13.11) and increased orientational ordering of water dipoles (saturation effect). Comparison between the predictions of the LPB model (Fig. 13.8) and the GI model shows a stronger decrease of relative permittivity of the electrolyte solution near the highly charged surface in the GI model, mainly due to depletion of water molecules in the vicinity of the charged surface.

In order to differentiate between the influence of the finite size of ions and the influence of the cavity field on the relative permittivity near the charged surface, the equations of the above described GI model are written in the limit of $\gamma \to 1$ and $n \to 1$ to get the Langevin–Bikerman equation (Gongadze et al., 2011c, 2013):

$$\nabla \cdot [\varepsilon_0 \, \varepsilon_r(x) \, \nabla \phi(x)] = -\rho_{\text{free}}(x), \tag{13.128}$$

where $\rho_{\text{free}}(x)$ is the macroscopic (net) volume charge density of coions and counterions:

$$\rho_{\text{free}}(x) = -2 \, e_0 \, n_s \, n_0 \, \frac{\sinh(e_0 \, \phi \, \beta)}{\mathcal{H}(\phi, \, E)}, \tag{13.129}$$

while $\varepsilon_r(x)$ is the relative permittivity (Gongadze et al., 2011c; Iglič et al., 2010):

$$\varepsilon_r(x) = 1 + n_{0w} n_s \, \frac{p_0}{\varepsilon_0} \, \frac{\mathcal{F}(p_0 \, E \, \beta)}{E \, \mathcal{H}(\phi, \, E)}, \tag{13.130}$$

where

$$\mathcal{H}(\phi, \, E) = 2 \, n_0 \, \cosh(e_0 \phi \beta) + \frac{n_{0w}}{p_0 \, E \, \beta} \, \sinh(p_0 \, E \, \beta). \tag{13.131}$$

Comparison between the space dependence of the relative permittivity within the GI model (Fig. 13.11) and within its limit model for $\gamma \to 1$, and $n \to 1$ (Gongadze and Iglič, 2012b; Gongadze et al., 2013) shows that consideration of the cavity field and electronic polarizability makes the reduction in permittivity of the electrolyte solution near the charged surface stronger (Gongadze and Iglič, 2012b). More importantly, in the limit of $\gamma \to 1$ and $n \to 1$ again the value $p_0 = 4.79$ D should be used (similarly, as in the LPB model) (Iglič et al., 2010) in order to get $\varepsilon_r(x \to \infty) = 78.5$, which shows the superiority of the GI model over its limit Langevin–Bikerman (LB) model for $\gamma \to 1$, and $n \to 1$ (Gongadze et al., 2011c, 2013; Iglič et al., 2010).

To conclude, in this section, it was shown that consideration of the cavity field of a single water molecule and the finite sized ions within the GI model results in an additional decrease of permittivity near the charged surface (see Gongadze et al., 2010, 2013; Iglič et al., 2010, and Fig. 13.10). The corresponding analytical expression for the spatial dependence of the relative permittivity of the electrolyte solution near the charged surface in the GI model is derived (Gongadze and Iglič, 2012a; Gongadze et al., 2011b, 2013).

Note that in the limit of $p_0 \to 0$, the particle distribution functions Eqs. (13.114) to (13.116) transform into Bikerman distribution functions (Eq. 13.64) (Bikerman, 1942; Dutta and Sengupta, 1954; Eigen and Wicke, 1954; Freise, 1952; Grimley, 1950; Grimley and Mott, 1947; Iglič and Kralj-Iglič, 1994; Kralj-Iglič et al., 1996; Wiegel and Strating, 1993):

$$n_+(x) = \frac{n_0\, n_s}{n_{0w}} \frac{e^{-e_0 \phi \beta}}{1 + (2\, n_0/n_{0w})\, \cosh(e_0\, \phi\, \beta)}, \quad (13.132)$$

$$n_-(x) = \frac{n_0\, n_s}{n_{0w}} \frac{e^{e_0 \phi \beta}}{1 + (2\, n_0/n_{0w})\, \cosh(e_0\, \phi\, \beta)}, \quad (13.133)$$

$$n_w(x) = \frac{n_s}{1 + (2\, n_0/n_{0w})\, \cosh(e_0\, \phi\, \beta)}, \quad (13.134)$$

while Eq. 13.128 transforms into the Bikerman equation (Eq. 13.66) (Bikerman, 1942; Dutta and Sengupta, 1954; Eigen and Wicke, 1954; Freise, 1952; Gongadze et al., 2011c; Grimley, 1950; Grimley and Mott, 1947; Iglič and Kralj-Iglič, 1994; Kralj-Iglič et al., 1996; Wiegel and Strating, 1993):

$$\nabla \cdot [\varepsilon_0\, \varepsilon_r\, \nabla \phi(x)] = -\rho_{\text{free}}(x), \quad (13.135)$$

where we made the transformation $\varepsilon_0 \to \varepsilon_r\, \varepsilon_0$ with $\varepsilon_r = 78.5$, while $\rho_{\text{free}}(x)$ is defined by Eq. 13.129.

13.8 Differential Capacitance

To ascertain whether the described GI mean-field approach which includes the orientational ordering of water, the cavity field, the electronic polarizability of water, and the finite size of molecules has improved the agreement between theory and experiments with respect to the classical GC model, one should compare the measured and predicted values of electric potential and differential capacitance of the EDL in both models. Using the GI model, the predicted values of the electric potential at higher surface charge densities σ are substantially more negative than the corresponding values within the GC model (see also Gongadze et al., 2013; Lockett et al., 2010, 2008, and references therein).

Within the GC model, we can estimate the electric potential ϕ_0 at the surface (of an electrode for example) by applying the Grahame equation (Butt et al., 2003; Gongadze et al., 2013):

$$\sigma = \sqrt{8 n_0 \varepsilon_0 \varepsilon_r / \beta} \cdot \sinh\left(\frac{e_0 \beta \phi_0}{2}\right), \qquad (13.136)$$

where ϕ_0 is the surface potential, that is, $\phi(x = 0)$. The corresponding GC differential capacitance is (Butt et al., 2003; Gongadze et al., 2013; Lockett et al., 2010):

$$C_{GC} = \frac{d\sigma}{d\phi_0} = \sqrt{2 e_0^2 \beta n_0 \varepsilon_0 \varepsilon_r} \cdot \cosh\left(\frac{e_0 \beta \phi_0}{2}\right). \qquad (13.137)$$

The GC model provides relatively good predictions for monovalent salts at concentrations below 0.2 mol/l in aqueous solutions and small magnitudes of the surface potentials (Butt et al., 2003).

As can be seen in Fig. 13.12, the GC differential capacitance C_{GC} monotonously increases as a function of the increasing surface potential ϕ_0. On the contrary, the differential capacitances calculated

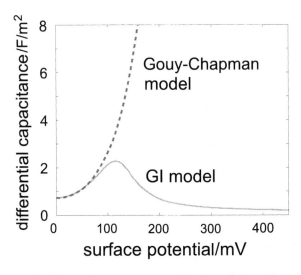

Figure 13.12 Differential capacitance as a function of the surface potential using Gouy–Chapman Eq. 13.137 (dashed line) and numerically by using GI Eq. 13.122 (full line). Figure adapted from Gongadze et al. (2013).

by the GI equation start to decrease after reaching a maximal value, as shown in Fig. 13.12. At high ϕ_0 values the calculated GI differential capacitance drop to very small values of the order of magnitude of $10\,F/m^2$ and smaller, in accordance with the experimental results (Lockett et al., 2010, 2008) (see also Bazant et al., 2009; Gongadze et al., 2013; Kornyshev, 2007).

The calculated dependences of $C_{\text{diff}}(\phi_0)$ in Fig. 13.12 are presented only for positive values of ϕ_0. The corresponding $C_{\text{diff}}(\phi_0)$ curves for negative values of ϕ_0 are the mirror images of the $C_{\text{diff}}(\phi_0)$ curves given in Fig. 13.12 (with respect to the vertical ($\phi_0 = 0$) axis). The GI $C_{\text{diff}}(\phi_0)$ curves therefore have a so-called camel (or saddle-like) shape, as also observed experimentally (Lockett et al., 2010, 2008), in Monte Carlo simulations (Fedorov et al., 2010) and in molecular dynamic simulations (Fedorov and Kornyshev, 2008).

Obviously, the GI model can also be applied at higher surface charge densities (i.e., high voltage), where the classical PB equation within the GC model completely fails, as the differential capacitance C_{GC} (unlike the experimental results (Lockett et al., 2010)) strongly and monotonously increases with increase in ϕ_0, while in this region of ϕ_0 the Bikerman equation predicts too high values of C_{diff} (Gongadze et al., 2013). To conclude, the GI differential capacitance decreases with increase in $\phi_0 > 0$ (after first reaching its maximum) and at large ϕ_0 attains the smaller values than other mean-field models (Gongadze et al., 2013), similar to that obtained experimentally.

Note that the predicted values of GI differential capacitance at high values of $|\phi_0|$ are also smaller than the corresponding values of C_{diff} predicted by the empirical formula for $\varepsilon(x)$ given in (Bazant et al., 2009). Moreover, if the GI model is modified by taking into account the distance of closest approach for ions (see also Gongadze et al., 2013; Nagy et al., 2011; Oldham, 2008), the predicted values of C_{diff} would even closely approach the experimental values.

Chapter 14

Attraction between Like-Charged Surfaces

14.1 Attraction between Like-Charged Surfaces Mediated by Spherical Macro-Ions

The outer surface of biological membranes is usually negatively charged (Cevc, 1990; Iglič et al., 1997; McLaughlin, 1989). Also, the outer membrane surface of the membrane daughter vesicles released from different kind of cells such as red blood cells (RBCs), platelets, and lymphocytes, as well as from apoptotic cells (with negatively charged cardiolipin and phosphatidylserine in the outer membrane layer) are negatively charged (Greenwalt, 2006; Hägerstrand and Isomaa, 1994; Hägerstrand et al., 1999; Martinez et al., 2005; Sorice et al., 2000).

In biological systems, charged membrane surfaces are surrounded by charged nanoparticle (proteins). Experiments with giant phospholipid vesicles (Fig. 14.1) indicate that certain plasma proteins (Frank et al., 2009; Urbanija et al., 2007, 2008b) and plasma itself (Frank et al., 2008; Perutková et al., 2010a) may induce the coalescence of like–like charged phospolipid vesicles (see also Chapter 18). In this chapter a mean-field theory is presented

---

Nanostructures in Biological Systems: Theory and Applications
Aleš Iglič, Veronika Kralj-Iglič, and Damjana Drobne
Copyright © 2015 Pan Stanford Publishing Pte. Ltd.
ISBN 978-981-4267-20-5 (Hardcover), 978-981-4303-43-9 (eBook)
www.panstanford.com

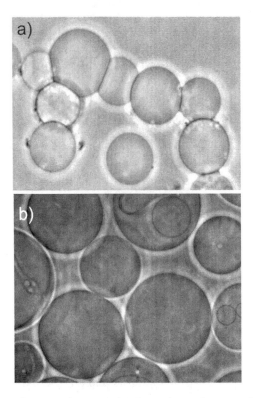

Figure 14.1 Adhesion of negatively charged membranes of giant phospholipid vesicles in the presence of a healthy donor plasma sample (a). Untreated giant phospholipid vesicles do not adhere (b). Reprinted with kind permission from Springer Science+Business Media: Perutková, Š., Frank, M., Bohinc, K., Bobojevič, K., Zelko, J., Rozman, B., Kralj-Iglič, V., and Iglič, A. (2010). Interaction between equally charged membrane surfaces mediated by positively and negatively charged nanoparticles. *J. Membr. Biol.*, 236, pp. 43–53.

to explain the observed charged nanoparticles-mediated attraction between the like-charged membrane surfaces.

Classical mean-field electric double layer (EDL) theories predict electrostatic repulsion between like-charged surfaces separated by a solution of dimensionless ions (point charges). The attractive interaction observed between like-charged surfaces (Fig. 14.1) could not be predicted for point charges (Evans and Wennerström, 1999;

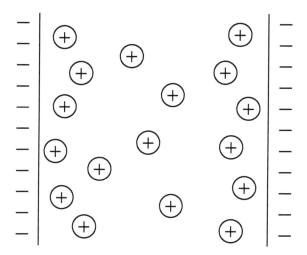

Figure 14.2 Two flat and equally charged surfaces immersed in a aqueous solution composed of counterions only.

Israelachvili, 1997; Sadar and Chan, 2000; Verwey and Overbeek, 1948).

As an illustrative example we first briefly consider a system composed of two flat and equally uniformly charged surfaces immersed in an aqueous solution composed of point-like counterions only (Fig. 14.2). The surface charge density of each surface is σ. The first charged surface is located at $x = 0$, while the second at $x = D$, where x is the coordinate perpendicular to the charged surfaces.

The electrostatic potential $\phi(x)$ is calculated by solving numerically the Poisson–Boltzman equation for counterions only (Eq. 13.51):

$$\frac{d^2\phi(x)}{dx^2} = -\frac{e_0}{\varepsilon_r \varepsilon_0} n_0 e^{-e_0 \phi(x)/kT}, \qquad (14.1)$$

taking into account the boundary condition :

$$\left.\frac{d\phi(x)}{dx}\right|_{x=0} = -\frac{\sigma}{\varepsilon_r \varepsilon_0}, \qquad (14.2)$$

assuming the electro-neutrality of the system and

$$\left.\frac{d\phi(x)}{dx}\right|_{x=\frac{D}{2}} = 0, \qquad (14.3)$$

taking into account the symmetry of the system with respect to the plane $x = D/2$

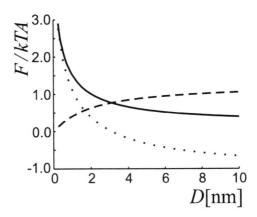

Figure 14.3 Free energy (full line), electrostatic energy (dashed line), and configurational entropy (dotted line) as a function of the distance between the equally charged surfaces D. Parameters of PB equation and corresponding free energy expression are: $|\sigma| = 0.1$ As/m^2 and $v_0 = 5$ nm^3.

Then, the number density of counterions $n(x)$ is determined using Eq. 13.50. Finally, the electrostatic free energy of the system $F = F_{el} + F_{ent}$ is calculated in the limit of very dilute solution (see Eqs. 13.4 and 13.15):

$$F/A = \frac{1}{2}\varepsilon_r\varepsilon_0 \int_0^D \left(\frac{d\phi}{dx}\right)^2 dx + kT \int_0^D [n(x)\ln(n(x)v_0) - n(x)]\, dx.$$

Figure 14.3 shows the electrostatic free energy F (full line) as a function of the distance between the equally charged planar surfaces D. We see that the free energy F decreases with increase in distance between the surfaces D, which corresponds to the repulsive force between equally charged surfaces. This is the consequence of the decrease in the entropic contribution to the free energy with increase in D, which prevails over the increase of the electrostatic part of the free energy.

Attraction between like-charged surfaces may be driven by particle–particle correlations (i.e., inter-ionic correlations) (Carnie and McLaughlin, 1983; Kirkwood and Shumaker, 1952; Kjellander, 1996; Netz, 2001; Oosawa, 1968). Also, orientational ordering (intra-ionic correlation) of charged nanoparticles (counterions) with internal charge distribution may lead to attractive forces between like-charged surfaces (Bohinc et al., 2004; Kim et al., 2008; May et al., 2008; Urbanija et al., 2008b). A generalization of the mean-field theory of the electric double layer for the case of multivalent charged nanoparticles could be made by taking into account the internal space charge distribution of a single spheroidal multivalent nanoparticle (Jackson, 1999). A theoretical description of such large multivalent spheroidal nanoparticles between two planar charged surfaces that takes into account the internal charge distribution was proposed elaborated in (Perutková et al., 2010a; Urbanija et al., 2008b).

In this chapter, the attraction between like-charged membrane surfaces mediated by charged nanoparticles with internal charge distribution is described, using mean-field density functional theory. To assess the effect of the mean-field approximation that is introduced into the theoretical description, we also carried out Monte Carlo (MC) simulations. Charged nanoparticles are considered as spherical ions with two equal effective charges spatially separated by a fixed distance l inside the particles (Fig. 14.4). We calculate the equilibrium configuration of the system by minimizing the free energy. The results of solving the integro-differential equation and by performing the MC simulation are shown to be in excellent agreement.

14.1.1 *Counterions Only*

We consider the interaction between two charged surfaces in the presence of charged nanoparticles of a single species (i.e., counterions only) with internal charge distribution.

In the model, the two interacting electrical double layers are formed by two flat membrane surfaces, each of area A, separated by distance D. The surface area A is assumed to be large compared to the distance between surfaces D so that end effects can be neglected. Each surface bears uniformly distributed charge with surface charge density σ. The space between the charged surfaces is filled with a solution of nanoparticles of a single species (counterions).

In the model, the spheroidal-charged nanoparticle is described as a sphere of diameter l (globular protein) within which two

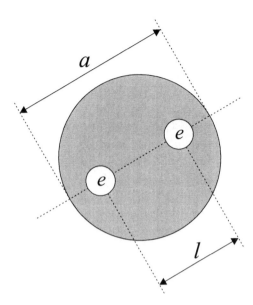

Figure 14.4 Schematic figure of a large spheroidal multivalent charged nanoparticle with net electric charge $2e$ and average diameter a. In the model, the space charge distribution of the multivalent ion is described by two effective poly-ions of charge $e = Ze_0$ located at different well-separated positions (i.e., at a distance $l \leq a$) (Urbanija et al., 2008b). The main axis of the nanoparticle coincides with the line connecting the two poly-ions.

equal positive point charges, each of valency Z ($e = Ze_0$), are separated by distance $l = a$ (Fig. 14.4). The theory presented can be generalized to include any separation between the charges within the spherical charged nanoparticle. The charged membrane surfaces are kept in the y–z plane and, hence the electrostatic field varies only in the x-direction. We assume that there are no external electric fields. The distance of closest approach of the spherical nanoparticles to the charged surface is taken into account, while the direct particle–particle hard core interactions are ignored in the model.

Charged nanoparticles are subject to positional and orientational degrees of freedom. For each macro-ion the centre of charge distribution (also its geometric centre) is located at x, $n(x)$ is the corresponding number density of nanoparticles. The two point

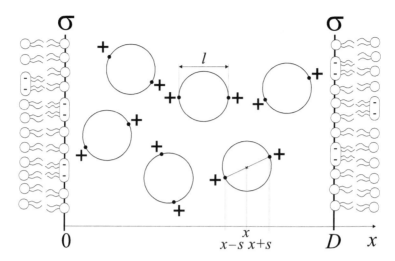

Figure 14.5 Schematic illustration of two negatively charged planar surfaces with surface charge density σ separated by a solution containing spherical charged nanoparticles (counterions) with spatially distributed positive charge. The charges within a counterion are separated by a fixed distance $l = a$, where a is the diameter of the nanoparticles. Reprinted with kind permission from Springer Science+Business Media: Perutková, Š., Frank, M., Bohinc, K., Bobojevič, K., Zelko, J., Rozman, B., Kralj-Iglič, V., and Iglič, A. (2010). Interaction between equally charged membrane surfaces mediated by positively and negatively charged nanoparticles. *J. Membr. Biol.*, 236, pp. 43–53.

charges are located at geometrically opposite points on the surface of the sphere such that, when projected on to the x-axis, their positions are at $x + s$ and $x - s$ respectively, as shown in Fig. 14.5.

Taking into account that the two point charges of the nanoparticle are indistinguishable, all possible orientations of the nanoparticle can be described by the values of s in the interval $0 < s < l/2$ (see Fig. 14.5). Therefore, the orientation of the spherical nanoparticle is specified by the conditional probability $p(s|x)$ which must satisfy the relation (Perutková et al., 2010a):

$$2/l \int_0^{l/2} p(s|x)\, ds = 1, \qquad (14.4)$$

where $p(s|x) = 0$ for any x and $|s| > l/2$.

The free energy of the system per unit area, expressed in units of thermal energy kT is (Urbanija et al., 2008b):

$$f = \frac{F}{AkT} = \int_0^D dx \left[\frac{\Psi'(x)^2}{8\pi l_B} + [n(x) \ln (n(x) v_0) - n] \right.$$

$$\left. + n(x) \left\langle p(s|x) \ln p(s|x) \right\rangle \right], \quad (14.5)$$

where the first term is the electrostatic contribution to the free energy, $\Psi = e_0 \phi / kT$ is the reduced electrostatic potential and l_B is the Bjerrum length (Eq. 13.76). The prime denotes a derivative with respect to x. The second term is the contribution due to configurational entropy (Eq. 13.15), where v_0 is the volume of a single lattice site. The third term denotes the contribution of orientational ordering of the nanoparticles. The centres of the nanoparticles are allowed to be distributed in the region $\frac{l}{2} \leq x \leq D - \frac{l}{2}$, that is, the distance of closest approach is taken into account to ensure that the spheroidal nanoparticles are confined within the region defined by the charged walls. The average of an arbitrary function $g(x)$ is defined as

$$\langle g(x) \rangle = \frac{2}{l} \int_0^{l/2} g(x, s) \, ds. \quad (14.6)$$

In the following, the limits of integration in the free energy expression are extended to infinity in both directions:

$$f = \frac{F}{AkT} = \int_{-\infty}^{\infty} dx \left[\frac{\Psi'(x)^2}{8\pi l_B} + [n(x) \ln (n(x) v_0) - n] \right.$$

$$\left. + n(x) \left\langle p(s|x) \ln p(s|x) \right\rangle \right], \quad (14.7)$$

where the values of $n(x)$ and $\Psi'(x)$ are assumed to be zero outside the space between the two charged surfaces.

The equilibrium state of the system is determined by the minimum of the total free energy F, subject to the constraints that (a) the orientational probability of the spheroidal charged nanoparticles integrated over all possible projections (Eq. 14.4), is equal to one, and that (b) the total number of charged nanoparticles is conserved. To solve this variational problem, a functional $\int_{-\infty}^{\infty} \mathcal{F} dx$ is constructed:

$$\int_{-\infty}^{\infty} \mathcal{F} dx = \frac{F}{AkT} + \int_{-\infty}^{\infty} \lambda(x) n(x) \left(\frac{2}{l} \int_{0}^{l/2} p(s|x) ds - 1 \right) dx$$

$$+ \mu \int_{-\infty}^{\infty} n(x) dx, \qquad (14.8)$$

where $\lambda(x)$ and μ are the local and global Lagrange multipliers, respectively.

Taking into account Eq. 14.7, we can re-write Eq. 14.8 in the form:

$$\int_{-\infty}^{\infty} \mathcal{F} dx = \int_{-\infty}^{\infty} dx \left[\frac{\Psi'(x)^2}{8\pi l_B} + n(x) \ln(n(x) v_0) - n(x) \right.$$

$$\left. + n(x) \left\langle p(s|x) \ln p(s|x) \right\rangle \right] \qquad (14.9)$$

$$+ \int_{-\infty}^{\infty} dx\, n(x) \lambda(x) [\langle p(s|x) \rangle - 1] + \mu \int_{-\infty}^{\infty} n(x) dx.$$

In equilibrium, the first variation of the functional $\int_{-\infty}^{\infty} \mathcal{F} dx$ should be zero:

$$\delta \int_{-\infty}^{\infty} \mathcal{F} dx = \delta \left(\frac{1}{8\pi l_B} \int_{-\infty}^{\infty} \Psi'^2 dx \right) + \int_{-\infty}^{\infty} dx\, \delta n(x) \ln(n(x) v_0)$$

$$+ \int_{-\infty}^{\infty} dx\, \delta n(x) \left\langle p(s|x) \ln p(s|x) \right\rangle$$

$$+ \int_{-\infty}^{\infty} dx\, \delta n(x) \left\{ \lambda(x) \left(\langle p(s|x) \rangle - 1 \right) + \mu \right\} \qquad (14.10)$$

$$+ \int_{-\infty}^{\infty} dx \left\langle \delta p(s|x)\, n(x) [\ln p(s|x) + 1 + \lambda(x)] \right\rangle = 0.$$

We first perform variation of the electrostatic energy, that is, variation of the first term in Eq. 14.10:

$$\delta \left(\frac{1}{8\pi l_B} \int_{-\infty}^{\infty} \Psi'^2 dx \right) = \frac{1}{4\pi l_B} \int_{-\infty}^{\infty} \Psi' \delta \Psi' dx. \qquad (14.11)$$

Using per partes integration, the right-hand side of Eq. 14.11 can be transformed into:

$$\int_{-\infty}^{\infty} \Psi' \delta \Psi' dx = \int_{-\infty}^{\infty} (\Psi \delta \Psi')' dx - \int_{-\infty}^{\infty} \Psi \delta \Psi'' dx. \qquad (14.12)$$

The first integral on the right-hand side of Eq. 14.12 is zero:

$$\int_{-\infty}^{\infty} (\Psi \delta \Psi')' dx = \int_{-\infty}^{\infty} d(\Psi \delta \Psi') = \Psi \delta \Psi' \big|_{-\infty}^{\infty} = 0, \qquad (14.13)$$

where we took into account that outside the space between the charged surfaces Ψ is constant, so variation of the first derivatives of the potential in both limits is zero: $\delta \Psi'|_{x=-\infty} = 0$ and $\delta \Psi'|_{x=\infty} = 0$. Thus, Eq. 14.12 becomes

$$\int_{-\infty}^{\infty} \Psi' \delta \Psi' dx = - \int_{-\infty}^{\infty} \Psi \delta \Psi'' dx. \qquad (14.14)$$

From Eqs. 14.11 to 14.13 and the Poisson equation

$$\Psi''(x) = -\rho(x) \frac{4\pi l_B}{e_0}, \qquad (14.15)$$

it follows that

$$\delta \left(\frac{1}{8\pi l_B} \int_{-\infty}^{\infty} \Psi'^2 dx \right) = \int_{-\infty}^{\infty} \Psi(x) \delta \left(\frac{\rho(x)}{e_0} \right) dx. \qquad (14.16)$$

Using Eq. 14.16, we can re-write Eq. 14.10 in the form:

$$\delta \int_{-\infty}^{\infty} \mathcal{F} dx = \int_{-\infty}^{\infty} \Psi(x)\, \delta\left(\frac{\rho(x)}{e_0}\right) dx + \int_{-\infty}^{\infty} dx\, \delta n(x)\, \ln(n(x)\, v_0)$$

$$+ \int_{-\infty}^{\infty} dx\, \delta n(x) \left\langle p(s|x)\, \ln p(s|x) \right\rangle$$

$$+ \int_{-\infty}^{\infty} dx\, \delta n(x) \left\{ \lambda(x)(\langle p(s|x)\rangle - 1) + \mu \right\}$$

$$+ \int_{-\infty}^{\infty} dx \left\langle \delta p(s|x)\, n(x)\, [\ln p(s|x) + 1 + \lambda(x)] \right\rangle = 0\ . $$

(14.17)

The volume charge density due to the nanoparticles at coordinate x ($\rho(x)$) contains contributions from the charges of the nanoparticles having their centres located in the region $[x - l/2, x + l/2]$:

$$\rho(x)/Z\, e_0 = \left\langle n(x-s)\, p(s|x-s) + n(x+s)\, p(s|x+s) \right\rangle,\quad (14.18)$$

where $n(x-s, s) = n(x-s)\, p(s|x-s)$ is the contribution of charged nanoparticles with their centres located on the left side of x at the positions $(x - s)$, while $n(x + s, s) = n(x + s) p(s|x + s)$ is the contribution of charged nanoparticles with their centres located on the right side of x at the positions $(x + s)$. The function $n(x, s)$ is defined as:

$$n(x, s) = n(x)\, p(s|x),\quad |s| < l/2\ . \qquad (14.19)$$

The first variation of the volume charge density $\delta\rho(x)$ is:

$$\delta\rho(x)/Z\, e_0 = \left\langle \delta n(x-s)\, p(s|x-s) + n(x-s)\, \delta p(s|x-s) \right\rangle$$

$$+ \left\langle \delta n(x+s)\, p(s|x+s) + n(x+s)\, \delta p(s|x+s) \right\rangle.$$

(14.20)

Substituting Eq. 14.20 into first term of variation $\int_{-\infty}^{\infty} \Psi(x)\,\delta\left(\frac{\rho(x)}{e_0}\right) dx$, we get

$$\int_{-\infty}^{\infty} \Psi(x)\,\delta\left(\frac{\rho(x)}{e_0}\right) dx =$$

$$+ \int_{-\infty}^{\infty} \Psi(x)\, Z \left\langle \delta n(x-s)\, p(s|x-s) + \delta n(x+s)\, p(s|x+s) \right\rangle dx$$

$$+ \int_{-\infty}^{\infty} \Psi(x)\, Z \left\langle n(x-s)\delta p(s|x-s) + n(x+s)\delta p(s|x+s) \right\rangle dx.$$

(14.21)

By introducing new variables, Eq. 14.21 can be rewritten as

$$\int_{-\infty}^{\infty} \Psi(x)\,\delta\left(\frac{\rho(x)}{e_0}\right) dx =$$

$$+ \int_{-\infty}^{\infty} \left\langle \delta n(x)\, p(s|x)\, [Z\,\Psi(x+s) + Z\,\Psi(x-s)] \right\rangle dx$$

$$+ \int_{-\infty}^{\infty} \left\langle n(x)\,\delta p(s|x)\, [Z\,\Psi(x+s) + Z\,\Psi(x-s)] \right\rangle dx . \quad (14.22)$$

If we substitute Eq. 14.22 in Eq. 14.17, we get

$$\delta \mathcal{F} = \int_{-\infty}^{\infty} \left\langle \delta n(x)\, p(s|x)\, [Z\,\Psi(x+s) + Z\,\Psi(x-s)] \right\rangle dx$$

$$+ \int_{-\infty}^{\infty} \left\langle n(x)\,\delta p(s|x)\, [Z\,\Psi(x+s) + Z\,\Psi(x-s)] \right\rangle dx$$

$$+ \int_{-\infty}^{\infty} dx\,\delta n(x)\, \ln(n(x)\, v_0) + \int_{-\infty}^{\infty} dx\,\delta n(x) \left\langle p(s|x)\, \ln p(s|x) \right\rangle$$

$$+ \int_{-\infty}^{\infty} dx\, \delta\, n(x) \left\{ \lambda(x) \left(\langle p(s|x) \rangle - 1 \right) + \mu \right\}$$

$$+ \int_{-\infty}^{\infty} dx \left\langle \delta p(s|x)\, n(x) \Big[\ln p(s|x) + 1 + \lambda(x) \Big] \right\rangle = 0. \quad (14.23)$$

Equation 14.23 has to be fulfilled for variations $\delta p(s|x)$ and $\delta n(x)$. This means that the expressions multiplied by $\delta p(s|x)$ and $\delta n(x)$ in Eq. 14.23 have to be zero. First, we consider the term multiplied by $\delta p(s|x)$:

$$\ln p(s|x) + 1 + \lambda(x) + Z\, \Psi(x+s) + Z\, \Psi(x-s) = 0, \quad (14.24)$$

from which the conditional probability density can be calculated:

$$p(s|x) = \exp\left[-Z\, \Psi(x+s) - Z\, \Psi(x-s) - 1 - \lambda(x)\right]. \quad (14.25)$$

The normalization condition (Eq. 14.4) determines the local Lagrange parameter $\lambda(x)$ and Eq. 14.25 becomes

$$p(s|x) = \frac{e^{-Z\, \Psi(x+s) - Z\, \Psi(x-s)}}{\langle e^{-Z\, \Psi(x+s) - Z\, \Psi(x-s)} \rangle}. \quad (14.26)$$

We also consider the terms multiplied by $\delta n(x)$:

$$\ln(n(x)v_0) + \left\langle p(s|x) \left[Z\, \Psi(x+s) + Z\, \Psi(x-s) \right] \right\rangle$$

$$+ \left\langle p(s|x) \ln p(s|x) \right\rangle + \mu = 0. \quad (14.27)$$

By substituting Eq. 14.26 in Eq. 14.27, we obtain the equation for the number density:

$$n(x) = \frac{e^{-\mu}}{v_0} \langle e^{-Z\, \Psi(x+s) - Z\, \Psi(x-s)} \rangle. \quad (14.28)$$

Substituting Eqs. 14.28 and 14.26 in equation $n(x, s) = n(x)\, p(s|x)$ yields

$$n(x, s) = \frac{e^{-\mu}}{v_0}\, e^{-Z\, \Psi(x+s) - Z\, \Psi(x-s)}. \quad (14.29)$$

Using the definition $n(x, s) = n(x)\, p(s|x)$ the volume charge density (Eq. 14.18) reads

$$\rho(x)/Z\, e_0 = \left\langle n(x-s, s) + n(x+s, s) \right\rangle. \quad (14.30)$$

Substituting Eq. 14.29 in Eq. 14.30 yields

$$\rho(x) = \frac{Ze_0}{v_0} \left\langle e^{-Z\Psi(x)-Z\Psi(x-2s)-\mu} + e^{-Z\Psi(x)-Z\Psi(x+2s)-\mu} \right\rangle. \quad (14.31)$$

In the first term of Eq. 14.31, the variable $-s$ is replaced by s and then the two terms are added to get

$$\rho(x) = \frac{2Ze_0}{v_0} \left\langle e^{-Z\Psi(x)-Z\Psi(x+2s)-\mu} \right\rangle. \quad (14.32)$$

The averaging is performed over s. The derived expression Eq. 14.32 for the volume charge density $\rho(x)$ and the Poisson equation 14.15 yield the integro-differential equation for the reduced electric potential in the form:

$$\Psi''(x) = -\frac{8\pi l_B Z}{v_0} \left\langle e^{-Z\Psi(x)-Z\Psi(x+2s)-\mu} \right\rangle. \quad (14.33)$$

The boundary conditions for Eq. 14.33 at both charged surfaces $x = 0$ and $x = D$ are

$$\Psi'(x=0) = -\frac{4\pi l_B \sigma}{e_0}, \quad \Psi'(x=D) = \frac{4\pi l_B \sigma}{e_0}, \quad (14.34)$$

In this theoretical model, the finite size of charged nanoparticles is taken into account only by considering the distance of closest approach of the centre of the nanoparticles to the charged surface ($l/2$).

Equation 14.33 was solved numerically as described in May et al. (2008). The solution of the integro-differential Eq. 14.33 yields the equilibrium reduced potential $\Psi(x)$, and the corresponding equilibrium distribution $n(x)$ and probability density $p(s|x)$. When the charged nanoparticles are uniformly distributed between the charged surfaces, the free energy is independent of the distance between the charged surfaces and can therefore be taken as a reference value in determining the values of the equilibrium free energy. Figure 14.6 shows the electrostatic free energy (Eq. 14.7) as a function of the distance between the two negatively charged surfaces for two different surface charge densities and two different distances between the charges within a single nanoparticle ($l = 2$ nm and $l = 5$ nm) (see also Fig. 14.4). For small surface charge density $|\sigma|$ and small separation between the charges within the charged nanoparticle, the interaction is found to be repulsive for

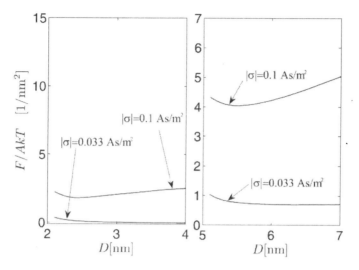

Figure 14.6 Normalized free energy f (Eq. 14.7) as a function of the distance between the negatively charged surfaces D for $Z = 1$, two different surface charge densities: $\sigma = -0.033$ As/m^2 and $\sigma = -0.1$ As/m^2, and two different distances between the charges within the nanoparticle: $l = 2$ nm (left left), $l = 5$ nm (right figure), $l_B = 0.7$ nm. Reprinted with permission from Urbanija, J., Bohinc, K., Bellen, A., Maset, S., Iglič, A., Kralj-Iglič, V., and Sunil Kumar, P. B. (2008b). Attraction between negatively charged surfaces mediated by spherical counterions with quadrupolar charge distribution. *J. Chem. Phys.*, 129, pp. 105101. Copyright 2008, AIP Publishing LLC.

all distances between the charged surfaces. However, large enough $|\sigma|$ and l yield non-monotonous behaviour of the free energy f with a minimum representing the equilibrium distance between the charged membrane surfaces.

We now discuss the results obtained from our theoretical analysis and MC simulations. MC simulations are widely used to describe solutions of point-like ions (Hatlo and Lue, 2009; Moreira and Netz, 2002), finite-sized ions (Bhuiyan and Outhwaite, 2009; Ibarra-Armenta et al., 2009; Tresset, 2008) or ions with internal charge distribution (Kim et al., 2008; May et al., 2008; Urbanija et al., 2008b) in contact with charged surface(s). In the MC simulation presented in this section, the standard MC Metropolis algorithm (Frenkel and Smith, 1996) with Lekner periodic boundary conditions (Lekner, 1991) in the directions parallel to the charged walls is used. A system of 100–200 spheres confined between two impenetrable charged surfaces is considered. As in the theory, the hard core interaction between the nanoparticles and charged walls is taken into account by means of the distance of closest approach ($l/2$), while the hard core interaction between charged nanoparticles is not considered. In each MC step, a spherical nanoparticle is chosen at random to be randomly rotated around its centre or linearly displaced. Selection of the type of move (orientational or translational move) has the same probability. Random linear displacement and random rotation ensure proper consideration of the translational and orientational entropy of the system (Frenkel and Smith, 1996). Computation of the potential in a periodic system with 2-D symmetry is performed by the Leckner–Sperb method (Leckner, 1991; Sperb, 1998), which is an alternative to Ewald summation (Ewald, 1921), whereas we use an implementation similar to that performed in (Moreira and Netz, 2002).

Figure 14.7 shows the results obtained from solutions of the integro-differential equation and MC simulations for the volume charge density $\rho(x)$ in a solution of divalent charged spherical nanoparticles ($Z = 1$) confined between two negatively charged planar surfaces separated by a distance D. For the D value which is comparable to the separation of charges within a single charged nanoparticle (l); that is, for $D = 2.5$ nm (squares), the charge density profile in the solution exhibits a single peak at each side indicating that the nanoparticles (on the average) orient to form bridging between the two charged planar surfaces. On the other hand, for somewhat larger distances ($D = 4$ nm) between the charged surfaces, we see a peak in the middle (triangles), which corresponds to overlapping of the ordered macro-ions (see Fig. 14.8). The charges on nanoparticles of both layers contribute to $\rho(x)$ at $x = D/2$, so a central peak in the volume charge density $\rho(x)$ is formed. For even larger distances ($D = 8$ nm), the profile exhibits twin-peaks close to both charged surfaces due to orientational ordering of nanoparticles having one charge close to the charged surface. The excellent agreement between the calculated volume charge density profiles (curves) and the results of MC simulations (points) can be seen.

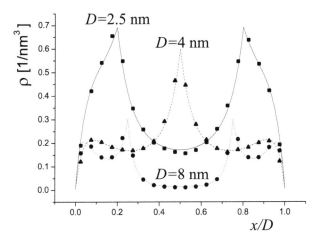

Figure 14.7 Profile of the volume charge density due to positively charged divalent nanoparticles ($Z = 1$) between two negatively charged surfaces. Lines represent the solutions of the integro-differential Eq. 14.33, points represent results of the MC simulations. Model parameters: $l = 2$ nm, $\sigma = -0.07$ As/m^2. Reprinted with permission from Urbanija, J., Bohinc, K., Bellen, A., Maset, S., Iglič, A., Kralj-Iglič, V., and Sunil Kumar, P. B., Attraction between negatively charged surfaces mediated by spherical counterions with quadrupolar charge distribution. *J. Chem. Phys.*, 129, pp. 105101. Copyright 2008, AIP Publishing LLC.

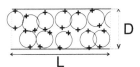

Figure 14.8 Schematic representation of spherical charged divalent nanoparticle positions and orientations at distance $D \simeq 4$ nm, where the diameter of the macro-ion is $l = 2$ nm. At the distance $D = 4$ nm, a peak in the density distribution of charges appears in the middle between the surfaces, as seen in Fig. 14.7.

Figure 14.9 shows the orientational order of the nanoparticles in terms of the nematic order parameter $S = \langle (3\cos^2(\vartheta) - 1)/2 \rangle$, where the angle ϑ describes the orientation of the axis connecting the two charges of the nanoparticle with respect to the x axis. $S = 0$ means that the nanoparticles are not oriented, while $S = 1$

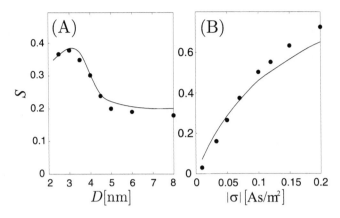

Figure 14.9 The average order parameter $S = \langle (3\cos^2\vartheta - 1)/2 \rangle$ describing the average orientation of divalent spherical nanoparticles ($Z = 1$), where ϑ is measured with respect to the x axis (A): as a function of the distance between the charged surfaces D for $Z = 1$, $l = 2$ nm, $\sigma = -0.07$ As/m^2 and (B): as a function of the surface charge density $|\sigma|$ for $Z = 1$, $l = 2$ nm, $D = 2.5$ nm. Lines: solutions of the integro-differential Eq. 14.33. Points: results of the MC simulations. Reprinted with permission from Urbanija, J., Bohinc, K., Bellen, A., Maset, S., Iglič, A., Kralj-Iglič, V., and Sunil Kumar, P. B., Attraction between negatively charged surfaces mediated by spherical counterions with quadrupolar charge distribution. *J. Chem. Phys.*, 129, pp. 105101. Copyright 2008, AIP Publishing LLC.

corresponds to the nanoparticles being fully oriented with respect to the reference axis.

The average orientation of the quadrupoles entrapped in the spherical nanoparticles is orthogonal to the charged surfaces, in contrast to the configuration of rod-like nanoparticles (May et al., 2008), which is mostly parallel. The order parameter S is sensitive to the charge density of the surface. As larger $|\sigma|$ gives a stronger field and a steeper gradient of the field in the vicinity of the charged surfaces, S increases with increase in $|\sigma|$. The dependence of S on D, however, exhibits a maximum close to an intercharge distance $D \approx l$ (Fig. 14.7).

The concept of free energy decrease due to orientational ordering was previously used in determination of the equilibrium shapes of phospholipid bilayers (Jorgačevski et al., 2010; Kralj-Iglič et al., 1999, 2006) (see also Sections 7.1 and 7.8), where it was shown that the in-plane orientational ordering of membrane constituents can decrease the free energy of a phospholipid vesicle by stabilizing shapes with larger area regions of unequal principal membrane curvatures. The in-plane ordering of membrane components was later generalized to 3-D ordering of ions in the electric double layer (May et al., 2008; Urbanija et al., 2008b). The results in this section show that internal degrees of freedom (orientational and positional ordering of constrained charges), coupled with a particular form of direct interaction between the charges (an imposed fixed distance within pairs of charges within nanoparticles), contribute to the decrease of the free energy of the system of spherical charged nanoparticles between two charged surfaces. Orientational ordering enables the nanoparticles to attain a configuration which is energetically most favourable. The effect is strong enough to cause an attractive interaction between like-charged surfaces. The origin of the bridging attraction in the system of spherical-charged nanoparticles with quadrupolar charge distribution (Urbanija et al., 2008b) is identical to that in the system of rod-like charged nanoparticles (Bohinc et al., 2004; Kim et al., 2008; May et al., 2008), namely the energetically favourable orientational ordering of the quadrupoles in the spatially varying electric field. However, in the system of spherical charged nanoparticles, the orientation of the quadrupoles is in effect orthogonal to the charged surfaces for all distances between the charged surfaces, while in the system of rod-like charged nanoparticles, the orientation of the rods is in effect parallel to the charged surfaces, except for distances D which are close to the charge separation within the rods l, where both the parallel and the orthogonal orientations are energetically favoured (Urbanija et al., 2008b).

It should be noted that the attractive interaction between like-charged surfaces described in this chapter is obtained within the density functional theory which is a mean-field approach (Fig. 14.6). This interaction vanishes when the two charges within a single nanoparticle are brought towards the centre of the ion, as is obtained in the the standard Gouy–Chapman theory, to which our equations reduce when the parameter l approaches zero (Urbanija et al., 2008b).

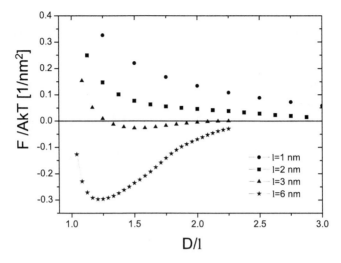

Figure 14.10 Normalized free energy $f = F/AkT$ as a function of the distance between the negatively charged surfaces D for four different extensions l between the charges within the charged nanoparticles. Other parameters are $Z = 1$, $\sigma = -0.033\,\text{As/m}^2$ and $l_B = 0.7\,\text{nm}$. Reprinted with permission from Urbanija, J., Bohinc, K., Bellen, A., Maset, S., Iglič, A., Kralj-Iglič, V., and Sunil Kumar, P. B. (2008b). Attraction between negatively charged surfaces mediated by spherical counterions with quadrupolar charge distribution. *J. Chem. Phys.*, 129, pp. 105101. Copyright 2008, AIP Publishing LLC.

Figure 14.10 shows that the interaction between the charged surfaces changes from attractive to repulsive as the distance between the charges in a single charged nanoparticle (l) decreases at a fixed surface charge density σ. Thus, the attraction between the like-charged surfaces shown in Fig. 14.6 does not derive from correlated interaction between the charged spherical nanoparticles. Instead, the attraction originates from intra-particle charge interactions, that is, an imposed inter-charged interaction expressed by a fixed distance between the charges within a single nanoparticle (Fig. 14.4). This effect may be also very important in DNA condensation by polyamines (Raspaud et al., 1998), since polyamines are water soluble linear molecules with monovalent charges separated at distance l in the nanometer range.

To conclude, it is shown in this section that the density functional theory (which does not include direct interactions between nanoparticles) and the MC simulation (which in contrast does include direct interactions between nanoparticles) show remarkably good agreement for the volume charge density profiles between charged surfaces (Fig. 14.7) and for the average orientational order parameter of the nanoparticles (Fig. 14.9). We thus argue that the bridging effect arising from the orientational ordering of nanoparticles with internal charge distribution is sufficient for attractive interaction between like-charged surfaces, as revealed within the mean-field approach (May et al., 2008; Urbanija et al., 2008b). The direct interaction between charged nanoparticles may give rise to additional effects.

14.1.2 *Counterions and Coions*

In the previous section, the functional density theory was used to describe attractive interactions between two negatively charged surfaces. However, Section 14.1.1 is limited to a system of two like-charged surfaces separated by a solution of multivalent counterions only. In order to describe theoretically the observed plasma-mediated (Fig. 14.1) or IgG antibody-mediated attractive interactions between negatively charged membranes (see Chapter 18 and Frank et al., 2008), this section is extended to the more general case of an solution composed of two kinds of charged nanoparticles, that is, positively and negatively charged multivalent charged nanoparticles. The results presented in this section indicate that in systems with both positive and negative nanoparticles (plasma (Fig. 14.1) or IgG antibody solutions) with internal charge distribution, attractive interactions between like-charged membranes can also occur. It is shown that the positional and orientational ordering of positive and negative nanoparticles with spatially distributed charges is crucial for this process (phenomenon).

The model is basically the same as described in the previous Section 14.1.1. In the model, the charge of a single-charged nanoparticle is composed of two negative or positive charges (each of the valency Z), separated by the distance l equal to the diameter of the nanoparticle. The solution of positive and negative

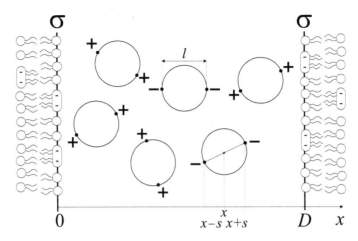

Figure 14.11 Schematic representation of two like-charged planar surfaces, interacting in an electrolyte solution that contains spherical positive and negative nanoparticles. The separation between the individual charges of each spherical nanoparticle is denoted by l, the distance between two surfaces is D. The position of each charge within the nanoparticle is described by the reference position of the centre (x) and the distance $|s| < l/2$. Reprinted with kind permission from Springer Science+Business Media: Perutková, Š., Frank, M., Bohinc, K., Bobojevič, K., Zelko, J., Rozman, B., Kralj-Iglič, V., and Iglič, A. (2010). Interaction between equally charged membrane surfaces mediated by positively and negatively charged nanoparticles. *J. Membr. Biol.*, 236, pp. 43–53.

nanoparticles is sandwiched between two large, planar negatively charged surfaces (Fig. 14.11) with surface charge density σ. The distance between the two charged surfaces is again denoted as D. As well as in the case of counterions only (Section 14.1.1), we assume here that there is no electric field behind the charged surfaces, which is equivalent to the condition of electroneutrality of the whole system. The electrostatic field varies only in the normal direction between the two charged surfaces (i.e., in the x-direction). The charged spherical nanoparticles are characterized by a positional and an orientational degree of freedom.

The number density $n_i(x)$ refers to the number density of nanoparticle centres. If the centre of the charged nanoparticle is located at position x, then the two point charges of the nanoparticle are located at geometrically opposite sides, that is, at $x + s$ and

$x - s$ with a certain probability density $p_i(s|x)$ for each value of s. Here, $i = +$ stands for positively charged nanoparticles and $i = -$ for negatively charged nanoparticles. Taking into account that the two point charges are indistinguishable, all possible orientations of a nanoparticle can be described by the values of s in the interval $0 < s < l/2$ (see Fig. 14.11). Therefore, the probability density should satisfy the conditions (Perutková et al., 2010a):

$$\frac{2}{l} \int_0^{l/2} ds \, p_i(s|x) = 1 \qquad (14.35)$$

and

$$p_i(s|x) = 0 \qquad (14.36)$$

for any x and $s > l/2$.

The free energy of the system (normalized per unit area of the charged surface A and thermal energy kT) is composed of the energy stored in the electrostatic field (first line) and the translational and orientational entropy (second and third line) of the charged spherical nanoparticle (Perutková et al., 2010a):

$$\frac{F}{AkT} = \frac{1}{8\pi l_B} \int_0^D dx \, \Psi'(x)^2$$

$$+ \int_0^D dx \left[\sum_{i=\pm} n_i(x) \ln \frac{n_i(x)}{n_0} + 2n_0 - \sum_{i=\pm} n_i(x) \right]$$

$$+ \int_0^D dx \sum_{i=\pm} n_i(x) \frac{2}{l} \int_0^{l/2} ds \, p_i(s|x) \ln p_i(s|x), \qquad (14.37)$$

where $\Psi(x)$ is the reduced electrical potential (Eq. 13.70), $n_i(x)$ is the number density of the centres of the macro-ions of type i, n_0 is the bulk number density of positive and negative macro-ions, and $l_B = 0.7$ nm is the approximate value of the Bjerrum length in water (Eq. 13.76). The second line in Eq. 14.37 describes the translational entropy of positively and negatively charged nanoparticles in the system in the limit of infinite dilution (Eq. 13.34). The third line in Eq. 14.37 is the orientational entropy of all nanoparticles in the system and is calculated by summation over all positive and negative nanoparticles in the space between the two charged surfaces, where the integral of $p_i(s|x) \ln p_i(s|x)$, running over all possible ds, gives the orientational entropy of a single nanoparticle at position x.

As in the previous Section 14.1.1, the centres of the nanoparticles are assumed to be restricted only to the region $l/2 \leq x \leq (D - l/2)$ (see Fig. 14.11), which ensures that the spherical nanoparticles cannot penetrate through the membrane surfaces. In thermal equilibrium, the free energy $F = F[n_i(x), p_i(s|x)]$ is minimal with respect to the functions $n_i(x)$ and $p_i(s|x)$. From a similar variational procedure as described in the previous section, taking into account the constraint (Eq. 14.35) and the constraints for conservation of the total numbers of positively and negatively charged nanoparticles, follows the expression for conditional probability (Perutková et al., 2010a):

$$p_i(s|x) = \frac{e^{-iZ\Psi(x+s)-iZ\Psi(x-s)}}{\langle e^{-iZ\Psi(x+s)-iZ\Psi(x-s)} \rangle}, \ i = +-, \tag{14.38}$$

and the number density of the centres of the positively and negatively charged nanoparticles (Perutková et al., 2010a):

$$n_i(x) = n_0 \langle e^{-iZ\Psi(x+s)-iZ\Psi(x-s)} \rangle, \ i = +, - \tag{14.39}$$

where $n_i(x)$ is defined only in the region $l/2 \leq x \leq (D - l/2)$ and the average value of an arbitrary function $g(x, s)$ in the region $0 \leq s \leq l/2$ is defined as in Eq. 14.6.

The magnitude of the local volume charge density due to the charged nanoparticles of i-th type at coordinate x ($\rho_i(x)$) contains the contribution from the charges of the nanoparticles of i-th type having their centres located in the region $[x - l/2, x + l/2]$:

$$\frac{\rho_i(x)}{Z e_0} = \langle n_i(x-s, s) + n_i(x+s, s) \rangle, \ i = +, -, \tag{14.40}$$

where $n_i(x - s, s) = n_i(x - s) p_i(s|x - s)$ is the contribution of the nanoparticles with their centres located on the left side of x at the positions $(x - s)$, while $n_i(x + s, s) = n_i(x + s) p_i(s|x + s)$ is the contribution of the nanoparticles with their centres located on the right side of x at the positions $(x + s)$. The function $n_i(x, s)$ is defined in the same way as in the previous section:

$$n_i(x, s) = n_i(x) p_i(s|x). \tag{14.41}$$

Substituting Eqs. 14.38 and 14.39 into Eq. 14.40 yields the total charge density $\rho(x)$ in the form:

$$\frac{\rho(x)}{Z\,e_0} = \sum_{i=\pm} i\,\frac{\rho_i(x)}{Z\,e_0} = 2\,n_0 \sum_{i=\pm} i\,\langle e^{-i\,Z\,\Psi(x) - i\,Z\,\Psi(x+2s)} \rangle, \quad (14.42)$$

where Eqs. 14.38 and 14.39 were taken into account.

By substituting $\rho(x)$ from Eq. 14.42 into the Poisson equation $\Psi''(x) = -4\pi\,l_B\,\frac{\rho(x)}{e_0}$, we obtain the integro-differential equation for the reduced electric potential:

$$\Psi''(x) = -8\pi\,l_B\,Z\,e_0\,n_0 \sum_{i=\pm} i\,\langle e^{-i\,Z\,\Psi(x)-i\,Z\,\Psi(x+2s)} \rangle. \quad (14.43)$$

The boundary conditions at both charged surfaces are given by Eqs. 14.34. The numerical solution of Eq. 14.43, taking into account the boundary conditions (Eq. 14.34) yields the equilibrium potential $\Psi(x)$, the equilibrium number density $n_i(x)$ (Eq. 14.39) and the probability densities $p_i(s|x)$ (Eq. 14.38) for different values of the charge parameter

$$P = 2\sigma\pi\,l_B\,l_D/e_0, \quad (14.44)$$

where $l_D = (\varepsilon_r\,\varepsilon_0\,k\,T/8\,e_0^2\,n_0)^{1/2}$ is the Debye length. This definition of the Debye length is equivalent to that of a 2:2 electrolyte, containing divalent point-like ions, where valency $Z = 2$ (Eq. 13.71).

The density profile of the charge between two negatively charged surfaces is depicted in Figs. 14.12 and 14.13 for different values of charge parameter P (Eq. 14.44) and different distances between the charged surfaces D. For comparison, the calculated number densities $n_i(x)$ and corresponding volume charge density $\rho_i(x)$ between the charged surfaces are also determined by MC simulations.

The standard Metropolis algorithm was used in the MC simulations (Metropolis et al., 1953) as described in the previous Section 14.1.1 for the model schematically shown in Fig. 14.11. The canonical system consisted of a mixture of positively and negatively charged spheres (there were between 100 and 178 spheres in a box with volume AD, where D is the distance between two negatively charged surfaces with area A). The shortest distance between positive and negative charges was set to be of the magnitude of the Bjerrum length ($l_B = 0.7\,\text{nm}$) to avoid agglutination of opposite

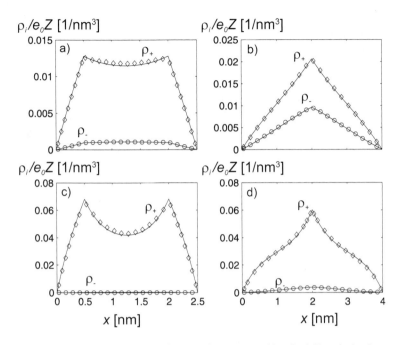

Figure 14.12 The volume charge density profile ($\rho_i(x)$) of divalent spherical nanoparticles ($l = 2$ nm, $Z = 1$) between two negatively charged surfaces calculated for two different values of charge parameter P and two different distances D: (a) $P = -0.1$, $D = 2.5$ nm; (b) $P = -0.1$, $D = 4$ nm; (c) $P = -0.5$, $D = 2.5$ nm; (d) $P = -0.5$, $D = 4$ nm. Theoretical predictions of $\rho_i(x)$ (lines) are compared to corresponding MC results (diamonds and circles). Reprinted with kind permission from Springer Science+Business Media: Perutková, Š., Frank, M., Bohinc, K., Bobojevič, K., Zelko, J., Rozman, B., Kralj-Iglič, V., and Iglič, A. (2010). Interaction between equally charged membrane surfaces mediated by positively and negatively charged nanoparticles. *J. Membr. Biol.*, 236, pp. 43–53.

charges to each other, and consequently to retain random movement of the particles. Due to repulsive forces, the distance between equal charges was considered to be arbitrary. The number of positively and negatively charged nanoparticles (N_+, N_-) was determined in accordance with theoretical predictions so that the system was kept electroneutral by the relation: $A^{1/2} = ((N_+ - N_-)e_0/\sigma)^{1/2}$. From MC simulations it was then possible to obtain the volume charge

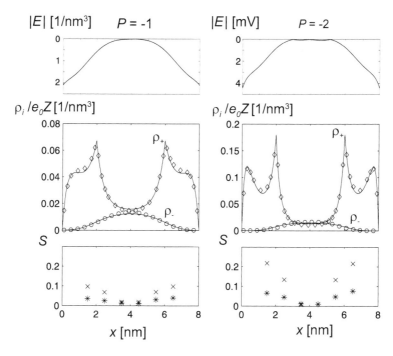

Figure 14.13 The spatial dependence of the magnitude of electric field strength (first row), the volume charge density of the positively charged nanoparticles (counterions) and negatively charged nanoparticles (coions) (second row), and the average order parameter S computed in six slices along the x-axis (positive nanoparticles: crosses, negative nanoparticles: stars) (third row) in the space between the two charged surfaces at the distance $D = 8$ nm. The value of the charge parameter: $P = -1$ (first column), $P = -2$ (second column). The values of other model parameters: $l = 2$ nm, $Z = 1$. Reprinted with kind permission from Springer Science+Business Media: Perutková, Š., Frank, M., Bohinc, K., Bobojevič, K., Zelko, J., Rozman, B., Kralj-Iglič, V., and Iglič, A. (2010). Interaction between equally charged membrane surfaces mediated by positively and negatively charged nanoparticles. *J. Membr. Biol.*, 236, pp. 43–53.

densities of the positive and negative nanoparticles between the negatively charged surfaces ($\rho_i(x)$) as well as their orientation.

The very good agreement between the theoretical prediction and MC simulations can be seen in Figs. 14.12 and 14.13 for low values of $|P|$ (i.e., low $|\sigma|$), as well as for higher values of $|P|$ (i.e., higher $|\sigma|$).

Figure 14.13 shows the dependence of the average order parameter $S = \langle (3\cos^2(\vartheta) - 1)/2 \rangle$ on position in the space between the charged surfaces. The average order parameter $S = \langle (3\cos^2(\vartheta) - 1)/2 \rangle$ within the slices of thickness $l/2 = 1$ nm along the x axis direction was calculated to find the orientation of the nanoparticles as a function of variation of the electric field strength in the space between the two charged surfaces (Perutková et al., 2010a). For positively charged nanoparticles the average order parameter was defined with respect to the reference orientation along the x direction, while for the negatively charged nanoparticles with respect to the reference orientation along the y direction. The value $S = 0$ corresponds to random orientation of the macro-ions, while the value $S = 1$ coincides with fully oriented macro-ions along the reference axis. It can be seen in Fig. 14.13 that at $x = D/2$, where the magnitude of the electric field strength $E = 0$, the value of $S = 0$. As the absolute value of E increases in directions towards the two charged surfaces, the order parameter S also increases in these two directions (Fig. 14.13). Therefore, S has its highest value when the particle is in the close vicinity of the charged surface. The values of S for spherical nanoparticles near the charged surfaces increase with increase in surface charge density $|\sigma|$ (Gongadze et al., 2013; Perutková et al., 2010a). Such behaviour of the average orientations of the nanoparticles, together with the fact that the number density of their centres is usually the highest at the distance $l/2$ from the surface, contribute to the phenomenon that positively charged spherical nanoparticles try to bridge negatively charged surfaces at $D \cong l$, as shown in Fig. 14.14.

Figure 14.14 shows the equilibrium distances between the charged walls (D_{eq}) where the free energy $F(D)$ exhibits an absolute minimum. The values of D_{eq} are shown as a function of nanoparticle diameter l for different values of the charge parameter P. The results correspond to electrostatic bridging, as also predicted in Figs. 14.12 (a) and 14.12 (c). At large diameters the equilibrium distance D_{eq} is approximately equal to the diameters of the spherical macro-ions l.

As indicated in experimental studies of agglutination of charged giant phospholipid vesicles with physiologically relevant contents of negative charge in solutions with added blood plasma (Fig. 14.1) or added IgG antibodies (see Chapter 18), macro-ions with internal

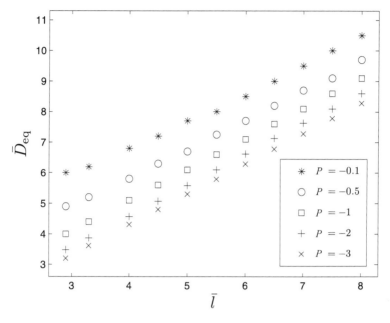

Figure 14.14 Stable equilibrium distances between the charged surfaces D_{eq} as a function of l for different charge parameters P, $Z = 1$. The values $\bar{D} = D/l_D$ and $\bar{l} = l/l_D$ are values of the distance between the two walls and the diameter of the spherical charged nanoparticles, respectively, normalized by the Debye length $l_D = 1$ nm. Reprinted with kind permission from Springer Science+Business Media: Perutková, Š., Frank, M., Bohinc, K., Bobojevič, K., Zelko, J., Rozman, B., Kralj-Iglič, V., and Iglič, A. (2010). Interaction between equally charged membrane surfaces mediated by positively and negatively charged nanoparticles. *J. Membr. Biol.*, 236, pp. 43–53.

charge distribution may indeed induce strong attractive interaction between two negatively charged membranes.

To conclude, using functional density theory and MC simulations it was shown in this section that spherical nanoparticles with distinctive internal charge distribution may be strongly oriented in the vicinity of oppositely charged surfaces which may lead to bridging (attractive) forces between like-charged membrane surfaces at small separation distances (see also Fig. 14.15). The predicted equilibrium distances between two negatively charged membrane surfaces (D_{eq}) are only slightly larger than the diameter of the charged nanoparticles. Consequently, at the equilibrium

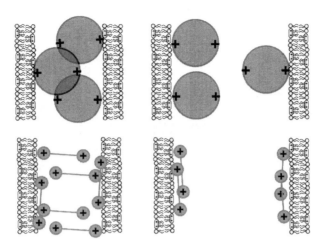

Figure 14.15 Schematic figure representing the different orientational ordering of rod-like and spherical macro-ions at small (left) and large (right) distance between two like-charged surfaces. Due to their stronger average orientation in the orthogonal direction spherical macro-ions are better mediators of attractive interactions between like-charged surfaces than rod-like macro-ions. Figure adapted from Gongadze et al. (2013).

distance between two negatively charged surfaces there is practically no space for negatively charged nanoparticles (coions) which are nearly completely excluded from the space between the charged membranes (see Figs. 14.12(a,c)) so that bridging attractive interactions mediated by positively charged nanoparticles (counterions) prevail.

The average orientation of macro-ions in the solution between two like-charged surfaces have a strong influence on the attractive–repulsive interaction between like-charged surfaces (Gongadze et al., 2013; Kim et al., 2008; May et al., 2008; Perutková et al., 2010a; Urbanija et al., 2008b). Stronger orientation of the macro-ions in the orthogonal direction with respect to the charged surface contributes to stronger attraction between the like-charged surfaces. Based on the results presented in (Gongadze et al., 2013; Kabaso et al., 2011b; Perutková et al., 2013; Urbanija et al., 2008b), Fig. 14.15 shows schematically the difference in orientational ordering between rod-like and spherical macro-ions for small and large distance between the two like-charged surfaces. For small distances some of the rod-like macro-ions are oriented orthogonally to the charged surfaces and some in a direction parallel to the charged surfaces (Fig. 14.15). On the other hand, for larger distances all rod-like macro-ions are oriented in a direction parallel to the charged surfaces (Gongadze et al., 2013; Perutková et al., 2013) (Fig. 14.15). In accordance with our observation, a rod-like macro-ion-mediated attractive interaction between two like-charged surfaces was predicted at small distances (Kim et al., 2008).

On the other hand, at high enough surface charge densities and macro-ion valency spherical macro-ions are mostly oriented orthogonally even for higher surface separations (Fig. 14.15) leading to the conclusion that spherical macro-ions are better mediators of attractive interactions between like-charged surfaces than rod-like macro-ions.

Excellent agreement between the results of functional density theory and MC simulations is predicted even at higher values of the coupling constant (Perutková et al., 2010a). This may be explained by the fact that at sufficiently large distances (l) between the two charges within a single charged divalent nanoparticle (see Fig. 14.11), the charge–charge correlation within the single-charged nanoparticle (i.e., intra-particle correlation) plays an important role. This is the main reason why the predictions of the functional density theory presented are in good agreement with the predictions of MC simulations over a large range of model parameters, in spite of the fact that the inter-particle (inter-ionic) correlations are neglected in the mean-field functional density theory. It is therefore expected that the agreement would not be so good for smaller distances between the charges l within a single nanoparticle (i.e., when the distances between the two charges would be smaller than the diameter of the nanoparticle) and especially for point-like nanoparticles where the distance between charges l would approach zero.

The above described theoretical analysis (Perutková et al., 2010a) involves a number of approximations, such as neglecting the image forces due to the different relative (dielectric) constant of a water solution of charged nanoparticles and the membrane. Also we totally neglected the short-range attractive van der Waals forces and the short range attractive or oscillatory hydration forces between charged surfaces which might be important if the sugar residues attached to proteins and lipids on the membrane surface do not eliminate them (Israelachvili, 1997).

Nevertheless, it is clearly evident (by functional density theory and MC simulations) that the adhesion between two equally charged surfaces can be driven by Coulombic interactions between the charged surfaces and spherical divalent positively and negatively charged nanoparticles (counterions and coions) (Perutková et al., 2010a). It is indicated that the charged nanoparticle-mediated attractive interaction between like-charged surfaces is primarily driven by orientational and positional ordering of divalent positively and negatively charged nanoparticles if the distance between the charges within the single nanoparticle is large enough (Perutková et al., 2010a).

14.2 Attraction between Negatively Charged Membrane Surfaces Mediated by Bound- Charged Proteins

In this section, we briefly discuss the possible physical origin of the attractive interactions observed between negatively charged membrane surfaces induced by binding of charged proteins to the membrane surface (see Fig. 14.16). Figure 14.17 shows an example of a rod-like (fish hook shape) β_2-GPI molecule (Bouma et al., 1999; Hagihara et al., 1995; Miyakis et al., 2004; Wang et al., 2002) bound to the surface of a negatively charged membrane. It was indicated that the specific spatial distribution of charge within the proteins (e.g., β_2-GPI) attached to the charged membrane surface may induce the attraction between like-charged membrane surfaces (Lokar et al., 2008; Urbanija et al., 2008a).

Atomic force microscopy revealed that bound β_2-GPI has a horizontal-like orientation on the bilayer surface (Gamsjaeger et al., 2005; Hamdan et al., 2007). However, the terminal charged groups of β_2-GPI are considered to participate in electrostatic bridging forces between two like-charged membrane surfaces where bound β_2-GPI molecules should have a vertical position with the positively charged first domain bound to the neighbouring membrane (Fig. 14.19 and (Hamdan et al., 2007; Lokar et al., 2008; Urbanija et al., 2008a).

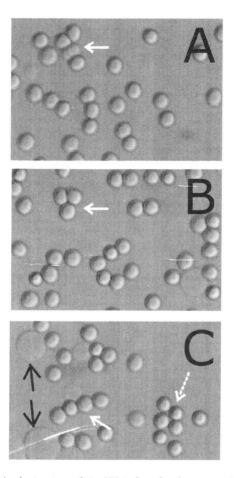

Figure 14.16 Agglutination of β_2-GPI-induced spherocytic RBCs at a low volume density of RBCs in the suspension. White arrows point to complexes of RBCs, that is, chains of self-assembled spherocytic RBCs. The dotted arrow points to RBCs which are not fully agglutinated, but are close together. Black arrows point to the negatively charged POPC-cardiolipin-cholesterol giant vesicles. Some spherocytic RBCs are attached to the giant phospholipid vesicle surface. Reprinted from Bioelectrochemistry, 73(2), Maruša Lokar, Jasna Urbanija, Mojca Frank, Henry Hägerstrand, Blaž Rozman, Malgorzata Bobrowska-Hägerstrand, Aleš Iglič, Veronika Kralj-Iglič, Agglutination of like-charged red blood cells induced by binding of β_2-glycoprotein I to outer cell surface, pp. 110–116, Copyright 2008, with permission from Elsevier.

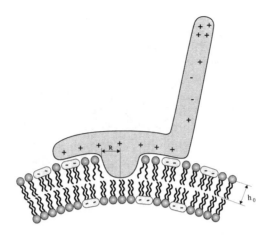

Figure 14.17 Schematic figure of a positively charged protein β_2-GPI attached in a vertical position to the outer surface of a negatively charged bilayer membrane. The hydrophobic protrusion of the attached protein is also shown embedded in the outer lipid layer. The electrostatic interactions of β_2-GPI with negatively charged membrane phospholipids are considered crucial for its physiological and pathogenic roles.

We suggest that β_2-GPI induces attraction between negatively charged membrane surfaces. This attraction is governed by electrostatic attraction between the positively charged first domain on the tip of the membrane-bound β_2-GPI and the negatively charged lipid headgroups of cardiolipin in the opposite membrane (Fig. 14.19).

For the sake of simplicity we assume that bound β_2-GPI is always in a vertical position (Fig. 14.17). The terminal (fifth and first) domains of β_2-GPI have net positive charge (Fig. 14.17). If the membrane is negatively charged, the fifth domain strongly binds to the membrane surface (see Fig. 14.17) because of electrostatic attraction and also because of insertion of the hydrophobic loop into the membrane (Bouma et al., 1999; Schwarzenbacher et al., 1999).

In the simplest theoretical model, we can consider two planar-charged lipid surfaces with an electrolyte (salt) solution between them (Fig. 14.18). The positively charged first domains of membrane-bound β_2-GPI create positively charged region approximately at the distance D of the β_2-GPI's length away from each surface (Fig. 14.18). In the model, the positive charge of the tips of

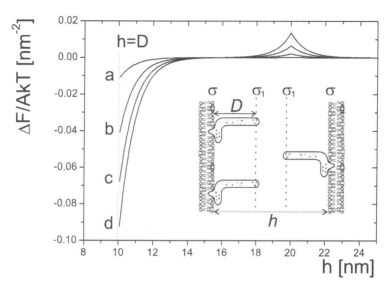

Figure 14.18 Free energy $\Delta F = F - F(h \to \infty)$ as a function of h for four different values of σ_1: 0.001 As/m² (a), 0.004 As/m² (b), 0.007 As/m² (c), 0.01 As/m². The length of the β_2-GPI molecule $D = 10$ nm. The surface charge density of both lipid surfaces and the buffer concentration are constant: $\sigma = -0.02$ As/m². The salt concentration in the bulk solution $n_0/N_A = 15$ mmol/l, where N_A is Avogadro's number.

the β_2-GPI molecules bound to both surfaces is represented by two charged surfaces (with surface charge densities σ_1) at the distance D from each of the lipid surfaces. The electric charge distribution of both lipid surfaces in the first approximation is described by the surface charge densities of both charged surfaces (σ), where the contribution due to fifth domain of bound β_2-GPI molecules is neglected.

Fig. 14.18 shows the free energy (F) of the system:

$$F = \int_0^h \left(\frac{1}{2}\varepsilon_r\varepsilon_0 \left(\frac{d\phi}{dx}\right)^2 + kT \sum_{i=+,-} \left(n_j \ln\left(\frac{n_j}{n_0}\right) - (n_j - n_0) \right) \right) A dx, \tag{14.45}$$

including the configurational entropy of the anions ($i = -$) and cations ($i = +$) (Eq. 13.34), as a function of the distance (h) between the two adjacent membrane surfaces with attached β_2-GPI molecules, calculated as described in (Lokar et al., 2008;

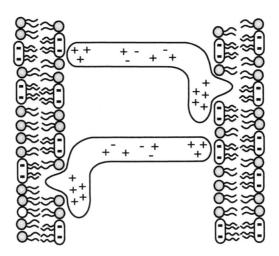

Figure 14.19 β_2-GPI protein-mediated attractive electrostatic interaction between negatively charged membrane surfaces.

Urbanija et al., 2008a). Here, n_j are the number densities of anions ($i = -$) and cations ($i = +$) in the salt solution between the charged membrane surfaces. As can be seen in Fig. 14.18, the free energy F first increases with decrease in intermembrane distance h and then decreases with decrease in h until the absolute minimum of F close to $h \cong D$ is reached. The results presented in Fig. 14.18 reflect the fact that two adjacent membranes without bound β_2-GPI molecules repel each other, while for a high enough concentration of membrane-bound β_2-GPI the force between two negatively charged cardiolipin-containing membranes becomes strongly attractive, leading to the equilibrium distance at $h \cong D$ (Fig. 14.18). The origin of the attractive interactions between two like-charged membrane surfaces is the electrostatic attraction between the positively charged first domain on the tip of the membrane-bound β_2-GPI and the negatively charged components of the opposite membrane (Perutková et al., 2013) (Fig. 14.19).

The strength of the β_2-GPI mediated electrostatic adhesion between negatively charged membrane surfaces ($|\Delta F(h \cong D)|/A$) (Fig. 14.18) strongly decreases with increase in the bulk salt concentration (n_0/N_A) (Lokar et al., 2008). This is in accordance with experimental observations which indicate that the capability of β_2-GPI to induce agglutination of negatively charged giant lipid vesicles or agglutination of negatively charged RBCs decreases with increase in ionic strength (Lokar et al., 2008; Sodin-Šemrl et al., 2008). The observed decreased degree of β_2-GPI-induced agglutination of RBCs at higher ionic strength (Lokar et al., 2008) may also be partially the consequence of altered (reduced) β_2-GPI binding to negatively charged RBCs at higher ionic strength (see also Wang et al., 1998).

In conclusion, in this section we described the attractive force between like-charged membrane surfaces mediated by bound charged proteins with a distinctive internal electric charge distribution. Theoretically, the β_2-GPI-mediated attraction between like-charged membrane surfaces was explained by bridging forces (Fig. 14.19) due to the specific spatial distribution of charge within the β_2-GPI molecules attached to the negatively charged membrane surfaces (Perutková et al., 2013).

14.3 Attraction between a Negatively Charged Nanostructured Implant Surface and Osteoblasts

The cell and tissue reactions to the composition of an implant, and especially to the chemical and physical features of the implant surface, ultimately determine the clinical success of an implant (Gongadze, 2011). The functional activity of cells in contact with the biomaterial is determined by the material characteristics of the surface, as well as by the surface topography (Gongadze et al., 2011a). The most widely used material in a gamut of medical applications is titanium, because it is non-toxic and is not rejected by the body.

In the past, different studies of implant surface modification have been performed at the micrometre scale level to improve the attachment of osteoblasts to the implant surface (Bobyn et al., 1980, 1982; Kabaso et al., 2011b). Recently, the titanium surface was modified by a self-assembled layer of vertically oriented TiO_2 nanotubes with diameters between 15 nm and 100 nm (Fig. 14.20) (Gongadze et al., 2012; Park et al., 2007). It was shown that adhesion, spreading, growth, and differentiation of cells on such vertically

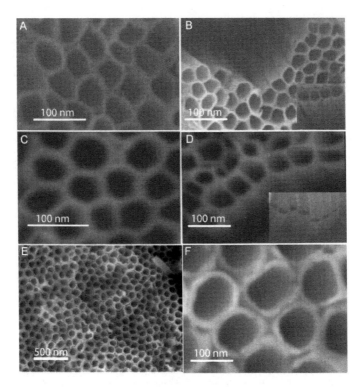

Figure 14.20 Electron microscope images of surface layers of self-assembled vertically aligned TiO$_2$ nanotubes synthesized by the anodization method. For preparation, an ethylene glycol solution with 0.3 wt. was used. The internal TiO$_2$ nanotube diameter is around 50–60 nm (A–D) and 100 nm (E–F), while the length could be up to 10 μm (B)Reprinted from Imani, R., Kabaso, D., Kreft, M. E., Gongadze, E., Penič, S., Elersič, K., Kos, A., Vŕranič, P., Zorec, R., and Iglič, A. Morphological alterations of T24 cells on flat end nanotubular TiO2 surfaces. *Croat Med. J.*, 53, pp. 577–585. Copyright © 2012 by the Croatian Medical Journal. All rights reserved.

aligned TiO$_2$ nanotube surfaces critically depend on the diameter of the nanotubes (Park et al., 2007). A nanotube diameter of 15 nm seemed to be more appropriate for differentiation of mesenchymal, endothelial cells, and smooth muscle cells in comparison to 70–100 nm nanotubes and to amorphous (smooth) TiO$_2$ surfaces (Park et al., 2009b). Moreover, on the 100 nm TiO$_2$ nanotube surface, a larger number of cells underwent apoptosis compared to the 15 nm nanotube surface (Park et al., 2009b). Also cells do not spread on the 100 nm TiO$_2$ nanotube surface but instead develop a morphology with long protrusions (Park et al., 2007).

Titanium oxide nanotube surfaces in the range of 15–20 nm diameter seem to provide optimal topographical properties to support the adhesion of cells. The optimal spacing of 15–20 nm could be determined by the size of the extracellular integrin domain (10–12 nm) which allows or induces clustering of integrins into focal adhesion complexes (Park et al., 2007, 2009b). A smaller spacing of around 10 nm seems to be too small to allow integrin clustering. In line with these results, it was recently shown that bone regeneration on titanium implants with 30 nm nanotube surface is very different from that without nanotubes (von Wilmowsky et al., 2009).

The above described results indicate that the surface nanostructure of the implant is a decisive factor for surface cell adhesion and growth. The topography of TiO$_2$ nanotube surfaces within the very narrow window of 15–20 nm is optimal for certain vital cell processes and is not confined to a specific cell type (Park et al., 2009a,b). In addition, the above mentioned findings seem not to be limited to TiO$_2$ nanotube surfaces only, but are valid more generally for cell response to other topographical nanorough surfaces (Park et al., 2007; Popat et al., 2007, 2006), and could therefore in the future have an important impact on the design and composition of metallic implant surfaces.

The optimum efficiency of cell adhesion and spreading on 15 nm TiO$_2$ nanotube surfaces can be partially explained by the dimensions of the integrin head (Park et al., 2007). Yet the increased adhesion of cells to the 15 nm TiO$_2$ nanotube surface compared to a smooth titanium surface (Park et al., 2007, 2009a,b) must also be connected to the different strength of attractive interactions per unit area.

In this section we show that the increased surface charge density and electric field strength at the highly curved edges of a charged nanostructured surface such as a vertically oriented TiO$_2$ nanotube surface can make the main contribution to the increased strength of osteoblast adhesion (Gongadze et al., 2011a). The proposed explanation is based on the mechanism of protein-mediated attractive interaction between a negatively charged metallic or TiO$_2$ surface and the negatively charged osteoblasts (Kabaso et al., 2011b), as well as on the cation-mediated binding of fibronectin (Heath et al., 2010). Therefore, the electric field strength near the highly curved edge of the metallic or TiO_2 surface is calculated, first in the limit of very sharp edges and finally within the Langevin–Bikerman model (see Section 13.7) for convex charged edges of finite curvature, where the spatial variation of permittivity near the metallic or TiO_2 surface is taken into account (Gongadze et al., 2011a).

14.3.1 Adhesion of Proteins to a Charged Surface

It was recently suggested that contact between the osteoblast membrane and the metallic or TiO_2 implant surface is established in two steps. Firstly, the osteoblast cell membrane makes a non-specific contact due to electrostatic forces (Kabaso et al., 2011b), followed by a second step, where specific binding involving integrin assembly into focal contacts takes place (Monsees et al., 2005; Park et al., 2007; Walboomers and Jansen, 2001).

Since osteoblasts are negatively charged (Smeets et al., 2009), they are electrostatically repelled by the negatively charged implant surface, unless some other attractive force is present in the system. Recently, a possible mechanism of osteoblast adhesion to the implant surface was proposed, assuming that positively charged proteins with internal charge distribution, attached to the negatively charged implant surface, serve as a substrate for the subsequent attachment of the negatively charged osteoblasts (Kabaso et al., 2011b; Smeets et al., 2009; Smith et al., 2004). In order to predict the orientation of such proteins near a charged implant surface, MC simulations of the distribution and the orientation of charged spheroidal proteins in the vicinity of the charged metallic or TiO_2 surface were performed (Gongadze et al., 2013; Kabaso et al., 2011b). It was shown (Gongadze et al., 2013; Kabaso et al., 2011b) that for high enough values of the charge density of the implant surface, the positively charged proteins with internal charge distribution are concentrated close to the charged implant surface and nearly completely oriented in a direction orthogonal to the charged surface (Figs. 14.21A and 14.15). It was also shown (Kabaso et al., 2011b) that at a high enough surface charge density of the implant surface and a distinctive internal charge distribution of the proteins, the

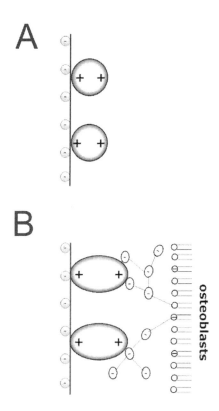

Figure 14.21 A: Schematic figure of the orientation of proteins with internal charge distribution, attached to a negatively charged metallic or TiO_2 surface (Gongadze et al., 2013; Perutková et al., 2013)(see also Fig. 14.15). For the sake of simplicity, in our model, the charge of a single spherical macro-ion is composed of two positive charges separated by a finite distance. B: Schematic figure of protein-mediated attraction between a negatively charged implant surface (left) and a negatively charged osteoblast surface (see also Gongadze et al., 2011a; Kabaso et al., 2011b). Two adjacent negatively charged implant and osteoblast surfaces without bound positively charged proteins repel each other, while for a high enough concentration of bound positively charged proteins with internal charge distribution the force between two negatively charged surfaces becomes strongly attractive (Gongadze et al., 2011a; Kabaso et al., 2011b), leading to an equilibrium distance approximately equal to the dimension of the proteins (see also Sections 14.1.1 and 14.2). Note that the positively charged proteins have a distinctive internal electric charge distribution.

positively charged proteins with internal charge distribution can turn the repulsive force between the negatively charged implant surface and the osteoblast surface into an attractive force. The corresponding attractive force is also called a bridging force (Kabaso et al., 2011b; Perutková et al., 2013). As described in Sections 14.1.1 and 14.2, the origin of the attractive interactions between two negatively charged surfaces is the electrostatic attraction between the positively charged domains on the tips of the titanium surface-bound proteins and the negative charges of the opposite osteoblast membrane (Fig. 14.21B). In accordance with the above suggested mechanism of protein-mediated interaction between negatively charged osteoblasts and the negatively charged implant surface, many studies in the past indicated that an increased negative surface potential on the implant promotes osteoblast adhesion and consequently, new bone formation (Gongadze et al., 2011a; Oghaki et al., 2001; Smeets et al., 2009; Teng et al., 2000).

In line with the predicted increase in strength of the protein-mediated attractive interaction between the negatively charged implant surface and osteoblast with increasing surface charge density (and electric field strength) (Kabaso et al., 2011b), we propose that the increased surface charge density and increased electric field strength at the sharp edges of the implant surface may promote protein-mediated adhesion of osteoblasts to the nanorough implant regions due to the increased accumulation of positively charged proteins with internal charge distribution (see Gongadze et al., 2011a, and Fig. 14.22A).

The increased electric field strength and surface charge density of nanorough implant regions with sharp edges and spikes may also promote the (divalent) cation-mediated adsorption of fibronectin to the negatively charged implant surface (Gongadze et al., 2012), and also in this way the integrin-mediated adsorption of cells to these implant regions. Fibronectin is an extracellular glycoprotein with a critical role in the process of cell adhesion (Gongadze et al., 2012; Heath et al., 2010). A hallmark of fibronectin function is its characteristic assembly into filaments and fibres to form an insoluble matrix which functions as a scaffold onto which extracellular domains of integrin molecules from the cell membrane are attached (Cooper, 2000; Nelea and Kaartinen, 2010). Fibronectin is negatively

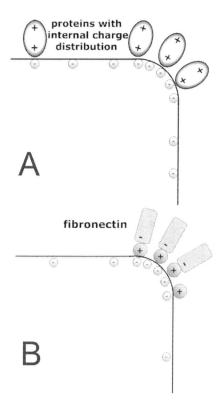

Figure 14.22 (A): Schematic figure of the adhesion of positively charged proteins at the sharp edge of a negatively charged metallic or TiO_2 surface. Due to internal charge distribution the proteins exhibit strong orientation in the direction of the surface normal vector (Gongadze et al., 2011a; Kabaso et al., 2011b). (B): Schematic figure of cation-mediated adhesion of negatively charged fibronectin molecules to the highly curved edge of the implant surface (Gongadze et al., 2012).

charged at physiological values of pH (Bouafsoun et al., 2007). An increase in salt concentration leads to a reduced electrostatic repulsion between fibronectin and the negatively charged implant surface (Heath et al., 2010). Study of the effect of some metal cations revealed an enhancement of fibronectin adsorption on a negatively charged mica surface (Heath et al., 2010). The origin of this effect may be bridging and direct interaction forces (Heath et al., 2010; Urbanija et al., 2008b; Zelko et al., 2010). Accordingly, it was indicated recently that increases in the negative net charge of a TiO_2 (implant) surface increases the fibronectin-mediated binding of osteogenic cell receptors (Rapuano and MacDonald, 2011). Moreover, it was also shown that a significantly higher amount of fibronectin was bound on 15 nm than on 100 nm TiO_2 nanotube surfaces (Gongadze et al., 2012). It was therefore proposed (Gongadze et al., 2011a, 2012) that the cation-mediated adhesion of fibronectin to the sharp edges of TiO_2 nanotubes is reinforced (Fig. 14.22B) by the increased electric field strength and increased surface charge density at sharp edges and spikes such as the edges of TiO_2 nanotube walls (Gongadze et al., 2012). In general, all these results suggest that the negatively charged implant surface plays a prominent role in the osseointegration of implant materials (Gongadze et al., 2011a; Rapuano and MacDonald, 2011).

To conclude, it was suggested that the increased electric field strength and corresponding surface charge density at the highly curved edges of vertically oriented 15 nm TiO_2 nanotubes or at the sharp edges of a rectangular titanium profile is important for efficient adhesion of cells (Gongadze et al., 2011a, 2012). In the case of TiO_2 of larger diameters nanotubes, the area density of the nanotube edge regions with high electric field is not optimal, that is, it is too small (Gongadze et al., 2011a, 2012). Similarly, in the case of wide ridges and grooves of a rectangular profile the area density of the edge regions with high electric field is also too small.

Based on the above arguments indicating the importance of the electric field strength and surface charge density of the implant surface in adhesion of cells, the electric field strength was calculated for different curvatures of sharp edges on the implant surface (Gongadze et al., 2011a) as described in the next subsection.

14.3.2 Electric Field Strength at Highly Curved Edges of the Implant Surface

In this subsection, the convex edge of the implant surface is first considered in the limit of very high curvature. Then, convex edges of finite curvature are also considered, where water ordering and the finite size of ions are also taken into account within the Langevin–Bikerman model (Section 13.7). For simplicity we assume that the

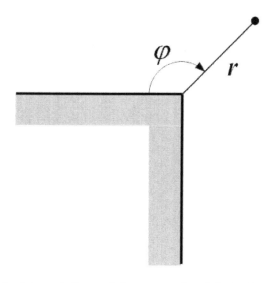

Figure 14.23 Schematic figure of the convex edge of the implant surface in the limit of very high curvature.

curvature of the implant surface in a perpendicular direction along the contour is constant. In order to estimate the electric potential near the convex implant metallic or TiO_2 surface, we solved the Laplace equation in cylindrical coordinates r and φ (Fig. 14.23):

$$\frac{\partial^2 \phi}{\partial r^2} + \frac{1}{r}\frac{\partial \phi}{\partial r} + \frac{1}{r^2}\frac{\partial^2 \phi}{\partial \varphi^2} = 0. \quad (14.46)$$

The solution of Eq. 14.46 in the limit of very high curvature of the convex edge, which mathematically represents a singularity, for small values of r (Fig. 14.23) up to the first order term gives the electric potential $\phi(r, \varphi)$ in the form $\phi = A r^{2/3} \sin(2\varphi/3)$, where A is a constant which can be determined from the additional boundary condition. The electric field strength $\mathbf{E} = -\nabla \phi = \frac{\partial \phi}{\partial r}\mathbf{e}_r + \frac{1}{r}\frac{\partial \phi}{\partial \varphi}\mathbf{e}_\varphi$ is (Gongadze et al., 2011a):

$$\mathbf{E} = -\frac{2A}{3}\frac{1}{r^{1/3}}\left(\sin(2\varphi/3)\mathbf{e}_r + \cos(2\varphi/3)\mathbf{e}_\varphi\right), \quad (14.47)$$

where $\mathbf{e}_r$ and $\mathbf{e}_\varphi$ are unit vectors. It can be seem from Eq. 14.47 that the electric field diverges at the surface edge ($r \to 0$) and then decreases with distance from the edge and the distance from the

Table 14.1 Comparison of the magnitude of the electric field strength at the top of the surface of the convex implant edge (E_{top}) in direction of the symmetry axis $\varphi = 3\pi/4$ (see also Fig. 14.22) calculated for different values of the edge curvature radius (R) within Langevin–Bikerman model

$R/$n m	$E_{\text{top}}/$(V/m)	$\sigma_{\text{top}}/$(As/m^2)
1.0	$4.58 \cdot 10^8$	-0.221
2.0	$4.38 \cdot 10^8$	-0.211
3.0	$4.30 \cdot 10^8$	-0.208
∞	$4.13 \cdot 10^8$	-0.200

Source: Gongadze et al. 2011a.

surface. The dependence of the electric field along the symmetry axis ($\varphi = 3\pi/4$) is (Gongadze et al., 2011a):

$$\mathbf{E}(\varphi = 3\pi/4) = -\frac{2A}{3}\frac{1}{r^{1/3}}\mathbf{e}_r. \qquad (14.48)$$

In the above theoretical consideration, the sharp implant edge mathematically represents a singularity. Yet no physical object has perfect corners but some degree of roundness. Therefore, the sharp edges were modelled as highly curved convex regions of different radii, where it was taken into account that the implant metallic or TiO$_2$ surface is in contact with an electrolyte solution (Gongadze et al., 2011a).

As shown in Table 14.1 (Gongadze et al., 2011a), the electric field strength is even higher if the curvature of the charged surface is increased. From the results summarized in Table 14.1, not only can we confirm high electric fields within the EDL, but also increased field strength on the convex part compared with the flat region ($R \to \infty$).

It can be seen in Table 14.1 that the calculated surface charge density at the surface of greatest curvature of the convex metallic or TiO$_2$ edge (σ_{top}) in the direction of the symmetry axis $\varphi = 3\pi/4$ (see also Fig. 14.23) increases with increase in curvature of the edge $1/R$, where R is the curvature radius. As a consequence the electric field at the top of the curved convex edges of the metallic or TiO$_2$ surface

(E_{top}) increases with increase in edge curvature (Table 14.1), that is, with decreased curvature radius R of the edge. This may explain why the cells are most strongly bound along the sharp convex edges or spikes of nanostructured titanium surfaces (Puckett et al., 2008), where the electric field strength and surface charge density are the highest. The results given in Table 14.1 offer a possible explanation for the increased cation-mediated fibronectin adhesion and charged protein-mediated adhesion of osteoblasts on vertically aligned TiO_2 15 nm nanotubes with respect to adhesion to a smooth titanium surface (Gongadze et al., 2012; Park et al., 2007, 2009a,b). These results can also provide a basic framework for understanding why the actin filaments are strongly oriented and accumulated at the edges of the titanium surface.

Note that in the case of vertically aligned 15 nm diameter TiO_2 nanotubes (Fig. 14.25), the radius of the curvature of the edges of the nanotube walls (R) is substantially smaller than 1 nm, which is the minimal value of R considered in Table 14.1. Therefore, the corresponding electric field at the 15 nm TiO_2 nanotube wall edge is considerably increased (as shown in Table 14.1 in a non-linear manner) with respect to the value for $R = 1$ nm given in Table 14.1.

14.3.3 Clustering of Integrin Molecules in Nanorough Surface Regions with Highly Curved Edges

In previous studies it has been shown that the integration of different cell types is more successful on small diameter (~15 nm) TiO_2 nanotubes than on large diameter (100 nm) nanotubes. It was suggested that due to the extracellular surface of the integrin molecule, the distance between the edges of small diameter nanotubes allows interaction between integrin molecules that are bound to neighbouring sharp edges. Consequently, the free energy of the system is reduced, overcoming the loss of configurational entropy by the aggregation of integrin molecules (Gongadze et al., 2011a). Yet, the underlying mechanisms that drive the adhesion of a cell membrane to the sharp nanotube edges are not fully clear.

Above, in Sections 14.3.1 and 14.3.2, it is suggested that due to the increased electric field strength and increased surface charge density at sharp edges and spikes of different metallic profiles or

TiO$_2$ nanotube surfaces, the cation-mediated adhesion of fibronectin is increased (Fig. 14.22B). The increased fibronectin accumulation in the nanorough regions of metallic surface (Gongadze et al., 2012) with increased electric field strength and increased surface charge density can facilitate the adhesion and aggregation of integrin molecules and therefore induce the formation of focal adhesion complexes (Cooper, 2000).

As was shown in Table 14.1, the electric field strength on the convex metallic surface regions increases with the curvature of the surface, that is, with decreasing radius of curvature. Based on the calculated electric field strength of a curved metallic or TiO$_2$ surface, it was suggested that nanorough regions due to the many highly curved nanoscale protrusions and/or edges have increased electric field strength and surface charge density (Gongadze et al., 2011a). The increased electric field strength and surface charge density of such nanorough regions promote the (divalent) cation-mediated adsorption of fibronectin to the negatively charged surface (Gongadze et al., 2012; Heath et al., 2010) and protein-mediated adhesion of osteoblasts to the negatively charged metallic or TiO$_2$ surface (Kabaso et al., 2011b), both leading to more efficient adhesion of osteoblasts to the nanorough surface (Fig. 14.24 and Gongadze et al., 2011a).

Experimentally, a nanorough region could be obtained using various experimental procedures, for example, by the construction of vertically aligned TiO$_2$ nanotubes (Fig. 14.20). The results of this electrostatic consideration in equilibrium conditions explain the strong attraction of integrin molecules to the sharp edges of the surface, for example, to the edges of the TiO$_2$ nanotube surface (Gongadze et al., 2012).

In accordance with these theoretical predictions, it has been shown recently (Puckett et al., 2008) that a decrease in the width of nanorough regions from 80 μm and 48 μm to 22 μm resulted in significant reduction in the number of osteoblast cells adhering to the structured surface. Osteoblast morphology in the smallest nanorough region (22 μm) was rounder and had less diffuse f-actin filaments, while filopods extending from the cells remained near their origin. It was hypothesized that osteoblasts recognize different surface roughness through the interaction of proteins in

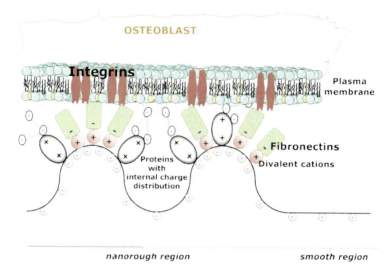

Figure 14.24 The protein-mediated adhesion of osteoblasts to negatively charged nanorough regions of metallic or TiO_2 surfaces is facilitated due to the increased electric field strength and surface charge density at highly curved convex edges and spicules. Republished with permission of DOVE Medical Press, from Gongadze, E., Kabaso, D., Bauer, S., Slivnik, T., Schmuki, P., van Rienen, U., and Iglič, A. (2011). Adhesion of osteoblasts to a nanorough titanium implant surface. *Int. J. Nanomed.*, 6, pp. 1801–1816.; permission conveyed through Copyright Clearance Center, Inc.

the extracellular matrix, which was confirmed in (Gongadze et al., 2011a, 2012). In another study (Lamers et al., 2010), it was shown that osteoblasts are responsive to small nanopatterns of length scale below 100 nm in groove width and depth, as detected by the deposition of minerals (e.g., hydroxypatite) along the nanosize patterns. As already mentioned, the nanorough surface of vertically aligned TiO_2 nanotubes facilitates the adhesion of osteoblasts and other cells compared to the adhesion to a smooth titanium surface (Park et al., 2007, 2009a,b).

Recent experimental data has revealed that the growth and differentiation of osteoblast cells on small diameter (∼15 nm) vertically aligned TiO_2 nanotubes is substantially greater than on large diameter (100 nm) nanotube surfaces (see Fig. 14.25). It has been proposed that the observed aggregation of integrin molecules

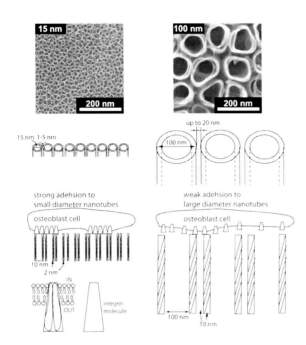

Figure 14.25 Hypothetical model explaining the observed differences in the binding strength of small and large diameter TiO$_2$ nanotubes. Electron microscope images of surfaces of vertically aligned TiO$_2$ nanotubes. Note that the small diameter (15 nm) nanotubes are much more closely packed than the large diameter (100 nm) TiO$_2$ nanotubes. The inner and outer diameter of a small diameter nanotube are approximately 10 nm and 15 nm, and the respective dimensions of a large diameter nanotube are approximately 80 nm and 100 nm. The small diameter nanotube surface has a significantly larger proportion of strong integrin binding regions (due to the larger area density of highly curved nanotube edges) than the large diameter nanotube surface. In addition, the extracellular part of the integrin molecules (of conical shapes) could bind to neigbouring nanotubes on the small diameter nanotube surface, which is not possible on a nanotube surface having too large a hollow interior space, since the interacting integrin molecules are in contact with the nanotube edges. Reprinted from Gongadze, E., Kabaso, D., Bauer, S., Park, J., Schmuki, P., and Iglič, A. (2012). Adhesion of Osteoblast to a Vertically Aligned TiO$_2$ Nanotube Surface. *Mini-Reviews in Medicinal Chemistry*. 13, 194–200, by permission of Eureka Science Ltd., copyright 2012, and republished with permission of DOVE Medical Press, from Gongadze, E., Kabaso, D., Bauer, S., Slivnik, T., Schmuki, P., van Rienen, U., and Iglič, A. (2011). Adhesion of osteoblasts to a nanorough titanium implant surface. *Int. J. Nanomed.*, 6, pp. 1801–1816.; permission conveyed through Copyright Clearance Center, Inc.

forming focal adhesion is enhanced on small diameter nanotubes because the extracellular part of the integrin molecule is of a similar size, enabling cross-binding over the edges of neighbouring nanotubes and over the hollow interiors of vertically oriented TiO_2 nanotubes (Fig. 14.25). In the light of the results presented in this section, it was suggested (Gongadze et al., 2011a) that the enhanced growth of a cell membrane on a nanotube surface is also facilitated by the interaction of integrin molecules during the formation of focal adhesion (Fig. 14.25). Moreover, the fact that small diameter nanotubes on average present more surface edges with increased electric field strength and surface charge density, the binding affinity on the small diameter nanotube surface is expected to be increased (see Fig. 14.25) in accordance with the results presented in Section 14.3.2.

The surface of semiconductor TiO_2 has a certain number of surface titanium and oxygen dangling bonds and therefore at physiological pH some of the available OH^- and H^+ ions in the electrolyte can be chemisorbed to the TiO_2 nanotube surface (Goniakowski and Gillan, 1996). Also chemisorption or adsorption of other ion species present in the electrolyte in contact with the TiO_2 nanotube surface may take place (Ottaviani et al., 1985). In addition, the ions present in the electrolyte used for fabrication of anatase TiO_2 nanotubes by etching of titanium foil (Mohammadpour et al., 2010) can be chemisorbed or adsorbed on the TiO_2 nanotube surface. As a result, the local density of states of the electronic molecular orbitals of surface titanium and oxygen atoms is different from the bulk ones, and consequently, the distribution of electronic charge is different (Mullins, 1998). When the semiconductor TiO_2 is in contact with the electrolyte, in equilibrium the surface of TiO_2 can be positively or negatively charged, depending on the pH value (Fernfindez-Nives et al., 1988). The net exchange of conduction band electrons between TiO_2 and the surrounding electrolyte is possible until in the steady state, the Fermi energies of the semiconductor and electrolyte become equal (Memming, 2007). As a result, a non-zero TiO_2 nanotube surface charge density is established due to the excess/depletion of conduction electrons at the TiO_2 surface which are moved to (or from) the nanotube surface in order to equilibrate the Fermi levels at the TiO_2 nanotube surface, in the bulk of the TiO$_2$ nanotube walls and in the surrounding electrolyte. These conduction electrons (or valence holes in the second case) are free to move so they can be accumulated/depleted at sharp edges of the TiO$_2$ nanotube wall (Gongadze et al., 2012). Also, at the edges of the TiO$_2$ nanotube wall the initial value of the surface Fermi energy (i.e., the Fermi energy before the steady state is reached) may, due to their specific structure, that is, high curvature of the nanotube edge, be different from that in the other regions of the TiO$_2$ nanotube surface. And finally, anions and cations from the electrolyte can also be adsorbed on the TiO$_2$ nanotube surface in a curvature-dependent way (Gongadze et al., 2012). All these processes may contribute to an increased negative surface charge density at the edges of the TiO$_2$ nanotube wall (Gongadze, 2011; Gongadze et al., 2011a, 2012).

In conclusion, nanorough metallic or TiO$_2$ implant regions due to their many highly curved nanoscale protrusions and/or edges have an increased electric field strength and surface charge density (Gongadze, 2011; Gongadze et al., 2011a). The increased electric field strength and surface charge density of such nanorough regions may promote (divalent) cation-mediated adsorption of fibronectin to the negatively charged surface (Fig. 14.22B) (Gongadze et al., 2011a, 2012; Heath et al., 2010) and protein-mediated adhesion of osteoblasts to the negatively charged surface (Fig. 14.21B), both leading to more efficient adhesion and spreading of osteoblasts on the metallic or TiO$_2$ implant surface (Fig. 14.24) (Gongadze, 2011; Gongadze et al., 2011a, 2012).

Chapter 15

Encapsulation of Charged Nanoparticles (Macro-Ions)

Cellular membranes serve as a permeability barrier that large water-soluble charged nanoparticles (macro-ions) are unable to penetrate by simple diffusion. Intra- and extracellular transport of such macro-ions is still possible by a dynamic membrane shape transformation that involves a change of membrane curvature (encapsulation) (Hägerstrand et al., 1999). For example, clathrin-mediated endocytosis controls the curvature of the coated transport vesicles. Membrane vesiculation can also be induced by self-assembly of membrane-adhering choleratoxin molecules (Schara et al., 2009).

Membrane deformation may progress passively, that is, without employing an additional energy source, driven solely by the interaction between the membrane and the macro-ion. One example is the viral budding (Cooper et al., 2003). Another example involves the transfer of drug delivery vehicles into cells. The intracellular entry of genetic material in particular continues to receive considerable attention. To form sufficiently compact aggregates DNA can be complexed with cationic lipids or cationic polymers; both cases result in positively charged condensates that interact

---

Nanostructures in Biological Systems: Theory and Applications
Aleš Iglič, Veronika Kralj-Iglič, and Damjana Drobne
Copyright © 2015 Pan Stanford Publishing Pte. Ltd.
ISBN 978-981-4267-20-5 (Hardcover), 978-981-4303-43-9 (eBook)
www.panstanford.com

electrostatically with the plasma membrane (Lin et al., 2003) which can then be internalized via an encapsulation process which involves membrane bending deformation (Fošnarič et al., 2009; Hägerstrand et al., 1999).

Charged nanoparticles (macro-ions) enveloped by lipid membranes have also promising biotechnological applications (Troutier and Ladaviere, 2007). Yet the lipid shell often lacks stability limiting the control of surface properties. Recent research efforts have thus been directed towards introducing chemical modifications that improve the stability of lipid-coated macro-ions. In addition, physical properties such as the surface topography and particle size contribute to the properties of membrane–macro-ion complexes. Understanding the interplay of the membrane elastic and electrostatic energies of macro-ion–membrane complexes is a prerequisite towards improving complex stability.

To conclude, the encapsulation of a macro-ion (charged nanoparticle) by an oppositely charged membrane is a fundamental process with relevance for cellular drug uptake, viral budding, biotechnological applications and studying the interactions of inorganic nanoparticles with biological membranes.

Encapsulation (wrapping) of charged nanoparticles (macro-ions) by a cell or lipid membrane has been considered in the past by different authors. Harries et al. (2004) used the nonlinear Poisson–Boltzmann (Gouy–Chapman) model (Section 13.5) to investigate the envelopment of charged proteins by initially planar lipid membranes, thereby accounting for the protein-induced demixing of charged lipids in a binary membrane. A comparison of the free energies corresponding to the fully wrapped and unwrapped states suggests encapsulation occurs above a critical protein charge that the authors found compatible with typical charge densities of membrane-penetrating peptide shuttles. In another theoretical study, Fleck and Netz (2004) modelled electrostatic charged nanoparticle–membrane binding by minimizing the free energy of a homogeneously charged membrane with respect to the membrane shape. The authors found that complete encapsulation is possible only for intermediate salt concentrations. However, for small and large salt concentrations only a low degree of wrapping was predicted.

Deserno and coworkers (Deserno, 2004a,b; Deserno and Bickel, 2003) studied the encapsulation of charged nanoparticles for the case of short-range (adhesive) nanoparticle–membrane interactions, where the deformation of an initially flat membrane is determined by the interplay of bending energy and interfacial tension. A discontinuous wrapping transition from the partially to the completely wrapped state of the macro-ion was predicted. If the membrane contains a binary mixture of lipids with opposite spontaneous curvatures, wrapping is facilitated by local lipid demixing (Nowak and Chou, 2008).

Demixing of membrane components is also important if the macro-ion binds to mobile adhesion sites, as is the case in the receptor-mediated uptake of viruses (Gao et al., 2005). The cellular entry of viruses and charged inorganic nanoparticles through the encapsulation process provides a major motivation to further advance models of charged nanoparticle–membrane complexes (Chou, 2007; Fošnarič et al., 2009; Zhang and Nguyen, 2008). Recently, simulations of the encapsulation of charged macro-ions have been performed based on dissipative particle dynamics (Smith et al., 2007) and using a solvent-free coarse-grained membrane model (Reynwar et al., 2007).

In this short chapter we briefly describe the results of Monte Carlo (MC) simulations which were employed to investigate the ability of a charged lipid vesicle to adhere to and encapsulate an oppositely charged macro-ion (Fošnarič et al., 2009). The lipid vesicle contains mobile charged lipids that interact electrostatically with the oppositely charged macro-ion and also among themselves through a screened electrostatic potential. The electric charges of the macro-ion are considered to be immobile. Both migration of the charged lipids of the vesicle membrane and elastic deformations of the vesicle membrane contribute to optimization of the vesicle–macro-ion interaction. Hence, coupling of vesicle-shaped optimization and local-charged segregation at the macro-ion adhesion site was predicted (Fošnarič et al., 2009).

In the MC simulations used, the lipid vesicle was represented by a set of N beads that are linked by tethers of flexible length l so as to form a closed, randomly triangulated, self-avoiding network (Fošnarič et al., 2009; Gompper and Kroll, 2004). The same model has been used previously to study the shapes and fluctuations of one-component (Gompper and Kroll, 1997; Kroll and Gompper, 1992) and two-component (Kohyama et al., 2003; Kumar and Rao, 1998; Kumar et al., 2001) lipid vesicles.

In the MC model membrane, fluidity is maintained by flipping bonds within the triangulated network. That is, the bond between the four given beads of two neighbouring triangles is cut and then re-established between the previously unconnected two beads. For that reason in the MC routine N attempts to change the position of the bead area are also followed by N attempted bond flips (Fošnarič et al., 2009). At the same time, the out-of-plane mobility of the N beads also enables the vesicle to adjust its shape. The MC model also allows in-plane lateral redistribution of the charged lipids for any given vesicle shape. In this way the interaction of the charged lipid vesicle with the oppositely charged spherical nanoparticle is optimized with respect to both the lipid vesicle shape and distribution of charged vertices (charged lipids) (Fošnarič et al., 2009).

Figure 15.1 shows three typical conformations of the macro-ion–vesicle complex as obtained by MC simulations for three different values of the total number of charged lipids in the membrane (M) (Fošnarič et al., 2009). The snapshots of the MC simulations in Fig. 15.1 indicate an interplay between the degree of wrapping and demixing of the charged lipids in the vesicle membrane, that is, charge segregation in the vesicle membrane. All charged lipids are sequestered close to the macro-ion for $M = 15$; the macro-ion is adsorbed on the lipid vesicle but the degree of wrapping is small). The choice $M = 60$ corresponds to almost half the number $Z_{np} N_{np} = 2 \times 65 = 130$ of elementary charges on the macro-ion. Note that very few charges appear to have escaped the membrane-wrapping region due to thermal fluctuations; these charges move essentially unrestrictedly within the non-wrapping part of the vesicle surface. Finally, for $M = 150$ the vesicle charge over-compensates that on the macro-ion, leading to complete encapsulation and a residual fraction of charged lipids on the non-wrapping part of the vesicle surface.

Based on these results (Fig. 15.1), we may conclude that the encapsulation of a spherical macro-ion (charged nanoparticle) is driven by electrostatic interactions between the macro-ion and the oppositely charged vesicle membrane. Since only a fraction of the

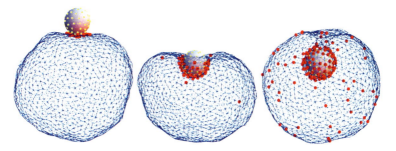

Figure 15.1 The wrapping of a spherical macro-ion. Snapshots of representative macro-ion–vesicle configurations obtained from MC simulations for different numbers of charged lipids (each bearing one unit charge) in the membrane: $M = 15$, $M = 60$, $M = 150$ (from left to right). The shape of the vesicle is represented by a triangulated surface, mobile charged lipids in the vesicle membrane and fixed charges on the macro-ion are indicated by dots. The right figure corresponds to the situation of complete encapsulation of the macro-ion. Model parameters: Debye length $l_D = 3\,l_B$, local membrane bilayer bending constant $k_c = 10\,kT$. The spherical macro-ion carries $N_{np} = 65$ uniformly distributed, point-like, positive charges of valence $Z_{np} = +2$ on its surface. Reprinted with permission from Fošnarič, M., Iglič, A., Kroll, D. M., and May, S. Monte Carlo simulations of complex formation between a mixed fluid vesicle and a charged colloid. *J. Chem. Phys.*, 131, pp. 105103. Copyright 2009, AIP Publishing LLC.

vesicle (mobile) lipids are charged, the encapsulation of the macro-ion is coupled to the lateral segregation of the vesicles charged lipids (Fig. 15.1).

Further, detailed analysis (Fošnarič et al., 2009) predicted a discontinuous wrapping transition from a partial to complete (or almost complete) degree of wrapping. The two energetically preferred states, partially and completely wrapped, can be separated by an energy barrier significantly larger than the thermal energy kT, implying the observation of hysteresis, depending on the initial conditions. Decreasing the local bending constant (k_c) of the vesicle membrane weakens the wrapping transition until a critical point is reached beyond which wrapping becomes a continuous process. The wrapping transition is inhibited if the intrinsic spontaneous curvature of the charged lipids penalizes migration from the bulk to the wrapping region of the vesicle. Interestingly, the preferred shape of the vesicle then becomes clamp-like, that is, non-axisymmetric (Fošnarič et al., 2009).

Chapter 16

Electrostatics and Mechanics of Hydrophilic Pores

The cell membrane is a semi-permeable barrier between the cell interior and its surroundings. One of the mechanisms for transmembrane transport involves the presence of pores in the lipid bilayer, through which a substantial flow of material can take place. For example, pores were observed in red blood cell ghosts (Lew et al., 1982; Lieber and Steck, 1982a,b), where the pore size depends on the ionic strength of the surrounding fluid (Lieber and Steck, 1982a).

The formation of pores in biological membranes can be induced by application of high intensity electric pulses of short duration (Abidor et al., 1979). This phenomenon is known as electroporation and has become widely used in medicine and biology (Lee and Kolodney, 1987; Maček-Lebar et al., 2002a,b; Neumann et al., 1989; Pavlin et al., 2005; Wolf et al., 1994). A number of theoretical studies have been made to understand the physical basis of electroporation (Crowley, 1973; Isambert, 1998). However, the mechanisms responsible for the energetics and stability of membrane pores still require further clarification.

Nanostructures in Biological Systems: Theory and Applications
Aleš Iglič, Veronika Kralj-Iglič, and Damjana Drobne
Copyright © 2015 Pan Stanford Publishing Pte. Ltd.
ISBN 978-981-4267-20-5 (Hardcover), 978-981-4303-43-9 (eBook)
www.panstanford.com

The formation of a hydrophilic pore in a lipid bilayer implies that the lipid molecules near the edge of the pore rearrange themselves in such a way that their polar head groups shield the hydrocarbon tails from water (Chernomordik et al., 1985; Litster, 1975). In the model, the excess energy due to modified packing of the phospholipid molecules at the edge of the pore is described by the line tension which makes the hydrophilic membrane pore energetically unfavourable. On the other hand, there are various examples where membrane pores live long enough to be observed experimentally (Huang, 2000; Karatekin et al., 2003; Lieber and Steck, 1982a). The question arises what mechanisms could be responsible for the stabilization of pores.

A possible mechanism has been suggested by Betterton and Brenner (Betterton and Brenner, 1999) for charged membranes based on competition between line tension and electrostatic repulsion between the opposed membrane rims within the pore. An analysis based on a linearized Gouy–Chapman model (Section 13.5) showed that for certain combinations of model parameters the pore becomes energetically stabilized. However, the depth of the minimum is below kT so that additional stabilizing effects are required to explain the existence of experimentally observed pores (Betterton and Brenner, 1999).

In this chapter, we describe a possible mechanism for the stabilization of pores in charged bilayer membranes, that is, the non-homogeneous lateral distribution and average orientational ordering of anisotropic membrane constituents (molecules, nano-domains), that is, their accumulation and orientation at the edge of the pore (Fošnarič et al., 2003; Kandušer et al., 2003). An anisotropic membrane component (molecule, nanodomain) (Fournier, 1996; Kralj-Iglič et al., 1996, 1999) may be a single molecule (Fig. 7.1) or a small complex of molecules (nanodomain) (Chapter 8). Isotropic and anisotropic membrane constituents (molecules, nanodomains) may laterally distribute in such way as to minimize the membrane free energy (Aranda-Espinoza et al., 1996; Bobrowska et al., 2013; Kralj-Iglič et al., 1996, 2005; Kumar et al., 2001; Laradji and Kumar, 2004; Lipowsky and Dimova, 2003; Markin, 1981; Sackmann, 1994). The lateral distribution of membrane constituents and in-plane average orientational ordering of anisotropic membrane constituents can be considered theoretically (Bobrowska et al., 2013; Fournier, 1996; Iglič et al., 2004b; Jorgačevski et al., 2010; Kralj-Iglič et al., 2006) as described in details in Sections 7.1 and 9.1 (see also Fig. 7.2). Non-homogeneous lateral and orientational distributions of anisotropic membrane constituents represent internal degrees of freedom. A method has been described in previous chapters starting from a microscopic description of the membrane constituents and applying the methods of statistical mechanics to obtain the membrane free energy (Chapter 9.1). To obtain the equilibrium configuration of the membrane, the membrane free energy was minimized taking into account the relevant geometrical constraints. The intrinsic properties of membrane constituents and interactions between them are thereby revealed in the equilibrium shape of the lipid vesicles (Section 7.8) and biological membranes (Section 9.1 and Božič et al., 2006; Bobrowska et al., 2013; Iglič et al., 2004b; Jorgačevski et al., 2010; Kralj-Iglič et al., 2006; Lipowsky and Dimova, 2003; Markin, 1981; Urbanija et al., 2008a).

In this chapter, we describe the effect of the intrinsic shape of anisotropic membrane constituents and the ionic strength on the stability of pores in lipid bilayers. The model presented is based on minimization of the free energy which involves three contributions: the energy due to the line tension of the lipid bilayer at the rim of the pore, the electrostatic energy of the charged membrane with the pore, and the energy of anisotropic membrane constituents (molecules, nanodomains). In order to calculate the electrostatic energy of the membrane with the pore, the electric potential in the vicinity of an infinite, uniformly charged plate with a circular pore is calculated analytically.

Anisotropic membrane constituents (Figs. 7.1, 8.2 and 8.6) are of special interest for the formation of membrane pores since the anisotropic pore rim (Fig. 16.1) provides a geometry with which anisotropic membrane constituents favourably interact. Of particular interest in this respect are peptide (Lin and Baumgaertner, 2000; Sperotto, 1997; Zemel et al., 2003; Zuckermann and Heimburg, 2001) or detergent (Kandušer et al., 2003; Troiano et al., 1998) stabilization of the membrane pore. Detergents and certain antimicrobial peptides are amphiphilic, often exhibiting their lytic

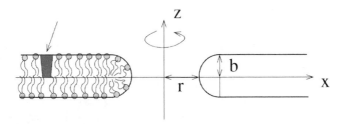

Figure 16.1 A planar lipid bilayer with a pore of radius r in the centre. The figure shows the cross-section in the x–z plane. Rotational symmetry around the z-axis is indicated. On the left side, the packing of lipid molecules is shown schematically. The head-groups of lipid molecules are represented by circles. The arrow denotes a membrane inclusion (single molecule or nanodomain) which is shown schematically. The local geometry within the rim is saddle-like everywhere. The semi-toroidal shape of the pore rim is an assumption; alternative pore shapes could be considered, but are not expected to alter the main conclusions of the theoretical analysis. Reprinted with permission from Fošnarič, M., Kralj-Iglič, V., Bohinc, K., Iglič, A., and May, S. Stabilization of pores in lipid bilayers by anisotropic inclusions. *J. Phys. Chem. B.*, 107, pp. 12519–12526. Copyright 2003, American Chemical Society.

activity (Hägerstrand et al., 2004; Huang, 2000; Shai, 1999), through the formation of membrane pores.

Antimicrobial peptides are typically elongated in shape rendering their interaction with curved membranes highly anisotropic. Also detergents or small complexes of a detergent with the surrounding membrane molecules may be anisotropic with a preference for high curvature of the pore rim due their large hydrophilic part (Hägerstrand et al., 2004; Kandušer et al., 2003). As already mentioned in previous chapters, examples of anisotropic membrane inclusions (molecules,nanodomains) also include various lipids (Chanturiya et al., 2003; Kralj-Iglič, 2002; Kralj-Iglič et al., 2006), glycolipids or lipoproteins (Malev et al., 2002) and gemini detergents (Kralj-Iglič et al., 2000).

In this chapter, we present an analysis of the energetics of a single membrane pore in a binary lipid membrane, consisting of (charged) lipids and anisotropic membrane inclusions (molecules, nanodomains) (see Fošnarič et al., 2003; Kandušer et al., 2003, and Fig. 16.1). The free energy of the inclusion-doped membrane consists of the line tension contribution, the interaction energy between the anisotropic inclusions and the membrane, and the electrostatic energy of the charged lipids (Fošnarič et al., 2003; Kanduušer et al., 2003).

We consider a planar lipid bilayer membrane that contains a single pore of aperture radius r, as shown schematically in Fig. 16.1. We locate a Cartesian coordinate system at the pore centre with the axis of rotational symmetry (the z-axis) pointing normal to the bilayer midplane. Even though experimental obtained evidence is currently not available, it seems a reasonable approximation to assume that the lipids within the rim assemble into a semi-toroidal configuration in order to shield the hydrocarbon chains from contact with the aqueous environment. The bilayer thickness is $2b$.

To obtain the equilibrium size of the pore, the overall free energy, F, of the pore is minimized. We assume that F is the sum of three contributions:

$$F = W_{\text{edge}} + U_{\text{el}} + F_i, \qquad (16.1)$$

where W_{edge} is the energy due to the line tension of the lipid bilayer without the inclusions, U_{el} is the electrostatic energy of the charged lipids and F_i is the energy due to the interactions between the membrane inclusions and the host membrane. We note that F is the *excess* free energy, measured with respect to a planar, pore-free, membrane (Fošnarič et al., 2003).

For an inclusion-free membrane the energy W_{edge} is given by:

$$W_{\text{edge}} = 2\pi \Lambda r, \qquad (16.2)$$

where r is the radius of the circular membrane pore and Λ is the line tension, that is, the excess energy per unit length of the pore edge in the lipid bilayer. One can obtain a rough estimate for Λ on the basis of the elastic energy required to bend a lipid monolayer into a semi-cylindrical pore rim (Chernomordik et al., 1985; Kanduušer et al., 2003). Adopting the usual quadratic curvature expansion for the bending energy according to Helfrich (Eq. 7.30 and Helfrich, 1973), one finds (Chernomordik et al., 1985) $\Lambda = \pi k_c/2b$, where k_c is the lipid layers's bending rigidity. For $b = 2.5\,\text{nm}$ and $k_c = 10\,kT$, the value $\Lambda \approx 6\,kT/\text{nm} \approx 2 \times 10^{-11}\,\text{J/m}$ (at room temperature). This order of magnitude corresponds to experimental results for the line tension of lipid bilayers (Karatekin et al., 2003; Moroz and Nelson, 1997; Taupin et al., 1975).

If inclusions are present within the membrane pore they replace some lipids. The replaced lipids do no longer contribute to the line tension W_{edge}. We account approximately for this reduction in line tension by writing:

$$W_{edge} = 2\Lambda\,(\pi r - N_P\,R_i)\,, \qquad (16.3)$$

where N_P denotes the number of inclusions within the pore rim and $2\,R_i$ is the lateral extension of the cross-sectional shape of the inclusions. Steric interactions limit the number of inclusions within the membrane rim; $N_P \leq N_P^{max} = \pi r/R_i$. Thus $W_{edge} \geq 0$, and the line tension always provides a tendency of the pore to shrink.

Calculation of the electrostatic energy of the membrane pore follows Betterton and Brenner (Betterton and Brenner, 1999) who derived an expression valid for a very thin membrane ($b \to 0$) within the Gouy–Chapman theory using the linearized Poisson–Botzmann (PB) equation (see Section 13.5). To keep our model traceable, we therefore solve the linearized PB equation (Eq. 13.73):

$$\nabla^2\,\phi = \kappa^2\,\phi\,, \qquad (16.4)$$

which determines the electric potential ϕ (measured in Volts) at a given Debye length $l_D = \kappa^{-1} = \sqrt{\epsilon\,\epsilon_0\,kT/(2\,c_0\,N_A\,e_0^2)}$ (Eq. 13.71). Here, $c_0 = n_0/N_A$ is the ionic strength of the surrounding electrolyte solution (i.e., the bulk salt concentration; assuming a 1:1 salt such as NaCl), n_0 is the number density of salt cations and anions in the bulk (see Eq. 13.72) and N_A is Avogadro's number.

The solution of the linearized PB equation for the case of an infinite flat surface without a pore (i.e., the electric potential ϕ_∞), which satisfies the boundary conditions

$$\phi(z \to \infty) = 0, \qquad (16.5)$$

$$\frac{d\phi}{dz}(z=0) = -\frac{\sigma}{\varepsilon_r\,\varepsilon_0}\,, \qquad (16.6)$$

can be written in the form (see Eqs. 13.74 and 13.75):

$$\phi_\infty(z) = \frac{\sigma}{\varepsilon_r\,\varepsilon_0\,\kappa}\,e^{-\kappa z}\,, \qquad (16.7)$$

where σ is the surface charge density.

The solution of the linearized PB equation for a planar lipid bilayer with a pore of radius r can then be written as the difference between the electrostatic potential of a flat infinite pore-free membrane (ϕ_∞) and the electrostatic potential of a circular flat membrane segment with radius r (ϕ_p), both having a constant surface charge density σ (Iglič et al., 2004a):

$$\phi(x, z) = \phi_\infty(z) - \phi_p(x, z). \qquad (16.8)$$

The electrical potential of the circular flat membrane segment with a surface charge density σ and radius r is calculated using cylindrical coordinates. For the axisymmetric case the linearized PB equation in cylindrical coordinates reads:

$$\frac{1}{x}\frac{\partial}{\partial x}\left(x\frac{\partial \phi_p}{\partial x}\right) + \frac{\partial^2 \phi_p}{\partial z^2} = \kappa^2 \phi_p, \qquad (16.9)$$

where the origin of the coordinate system is located at the pore centre with the axis of rotational symmetry (the z-axis) pointing normal to the bilayer midplane (Fig. 16.1). We seek for the solution of Eq. 16.9 by the ansatz

$$\phi_p(x, z) = R(x) Z(z), \qquad (16.10)$$

where $R(x)$ is a function of x and $Z(z)$ is a function of z. In this way, the Eq. 16.9 yields:

$$\frac{1}{R(x)}\frac{1}{x}\frac{\partial}{\partial x}\left(x\frac{dR(x)}{dx}\right) + \frac{1}{Z(z)}\frac{d^2 Z(z)}{dz^2} = \kappa^2. \qquad (16.11)$$

Since the first term in Eq. 16.11 depends solely on the coordinate x, while the second term is a function of coordinate z only, the sum of both terms can always be equal to the constant κ^2 only if both terms are also constant. We take

$$\frac{1}{Z(z)}\frac{d^2 Z(z)}{dz^2} = \kappa^2 + k^2, \qquad (16.12)$$

$$\frac{1}{R(x)}\frac{1}{x}\frac{d}{dx}\left(x\frac{dR(x)}{dx}\right) = -k^2. \qquad (16.13)$$

The general solution of Eq. 16.12 has the form (Arfken and Weber, 1995):

$$Z(z) = C\, e^{-\sqrt{\kappa^2+k^2}\,z} + C_1\, e^{\sqrt{\kappa^2+k^2}\,z}. \qquad (16.14)$$

By taking into account the boundary condition $\phi_p(z \to \infty) = 0$, we chose $C_1 = 0$, therefore:

$$Z(z) = C\, e^{-\sqrt{\kappa^2 + k^2}\, z}. \tag{16.15}$$

Equation 16.13 is rewritten in the form:

$$x^2 \frac{d^2 R}{dx^2} + x \frac{dR}{dx} + k^2 x^2 R = 0. \tag{16.16}$$

The regular solution of differential Eq. 16.16 is a Bessel function of the first kind (Arfken and Weber, 1995)

$$R = C\, J_0(kx). \tag{16.17}$$

The solution of Eq. 16.9 in the form of $\phi_p(x, z) = R(x)\, Z(z)$ (see Eq. 16.10) is therefore

$$\phi_p(x, z) = C(k)\, J_0(kx)\, e^{-\sqrt{\kappa^2 + k^2}\, z}. \tag{16.18}$$

The *general* solution of Eq. 16.9 is thus

$$\phi_p(x, z) = \int_0^\infty dk\, C(k)\, J_0(kx)\, e^{-\sqrt{\kappa^2 + k^2}\, z}. \tag{16.19}$$

In the following, Eq. 16.19 is first differentiated with respect to the coordinate z:

$$\frac{\partial \phi_p}{\partial z} = \int_0^\infty dk\, (-\sqrt{\kappa^2 + k^2})\, C(k)\, J_0(kx)\, e^{-\sqrt{\kappa^2 + k^2}\, z}. \tag{16.20}$$

At $z = 0$, it follows from the above equation (Iglič et al., 2004a):

$$\frac{\partial \phi_p}{\partial z}\bigg|_{z=0} = \int_0^\infty dk\, (-\sqrt{\kappa^2 + k^2})\, C(k)\, J_0(kx). \tag{16.21}$$

Using the Hankel transformation (Arfken and Weber, 1995), the values of coefficients $C(k)$ can be calculated from Eq. 16.21 as follows:

$$C(k) = -\frac{k}{\sqrt{\kappa^2 + k^2}} \int_0^\infty dx\, x\, J_0(kx) \frac{\partial \phi_p}{\partial z}\bigg|_{z=0}. \tag{16.22}$$

Integration of Eq. 16.22 is divided in two parts (Iglič et al., 2004a):

$$C(k) = -\frac{k}{\sqrt{\kappa^2 + k^2}} \left(\int_0^r dx\, x\, J_0(kx) \frac{\partial \phi_p}{\partial z}\bigg|_{z=0} \right.$$

$$\left. + \int_r^\infty dx\, x\, J_0(kx) \frac{\partial \phi_p}{\partial z}\bigg|_{z=0} \right). \tag{16.23}$$

Taking into account the boundary conditions:

$$\frac{\partial \phi_p}{\partial z}(z=0) = -\frac{\sigma}{\varepsilon_r \varepsilon_0}, \quad x < r, \quad (16.24)$$

$$\frac{\partial \phi_p}{\partial z}(z=0) = 0, \quad x \geq r, \quad (16.25)$$

it follows that

$$C(k) = \frac{\sigma}{k \varepsilon_r \varepsilon_0 \sqrt{\kappa^2 + k^2}} \int_0^r d(kx) \, kx \, J_0(kx). \quad (16.26)$$

Considering the relations (Arfken and Weber, 1995)

$$kr J_1(kr) = \int_0^r d(kx) \, kx \, J_0(kx), \quad (16.27)$$

it follows from Eq. 16.26 that

$$C(k) = \frac{\sigma r J_1(kr)}{\varepsilon_r \varepsilon_0 \sqrt{\kappa^2 + k^2}}. \quad (16.28)$$

If the expression calculated for $C(k)$ is inserted in Eq. 16.19, the electric potential $\phi_p(x, z)$ can be written as (Iglič et al., 2004a)

$$\phi_p(x, z) = \frac{\sigma r}{\varepsilon_r \varepsilon_0} \int_0^\infty dk \frac{J_0(kx) J_1(kr)}{\sqrt{\kappa^2 + k^2}} e^{-\sqrt{\kappa^2 + k^2} z}, \quad (16.29)$$

where J_0 and J_1 are Bessel functions. Using Eqs. 16.7, 16.8 and 16.29, we can determine the expression for the electric potential of a flat charged membrane with a circular pore of radius r, in contact with an electrolyte solution (Betterton and Brenner, 1999):

$$\phi(x, z) = \frac{\sigma}{\varepsilon_r \varepsilon_0 \kappa} e^{-\kappa z} - \frac{\sigma r}{\varepsilon_r \varepsilon_0} \int_0^\infty dk \frac{J_0(kx) J_1(kr)}{\sqrt{\kappa^2 + k^2}} e^{-\sqrt{\kappa^2 + k^2} z}. \quad (16.30)$$

Finally, the electrostatic free energy of the system can be derived via a charging process (Andelman, 1995; Verwey and Overbeek, 1948):

$$U_{el, tot} = 2\pi \int_0^\infty \sigma(x) \phi(z=0) \, x \, dx. \quad (16.31)$$

Equation 16.31 is processed analytically using Eq. 16.30. By subtracting the electrostatic energy of the charged pore-free membrane, one obtains an explicit expression for the excess electrostatic energy of the pore (Betterton and Brenner, 1999; Fošnarič et al., 2003):

$$U_{el} = -\frac{\pi \sigma^2 r^2}{\varepsilon_r \varepsilon_0 \kappa} + \frac{2\pi \sigma^2 r^3}{\varepsilon_r \varepsilon_0} \int_0^\infty \frac{J_1(x)^2}{x \sqrt{x^2 + \kappa^2 r^2}} \, dx. \quad (16.32)$$

The energy of a single anisotropic membrane constituent (molecule, nanodomain) can be expressed as (see Eqs. 7.4 and 8.4):

$$E(\omega) = (2 K_1 + K_2)(H - H_m)^2 - K_2 (D^2 - 2 D D_m \cos(2\omega) + D_m^2), \quad (16.33)$$

where $H = (C_1 + C_2)/2$ and $H_m = (C_{1\,m} + C_{2\,m})/2$ are the respective mean curvatures, while $D = |C_1 - C_2|/2$ and $D_m = |C_{1\,m} - C_{2\,m}|/2$ are the curvature deviators. Here C_1 and C_2 are the two principal curvatures (for the definition see Fig. 5.2), while $C_{1\,m}$ and $C_{2\,m}$ are the two intrinsic principal curvatures of the inclusion. The intrinsic curvature deviator D_m describes the intrinsic anisotropy of a single membrane inclusion (Figs. 7.1 and 8.6), while K_1 and K_2 are interaction constants (Kralj-Iglič et al., 2006). The inclusions can rotate around the axis defined by the membrane normal at the site of the inclusion. The time scale for orientational changes of the anisotropic inclusions is usually small compared to shape changes of the lipid bilayer. Therefore the corresponding partition function, q, of a single inclusion is (see Eqs. 9.3 or 7.9):

$$q = \frac{1}{\omega_0} \int_0^{2\pi} \exp\left(-\frac{E(\omega)}{kT}\right) d\omega, \quad (16.34)$$

where ω_0 is an arbitrary angle quantum. Inclusions (molecules, nanodomains) can also move laterally over the membrane bilayer, so that they can distribute laterally over the membrane in a way that is energetically the most favourable (see Chapter 9). The expression for the contribution of the inclusions to the membrane free energy can be derived, based on Eqs. 16.33 and 16.34 (Fošnarič et al., 2003):

$$\frac{F_i}{kT} = -N \ln \left[\frac{1}{A} \int_A q_c \cdot I_0 \left(\frac{2 K_2}{kT} D D_m \right) dA \right], \quad (16.35)$$

where N is the total number of inclusions in the membrane segment, while q_c is defined as

$$q_c = \exp\left(-\frac{2 K_1 + K_2}{kT}(H^2 - 2 H H_m) + \frac{K_2}{kT} D^2\right), \quad (16.36)$$

and I_0 is the modified Bessel function. Integration in Eq. 16.35 is performed over the whole area of the membrane (A). For a large planar bilayer membrane that contains a single pore only, those inclusions contribute to F_i that are located directly in the pore rim.

In this case Eq. 16.35 can be rewritten in the form (Fošnarič et al., 2003):

$$\frac{F_i}{kT} = n \int_{A_p} \left[1 - q_c \cdot I_0 \left(\frac{2 K_2}{kT} D D_m \right) \right] dA_P, \quad (16.37)$$

where $n = N/A$ is the average area density of the inclusions in the membrane, and where integration extends only over the area of the membrane rim (A_P). The influence of the inclusion's anisotropy (Figs. 7.1 and 8.6) is contained in the Bessel function $I_0(2 D D_m K_2/kT)$. Because $I_0 \geq 1$ we see from Eq. 16.37 that anisotropy of inclusions always tends to lower F_i. Whether the inclusions lower or increase F_i depends crucially on D_m and H_m, and on the interaction constants K_1 and K_2. The number of inclusions within the pore rim is (Fošnarič et al., 2003):

$$N_P = n \int_{A_P} q_c I_0 \left(\frac{2 K_2}{kT} D D_m \right) dA_P. \quad (16.38)$$

If the inclusions have no preference for partition into the pore rim ($q_c I_0 = 1$), then Eq. 16.38 predicts $N_P/A_P = n$. Combination of Eqs. 16.37 and 16.38 yields (Fošnarič et al., 2003)

$$\frac{F_i}{kT} = n A_P - N_P. \quad (16.39)$$

Hence, inclusions that enter the membrane pore (at a density that exceeds the bulk density) contribute one kT per inclusion to the free energy. If the density of the inclusions within the pore region greatly exceeds the bulk density, then $n A_P \ll N_P$ and thus, $F_i \approx -N_p kT$ (Fošnarič et al., 2003). The inclusion size determines the maximal number of inclusions, N_P^{max}, that can enter the pore rim. For rather large inclusions $R_i \approx b$ and small pores $r \approx b$ we expect that N_P^{max} is quite small, of the order of a very few inclusions (Fošnarič et al., 2003). Below, it is shown that for charged bilayer membranes, anisotropic inclusions can dramatically reduce the total free energy F (much more than $-N_p kT$).

In the case of lipid molecules, the interaction constants, K_1 and K_2 can be estimated using Eqs. 7.5 and 7.31, which yield $K_1 \sim -K_2 \sim k_c a_0$. Assuming $k_c \approx 10 kT$ for the bending constant of nearly flat lipid monolayer and $a_0 \sim 1 \text{ nm}^2$ for the cross-sectional area per lipid, we get $K_1 \sim -K_2 \sim 10\,kT\,\text{nm}^2$ for lipid molecules in a nearly flat lipid monolayer. However, it is expected that the value $K_1 \sim 10\,kT\,\text{nm}^2$ is at least an order of magnitude smaller than the interaction constant K_1 in the expression for the single-inclusion energy in a strong curvature field (Eq. 16.33). Hence, sufficiently large and anisotropic membrane inclusions are expected to strongly partition into appropriately strongly curved membrane regions like the rim of a hydrophilic pore in a membrane bilayer.

We note that partitioning of membrane inclusions into the rim of a membrane pore replaces some structurally perturbed lipids (besides causing an extra (excess) splay). These lipids no longer contribute to the energy of the pore. The corresponding energy gain is not contained in F_i because we took it into account already in W_{edge} (see Eq. 16.1).

All the following results are presented for a thickness of the lipid layer $b = 2.5$ nm, for a line tension of $\Lambda = 10^{-11}$ J/m, and for a surface charge density $\sigma = -0.05$ A s/m^2 of the lipid layer (Fošnarič et al., 2003). Taking into account the cross-sectional area per lipid of $a_0 = 0.6 - 0.8\,\text{nm}^2$, the value for σ would correspond roughly to a 1:4 mixture of (monovalent) charged and uncharged lipids. This is a common situation in biological and model bilayer membranes.

In the case of and inclusion-free membrane (Betterton and Brenner, 1999), the total membrane free energy consists only of the line tension contribution (Eq. 16.1) and the electrostatic free energy (Eq. 16.32). The former favours shrinking, the latter widening (growing) of the membrane pore. For small values of the Debye length l_D the pore closes, for large l_D the pore grows. Betterton and Brenner (Betterton and Brenner, 1999) showed that for intermediate values of l_D there exists a very shallow local minimum of total membrane free energy F as a function of the radius r of the pore. As an illustration, Fig. 16.2 shows the function $F(r)$ for three different values of $l_D = 2.6$ nm (a), 2.8 nm (b) and 3.0 nm (c). A local minimum of $F(r)$ is present only in curve (b). Figure 16.2 exemplifies a general finding for an inclusion-free isotropic and uniformly charged bilayer membrane: the local minimum of the membrane free energy $F(r)$ is very shallow (below

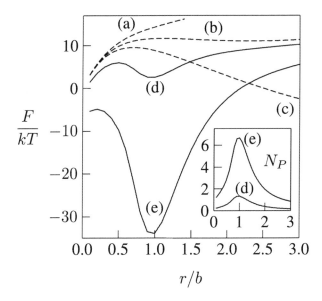

Figure 16.2 The pore free energy, F, as a function of the pore size r. The dashed lines correspond to a charged inclusion-free membrane of charge density $\sigma = -0.05\,\text{As}/\text{m}^2$ with Debye length $l_D = 2.6$ nm (a), $l_D = 2.8$ nm (b), and $l_D = 3.0$ nm (c). The solid lines describe the effect of adding anisotropic inclusions (characterized by $K_1 = 98\,kT\,\text{nm}^2$, $K_2 = -65\,kT\,\text{nm}^2$, $C_{1m} = -C_{2m} = 1/b$) to the charged membrane with $\sigma = -0.1\,\text{As}/\text{m}^2$ and $l_D = 2.8$ nm. The average area density of inclusions n is $1/70000\,\text{nm}^2$ (d) and $1/14000\,\text{nm}^2$ (e). The inset shows the corresponding numbers, N_P, of inclusions within the membrane rim for curves (d) and (e). Reprinted with permission from Fošnarič, M., Kralj-Iglič, V., Bohinc, K., Iglič, A., and May, S. Stabilization of pores in lipid bilayers by anisotropic inclusions. *J. Phys. Chem. B.*, 107, pp. 12519–12526. Copyright 2003, American Chemical Society.

kT) and appears in the very narrow region of the values of Debye length l_D. Based on these results it can therefore be concluded that, a hydrophilic pore in an isotropic and uniformly charged bilayer membrane cannot be stabilized solely by competition between the system electrostatic free energy and the line tension energy of the pore rim (Betterton and Brenner, 1999; Fošnarič et al., 2003).

In order to illustrate the effect of anisotropy of the membrane inclusions, we choose an inclusion which favours a saddle shape $C_{1m} = -C_{2m} = 1/b$ (Fig. 8.6). Figure 16.2 shows $F(r)$ for two values of the average area density of inclusions (n): $1/70000\,\text{nm}^2$ (curve d) and $1/14000\,\text{nm}^2$ (curve e). The ability of anisotropic inclusions to lower the local minimum of the membrane free energy $F(r)$ can be clearly seen. The anisotropic inclusions tend to accumulate within the rim of the hydrophilic pore (Fošnarič et al., 2003). The number of inclusions within the rim of the pore (N_P) is estimated by Eq. 16.38. This number is plotted in the inset of Fig. 16.2 for $n = 1/70000\,\text{nm}^2$ (d) and $n = 1/14000\,\text{nm}^2$ (e).

The depth of the minimum of $F(r)$ for $n = 1/14000\,\text{nm}^2$ (curve e in Fig. 16.2) is approximately $30kT$. It arises predominantly from the accumulation of anisotropic membrane inclusions in the region of the pore rim. On the other hand, Eq. 16.39 predicts that the inclusion energy $F_i \approx N_P\,kT$. The inset of Fig. 16.2 shows that $N_P \leq 6$, therefore the deep minimum of $F(r)$ cannot arise solely from the inclusion contribution F_i (Fošnarič et al., 2003). To explain the deep minimum in $F(r)$, we recall that in the inclusion-free membrane the electrostatic energy and the line tension nearly balance each other for small enough values of r/b. If inclusions enter the pore region they reduce the line tension (see Eq. 16.3). As a result U_{el} is no longer counterbalanced by positive W_{edge} and thus strongly lowers the total membrane free energy F (Fošnarič et al., 2003).

The minimum of $F(r)$ in Fig. 16.2 occurs at $r \approx b$ (see curves (d) and (e)). This reflects our choice of a saddle shape for the anisotropic inclusion: $C_{1m} = 1/b$, $C_{2m} = -1/b$ (see also Figs. 16.5 and 8.6). In fact, for $r = b$ the principal curvatures of the pore rim at the equatorial plane are $C_1 = 1/b$ and $C_2 = -1/b$, coinciding with the inclusion's principal curvatures. This observation suggests the possibility of increasing the optimal size of the pore by altering the shape of the membrane inclusions from saddle-like ($C_{1m} = 1/b$, $C_{2m} = -1/b$) towards more wedge-like ($C_{1m} = 1/b$, $C_{2m} \approx 0$, see also Fig. 8.6 and (Fošnarič et al., 2003). The smaller the magnitude of $|C_{2m}|$, the larger should be the preferred pore size (see also the inset in Fig. 16.3). Regarding the principal curvatures at the waist of the rim, $C_1 = 1/b$ and $C_2 = -1/r$, one would expect that the optimal pore size (r^{opt}) is approximately determined by $C_{2m} = -1/r^{opt}$ and $C_{1m} = C_1 = 1/b$, leading to the approximate relation (Fošnarič et al., 2003):

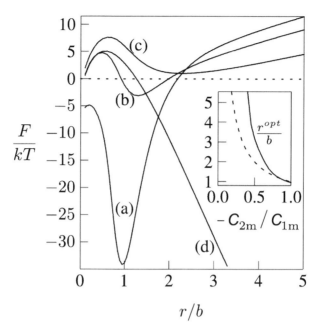

Figure 16.3 The free energy of the pore (F) as a function of the pore size r for differently shaped, anisotropic inclusions: $C_{2m}/C_{1m} = -1$ (a), $C_{2m}/C_{1m} = -0.8$ (b), $C_{2m}/C_{1m} = -0.6$ (c), and $C_{2m}/C_{1m} = 0$ (d). In all cases, the membrane is charged ($\sigma = -0.05$ A s/m^2, $l_D = 2.8$ nm), $C_{1m} = 1/b$ and $n = 1/14000$ nm^2. The inset shows the position of the local minimum, r^{opt}, as a function of C_{2m}/C_{1m} (solid line). The dashed line in the inset corresponds to $-C_{2m}/C_{1m} = b/r^{opt}$. Reprinted with permission from Fošnarič, M., Kralj-Iglič, V., Bohinc, K., Iglič, A., and May, S. Stabilization of pores in lipid bilayers by anisotropic inclusions. *J. Phys. Chem. B.*, 107, pp. 12519–12526. Copyright 2003, American Chemical Society.

$$-\frac{C_{2m}}{C_{1m}} \approx \frac{b}{r^{opt}}. \quad (16.40)$$

In Figs. 16.3 and (Fošnarič et al., 2003), we consider anisotropic inclusions with an intrinsic shape characterized by $C_{1m} = 1/b$ and C_{2m}/C_{1m}: -1 (a), -0.8 (b), -0.6 (c) and 0 (d). As can be seen in Fig. 16.3, the local minimum of $F(r)$ shifts to larger pore sizes as the inclusions become more wedge-shaped (compare the position of the local minimum of curves (a)–(c)). The solid line in the inset of Fig. 16.3 shows how the optimal pore radius r^{opt} changes with C_{2m}/C_{1m}. The broken line in the inset displays the prediction of

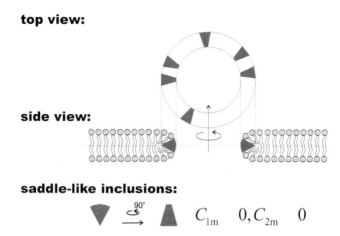

Figure 16.4 Schematic representation of the stabilization of a hydrophilic pore in a bilayer membrane by anisotropic saddle-like membrane inclusions.

the approximate Eq. 16.40. Figure 16.3 also shows that below some critical values of the ratio $|C_{2m}/C_{1m}|$, the local minimum in $F(r)$ disappears (in Fig. 16.3 for $|C_{2m}/C_{1m}| < 0.4$), which means that the pore becomes unstable and starts to grow in a process which never stops. It should also be stressed that for isotropic inclusions where $C_{1m} = C_{2m}$ (see Fig. 8.6), we do not find energetically stabilized pores. The stabilization of a pore derives from the matching of the rim geometry with the inclusion's preference (Fig. 16.4). The pore rim provides a saddle-like geometry with different signs of C_1 and C_2 (see also Fig. 5.2). Consequently, saddle-like inclusion geometry (i.e., different signs of C_{1m} and C_{2m}) is needed to stabilize the pore (Fošnarič et al., 2003). Possible candidates for saddle-like inclusions include strongly anisotropic lipid molecules (Fig. 16.5).

In all the examples presented in Fig. 16.3, we added anisotropic inclusions (single molecules or nanodomains) to charged membranes with a specifically selected Debye length $l_D = 2.8$ nm (Fošnarič et al., 2003) (the Debye length l_D is inversely proportional to the square root of the ionic strength $c_0 = n_0/N_A$, see Eq. 13.71). We recall from Fig. 16.2 that this was the choice for which an inclusion-free membrane exhibits a very shallow minimum in $F(r)$ (see the dashed curve (b) in Fig. 16.2). The question arises whether pores

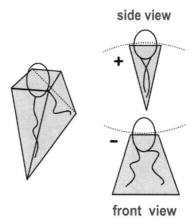

Figure 16.5 Saddle-like membrane inclusions with $C_{1m} > 0$ and $C_{2m} < 0$ may also be lipid molecules. Figure adapted from Rappolt (2012).

in a membrane with anisotropic inclusions can also be stabilized for other electrostatic conditions (i.e., other values of the ionic strength). In this respect, it is interesting to compare our theoretical predictions with the experimental observation of stable pores in red blood cell ghosts for which data exist on the optimal pore radius r^{opt} as a function of the salt concentration c_0 (Lieber and Steck, 1982a). Our theoretical approach (Fošnarič et al., 2003) is able to reproduce this experimental data as presented in Fig. 16.6. Figure 16.6 shows the calculated and experimentally determined stable pore radius as a function of the salt concentration (ionic strength) in a suspension of red blood cell ghosts (Fošnarič et al., 2003). The inset of Fig. 16.6 shows the corresponding number of inclusions in the rim of the pore (N_P) (solid line), as well as the maximal possible number of inclusions in the rim of the pore $N_P^{max} = \pi r^{opt}/R_i$ (broken line) at which the inclusions would sterically occupy the entire rim. The observation $N_P < N_P^{max}$ indicates the applicability of our approach for the selected average area density of inclusions in the membrane. Nevertheless, Fig. 16.6 should be understood only as an illustration of the principal ability of anisotropic membrane inclusions to stabilize membrane pores under different electrostatic conditions.

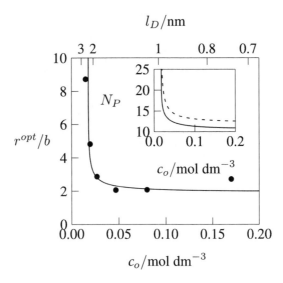

Figure 16.6 Optimal pore size r as a function of the ionic strength (salt concentration) of the surrounding electrolyte medium. The charge density of the membrane is $\sigma = -0.05\,\mathrm{As/m^2}$, the average area density of the inclusions is $n = 1/(2000\,\mathrm{nm^2})$, and the inclusion's preferred curvatures $C_{1m} = 1/b$ and $C_{2m}/C_{1m} = -0.4$. Experimental values (Lieber and Steck, 1982a) are also shown (●). The inset shows the actual number of inclusions, N_P, residing in the pore of optimal size, r^{opt} (solid line), and the maximal number, $N_P^{max} = \pi r^{opt}/R_i$ (broken line). Reprinted with permission from Fošnarič, M., Kralj-Iglič, V., Bohinc, K., Iglič, A., and May, S. Stabilization of pores in lipid bilayers by anisotropic inclusions. *J. Phys. Chem. B.*, 107, pp. 12519–12526. Copyright 2003, American Chemical Society.

Electroporation is a method for the artificial formation of pores in biological membranes by applying an electric field across the membrane (Maček-Lebar et al., 2002a,b). A problem in the electroporation of living tissue is that it often causes irreversible damage to the exposed cells and tissue (Lee and Kolodney, 1987). Increasing the amplitude of the electric field in electroporation diminishes cell survival rates (Wolf et al., 1994). On the other hand, if the applied electric field is too low, stable pores are not formed. A way to improve the efficiency of electroporation is chemical modification of the membranes by surfactants. Little is known about

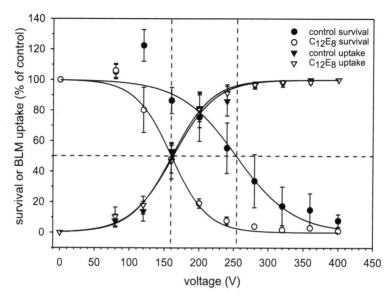

Figure 16.7 The effect of $C_{12}E_8$ on reversible electroporation (measured by bleomycin uptake) and irreversible electroporation measured by cell survival on the cell line DC3F. Reprinted from *Colloids and Surfaces A: Physicochemical and Engineering Aspects*, 214(1–3), Maša Kandušer, Miha Fošnarič, Marjeta Šentjurc, Veronika Kralj-Iglič, Henry Hägerstrand, Aleš Iglič, and Damijan Miklavčiča, Effect of surfactant polyoxyethylene glycol (C12E8) on electroporation of cell line DC3F, pp. 205–217, Copyright 2003, with permission from Elsevier.

the effect of surfactants on cell membrane fluidity and its relation to electroporation.

A recent electroporation experiment showed that the non-ionic surfactant (detergent) polyoxyethylene glycol $C_{12}E_8$ does not affect reversible electroporation, but it significantly increases irreversible electroporation. Irreversible electroporation occurs at a lower applied voltage in the presence of $C_{12}E_8$ (Fig. 16.7). The addition of $C_{12}E_8$ caused cell death at the same voltage at which reversible electroporation took place. This can be explained by the pore stabilization effect of $C_{12}E_8$ (Kandušer et al., 2003) taking into account the results of the theoretical study presented above on the influence of anisotropic membrane inclusions on the energetics and stability of hydrophilic membrane pores.

$C_{12}E_8$ is incorporated in the lipid bilayer with its polar detergent headgroup at the level of the polar phosphate headgroups and with the detergent chain inserted in between the acyl chains of fatty acids of the membrane phospholipids (Thurmond et al., 1994). Incorporation of $C_{12}E_8$ into the phospholipid bilayer leads to a decreased average chain length and an increased average area per chain, and considerable perturbation of the acyl chain ordering of neighbouring phospholipid molecules. Consequently, the effective shape of phospholipids around $C_{12}E_8$ changes from a cylinder to an inverted truncated cone (Thurmond et al., 1994). The cooperative interaction of one $C_{12}E_8$ molecule and some adjacent phospholipid molecules has been proposed (Heerklotz et al., 1998). Based on this experimental data, an anisotropic effective shape of the $C_{12}E_8$ phospholipid complex (nanodomain) has been suggested recently (Hägerstrand et al., 2004).

In accordance with our theoretical predictions (Figs. 16.2 and 16.3), we therefore suggested that $C_{12}E_8$ induces an anisotropic membrane nanodomain (inclusion) (Hägerstrand et al., 2004) which stabilizes the membrane hydrophilic pore by accumulating on the toroidally shaped rim of the pore and attaining a favourable orientation (Fig. 16.4 and Kandušer et al., 2003).

We presume that hydrophilic pores are formed at the voltages at which reversible electroporation takes place, and that these pores are a prerequisite for the access of bleomycin to the cell interior that causes cell death. On the other hand, cell death that is a consequence of irreversible electroporation is caused by the electric field itself provoking irreversible changes in the membrane. In control cells which were treated with $C_{12}E_8$ so that pore stabilization did not occur, 50 percent of the cells survived the application of pulses of an amplitude of 250 V. In these cells, resealing of the cell membrane took place, while in the $C_{12}E_8$ treated cells no cells survived the application of pulses of an amplitude of 250 V, as resealing was prevented by $C_{12}E_8$ (Fig. 16.7). In control cells, we observed 50 percent permeabilization as determined by bleomycin uptake at 160 V (Kandušer et al., 2003). At the same voltage in the $C_{12}E_8$ treated cells we observed 50 percent permeabilization and also only 50 percent of cell survival after treatment with the electric field (Fig. 16.7). This shows that the irreversible electroporation of the

$C_{12}E_8$ treated cells is shifted to the same voltage at which reversible electroporation occurs. In other words, electropermeabilization in the presence of $C_{12}E_8$ becomes irreversible as soon as it occurs. These results lead to the conclusion that stabilization of the hydrophilic membrane pores by $C_{12}E_8$ is induced by anisotropic membrane inclusions (nanodomains) (Figs. 16.2, 16.3 and 16.4).

To confirm this conclusion additional experiments were performed (Kandušer et al., 2003). Namely, from the above described experiments with $C_{12}E_8$, we could not distinguish between the pore stabilization effect of the $C_{12}E_8$-induced anisotropic membrane nanodomains (Fig. 16.4) and the possibility that $C_{12}E_8$ could be toxic when it has access to the cell interior. Therefore, in these additional experiments, the molecules of $C_{12}E_8$ were added after the application of the train of eight electric pulses. It was shown that $C_{12}E_8$ was not cytotoxic when it gained access to the cell interior (Fig. 16.8), as after electroporation the cell membrane remains permeable for relatively small molecules such as $C_{12}E_8$ (Kandušer et al., 2003). From these results we concluded (Kandušer et al., 2003) that the cell death observed in the previous experiments (Fig. 16.7) is caused by bleomycin which is transported into the cell through pores which are stabilized by $C_{12}E_8$ (Fig. 16.4). Also, it was concluded that in order to show this effect $C_{12}E_8$ has to be incorporated in the cell membrane prior to the application of the electric pulses.

The influence that membrane inclusions (single molecules or nanodomains) have on the energetics of membrane pores is often interpreted in terms of altering the mesoscopic elastic properties of the membrane. For example, the effect of surfactants is often described by the surfactant-dependent effective bending stiffness of the membrane bilayer and the effective membrane spontaneous curvature (Božič et al., 2006; Kralj-Iglič et al., 1996, 1999; Safinya et al., 1989). Accordingly, it is assumed that the presence of a cone-like or inverted cone-like membrane constituent (Fig. 8.6) can induce a shift in the spontaneous curvature (Božič et al., 2006; Bobrowska et al., 2013; Kralj-Iglič et al., 1996, 1999). This shift can be translated into a change of line tension which may provide a simplified basis for analysing the energetics of the membrane pore (Karatekin et al., 2003).

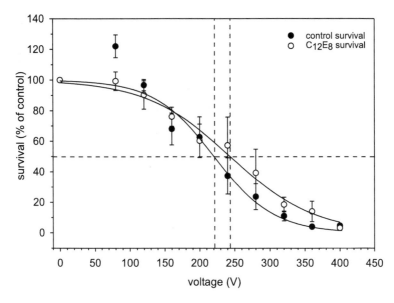

Figure 16.8 Effect of $C_{12}E_8$ added immediately after application of electric pulses on the survival of DC3F cells. Reprinted from *Colloids and Surfaces A: Physicochemical and Engineering Aspects*, 214(1–3), Maša Kandušer, Miha Fošnarič, Marjeta Šentjurc, Veronika Kralj-Iglič, Henry Hägerstrand, Aleš Igliča, and Damijan Miklavčiča, Effect of surfactant polyoxyethylene glycol (C12E8) on electroporation of cell line DC3F, pp. 205–217, Copyright 2003, with permission from Elsevier.

The theoretical approach presented in this chapter contains isotropic membrane constituents only as a special case, namely the membrane constituents are isotropic for $D_m = 0$ (see Fig. 8.6). Beyond the effect of cone-like and inverted cone-like membrane constituents, our present approach also allows analysis of other shapes, such as wedge- or saddle-like shape (Fig. 16.5). Such membrane constituents (see also Fig. 7.1) and nanodomains (Fig. 8.2) can be characterized by an appropriate combination of H_m and D_m (or equivalently C_{1m} and C_{2m}).

In the case of a homogeneous lateral distribution of membrane inclusions (single molecules or nanodomains), the intrinsic spontaneous mean curvature of the inclusions (H_m) renormalize the membrane spontaneous curvature (see also Božič et al., 2006; Kralj-Iglič et al., 1996, 1999). However, if the lateral distribution of inclusions is not homogeneous (Bobrowska et al., 2013; Hägerstrand et al., 2006; Iglič et al., 2004b; Tian and Baumgart, 2009), the effect of the membrane inclusions (e.g., surfactant-induced membrane nanodomains, rigid protein-induced nanodomains, etc.) on membrane elasticity cannot be described simply by renormalization of the membrane spontaneous curvature.

Adding the non-ionic surfactant octaethyleneglycol dodecylether ($C_{12}E_8$) (Kandušer et al., 2003; Troiano et al., 1998) to the outer solution of the phospholipid membrane or the cell membrane causes a decrease in the threshold for irreversible electroporation (i.e., $C_{12}E_8$ decreases the voltage necessary for reversible electroporation) (Fig. 16.7). In other words, $C_{12}E_8$ molecules make transient pores in the membrane more stable (Kandušer et al., 2003).

The theoretical approach presented in this chapter could also help to obtain a better understanding of the pore energetics as investigated by Karatekin et al. (2003). For example, the authors measured a dramatic increase of the transient pore lifetime induced by the detergent Tween 20 which has an anisotropic polar headgroup. The importance of anisotropy of polar heads of detergents for the stability of anisotropic membrane structures has been indicated recently. As already mentioned in Section 9.3, it has been shown that a single-chained detergent with an anisotropic dimeric polar head (dodecyl D-maltoside) may induce tubular nanovesicles (Bobrowska et al., 2013; Hägerstrand et al., 1999; Kralj-Iglič et al., 2005) in a way similar to that induced by strongly anisotropic dimeric detergents (Kralj-Iglič et al., 2000).

This approach could also add to better understanding of the pore formation induced by some antimicrobial peptides (Huang, 2000; Shai, 1999). These peptides have a pronounced elongated shape which arises from their alpha-helical backbone structure which renders them highly anisotropic. Some of these peptides are believed to self-assemble cooperatively into membrane pores. Thus, they can not only facilitate pore formation but also can actively induce it. Our model provides a simple way to describe the underlying physics of peptide-induced pore formation in lipid membranes, but it also involves a number of approximations (Fošnarič et al., 2003). For example, concerning the geometry of the membrane pore, its shape is assumed to be circular, covered by a semi-toroidal rim. Further, direct interactions between inclusions (Marčelja, 1976) (which can be included in our theoretical approach as described in Chapter 9) may become important for the inclusions distributed in the pore rim where the distance between neighbouring inclusions can be very small.

This theoretical approach takes into account the anisotropy of the membrane inclusions (single molecules or nanodomains) enabling us to describe various molecular shapes, such as cone-, inverted cone-, wedge-, and saddle-like inclusions (Figs. 8.6 and 7.1). In the model, the lateral density of anisotropic inclusions (single molecules or nanodomains) is not kept constant so the inclusions may be predominantly localized in energetically favourable regions (Bobrowska et al., 2013; Hägerstrand et al., 2006; Iglič et al., 2004b) such as pore edges. Our model is simple, but it provides a lucid framework to analyse the energetics of pore formation in bilayer membranes (Fošnarič et al., 2003) due to exogeneously bound molecules such as, for example, the detergent sodium cholate (Karatekin et al., 2003), the detergent $C_{12}E_8$ (Kandušer et al., 2003) or the protein talin (Saitoh et al., 1998).

To conclude, in this chapter it is shown that the optimal pore size in a charged bilayer membrane is determined by the ionic strength of the surrounding electrolyte solution and by the intrinsic shape of the anisotropic membrane inclusions (single molecules or nanodomains). Saddle-like membrane inclusions (Fig. 16.5) favour small pores, whereas more wedge-like inclusions (Fig. 7.5) give rise to larger pore sizes (Fošnarič et al., 2003). We showed theoretically that for an ionic strength below 0.05 $\mathrm{mol\,dm^{-3}}$, the optimal size of the pore strongly increases with decrease in ionic strength. In accordance with theoretical predictions, it is indicated experimentally that $C_{12}E_8$-induced anisotropic membrane inclusions may stabilize a hydrophilic pore in the membrane, presumably due to accumulation of $C_{12}E_8$ on the toroidally shaped rim of the pore (Kandušer et al., 2003).

Chapter 17

Membranous Nanostructures as *in vivo* Cell-to-Cell Transport Mechanisms

Recently, a new mechanism of cell-to-cell communication was proposed when thin tubular connections between membrane-enclosing compartments were discovered (Fig. 17.1). The basic research was first performed on liposomes where membranous tubes of thickness below a micrometre are commonly formed, especially if a mechanical or a chemical disturbance is introduced into the liposome system (Kralj-Iglič et al., 2001a; Kralj-Iglič, 2002; Mathivet et al., 1996). Such lipid bilayer nanotubes may connect two or more liposomes (Karlsson et al., 2001). It was observed (Iglič et al., 2003) that a dilatation of the tube forming a gondola may exist and travel along the tube (Fig. 17.2).

Based on the discovery of nanotubes and gondolas in artificial systems (Karlsson et al., 2001; Kralj-Iglič et al., 2001a; Kralj-Iglič, 2002) and the discovery of intra-tubular particle transport between two liposomes (Karlsson et al., 2001), it was suggested that similar mechanisms may also take place in cells (Iglič et al., 2003). In cells nanotubes and gondolas (forming an integral part of the nanotube) may constitute a transport system within and between the cells (Iglič et al., 2003; Karlsson et al., 2001). Transport to the target point

---

Nanostructures in Biological Systems: Theory and Applications
Aleš Iglič, Veronika Kralj-Iglič, and Damjana Drobne
Copyright © 2015 Pan Stanford Publishing Pte. Ltd.
ISBN 978-981-4267-20-5 (Hardcover), 978-981-4303-43-9 (eBook)
www.panstanford.com

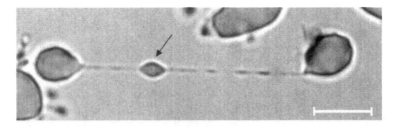

Figure 17.1 A micrograph showing two membrane-enclosed parts of a disintegrated red blood cell connected by long partially tubular membrane structure. The arrow points to a large prolate bleb which is an integral part of the membrane tube. The red blood cells were observed in isotonic physiological solution with added dibucaine at pH $\approx$ 8.5. Scale bar = 3 μm. Reprinted from *Physics Letters A*, 310(5–6), Aleš Iglič, Henry Hägerstrand, Malgorzata Bobrowska-Hägerstrand, Vesna Arrigler, and Veronika Kralj-Iglič, Possible role of phospholipid nanotubes in directed transport of membrane vesicles, pp. 493–497, Copyright 2003, with permission from Elsevier.

would be much more selective, if the motion of the vesicles could be directed by the nanotubes. Such nanotube-directed transport might have an important role in the selectivity of specific pathways in cellular systems where the transport vesicles move specifically from one membrane to another (Iglič et al., 2003).

After the discovery of nanotubes in liposome systems, the first indication that nanotubular structures might also be present in cellular systems came from experiments with manipulated erythrocytes. It was observed (Iglič et al., 2003) that small vesicles released from erythrocytes moved synchronously with the parent cell, and that these vesicles were connected to the cell by thin tubes (Fig. 10.9). Recently, thin membranous tubes, so-named tunnelling nanotubes (TNTs) that bridge distances up to a few 100 μm, have been discovered in different cellular systems (see Chinnery et al., 2008; Davis and Sowinski, 2008; Gerdes et al., 2007; Gerdes and Carvalho, 2008; Gimsa et al., 2007; Hurtig et al., 2010; Iglič et al., 2007b; Koyanagi et al., 2005; Önfelt et al., 2004; Rustom et al., 2004; Veranič et al., 2008; Vidulescu et al., 2004; Watkins and Salter, 2005). It was proposed that TNTs represent a new mode of cell-to-cell communication and that they might also enable direct transport of

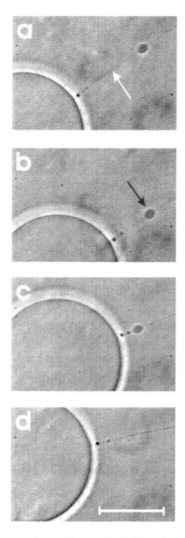

Figure 17.2 Transport of a small phospholipid prolate bleb (black arrow) along a thin phospholipid tube (white arrow) protruding from a liposome. Note that the bleb (gondola) is an integral part of the tube membrane. Scale bar, 10 μm. The vesicles were observed under an inverted microscope with phase contrast optics. Reprinted from *Physics Letters A*, 310(5–6), Aleš Iglič, Henry Hägerstrand, Malgorzata Bobrowska-Hägerstrand, Vesna Arrigler, and Veronika Kralj-Iglič, Possible role of phospholipid nanotubes in directed transport of membrane vesicles, pp. 493–497, Copyright 2003, with permission from Elsevier.

molecules and even organelles between the cells (Gerdes et al., 2007; Hurtig et al., 2010; Iglič et al., 2003; Koyanagi et al., 2005; Önfelt et al., 2004; Rustom et al., 2004; Veranič et al., 2008).

Nanotubes that bridge neighbouring cells (i.e., bridging nanotubes) were mostly found in cells that are weakly connected to each other or actively migrate and seek for bacteria or attachment to eukaryotic cells. However, bridging nanotubes also exist in cells with a limited ability of movement and strong intercellular connections (Rustom et al., 2004; Veranič et al., 2008). Nanotubes may also connect intracellular membranous compartments such as Golgi stacks (Iglič et al., 2004b; Mathivet et al., 1996) and references therein), and may be a part of the subjacent membrane pool which forms an infrastructure of the cell.

It was shown that there are at least two types of bridging nanotubes in different processes of formation, stability, cytoskeletal contents, and function (Veranič et al., 2008). Type I was classified as those membrane tubes which contain actin filaments and start growing as filopodia, but can become up to 30 µm long (Fig. 17.3). This type of tubular protrusion usually appears as bunches of several tubes which dynamically seek for connections with neighbouring cells (Veranič et al., 2008).

Protrusions remain stable even after disintegration of the actin filaments with cytochalasin D (Fig. 17.4). After reaching an appropriate neighbouring cell, the protrusions connect to the target cell (Fig. 17.3A) and remain connected for several tens of minutes. The tube may be attached to the plasma membrane of the target cell by an anchoring type of intercellular junction (Veranič et al., 2008). From the results of experiments with actin–GFP (Fig. 17.5), we know that there is also a cytosolic and not only a membrane connection between the two cells interconnected by type I nanotubes. We found the spread of actin–GFP via a tunnelling nanotube from one T24 cell with highly expressed actin–GFP to another cell which was devoid of actin–GFP (Fig. 17.5 A). The spreading of actin–GFP into the second cell is clearly visible as a cone of fluorescence at the connection point. To further confirm the connectivity of two cells, we screened multiple non-transfected cells which were connected to an actin–GFP overexpressing cell via type I nanotubes. Frequently, we observed diffraction-limited signals in the non-

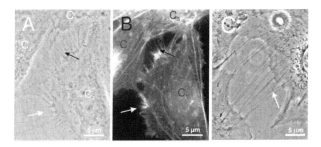

Figure 17.3 Type I nanotubes. Panel A is a phase contrast image of live T24 cells, while panel B is a fluorescence micrograph showing actin labelling of the same cells as in A, after 15 minutes of paraformaldehyde fixation. Cell C1 is approaching the cells C2 and C3. The white arrows in A and B indicate short and dynamic membrane protrusions with which the approaching cell explores its surroundings. The black arrow in A points at protrusions that have already connected to the target cell. In all these multiple tubular connections actin filaments are present (↑ in B). Bridging nanotubes of type I can be more than 20 μm long and occasionally bifurcations are seen (↑ in C). Reprinted from *Biophysical Journal*, 95(9), Peter Veranič, Maruša Lokar, Gerhard J. Schütz, Julian Weghuber, Stefan Wieser, Henry Hägerstrand, Veronika Kralj-Iglič, and Aleš Iglič, Different types of cell-to-cell connections mediated by nanotubular structures, pp. 4416–4425, Copyright 2008, with permission from Elsevier.

transfected cell, which moved with very high mobility, too fast to be traceable at a time-delay of 22 ms; the signal amplitudes concur with the brightness of a single or several GFP molecules (Fig. 17.5B). We interpret the signals as free actin–GFP monomers, or small associates that have dissociated from the actin filaments upon tube formation. We never observed such signals in non-transfected unconnected cells.

The exchange of lipid components of the plasma membrane between cells connected by nanotubes of type I seems to be nearly completely stopped at the junction between the nanotube and the neighbouring target cell (Fig. 17.6). The fluorescent lipid marker DiI did not pass the junction point even after 24 hours of co-cultivation of labelled T24 cells and non labelled cells (Fig. 17.6). Only some small spots of DiI were found on the non-labelled cells, which could also indicate vesiculation of the labelled cells and the fusion (or

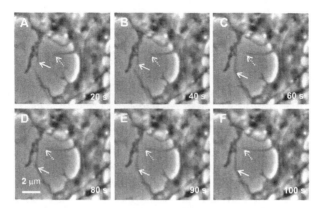

Figure 17.4 Stable membrane protrusions after cytochalasin D treatment of T24 cells can be seen by time-lapse phase-contrast microscopy. After incubation in cytochalasin D for 30 minutes, a time-lapse sequence was recorded. The white arrows point to the tips of two nanotubes that move passively. The times indicated in A–F are the times passed from the beginning of the time-lapse sequence. Reprinted from *Biophysical Journal*, 95(9), Peter Veranič, Maruša Lokar, Gerhard J. Schütz, Julian Weghuber, Stefan Wieser, Henry Hägerstrand, Veronika Kralj-Iglič, and Aleš Iglič, Different types of cell-to-cell connections mediated by nanotubular structures, pp. 4416–4425, Copyright 2008, with permission from Elsevier.

adhesion) of the released vesicles with the membranes of the non-labelled cells.

Type II bridging nanotubes have cytokeratin filaments and are mainly located more appically on the cell (Fig. 17.7). These nanotubes start to grow as the cells move apart (Fig. 17.8). At the very beginning of tube formation some actin is still present at the entry point of the tubes. As the tube extends, the actin gradually disappears and only cytokeratin filaments remain. After the dissociating cells reach a distance of 30 to 40 µm only one such cytokeratin-containing nanotube remains as a link between the two cells. These longer tubes, which can be up to several 100 µm long, can connect dissociating cells for more than 2 hours (Figs. 17.7 and 17.8).

On many nanotubes that connect neighbouring urothelial cells, vesicular dilatations were found (Fig. 17.9). Vesicular dilatations can be seen in both types of bridging nanotubes. The dilatations

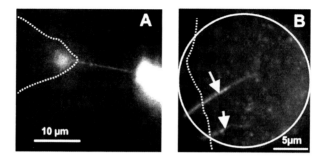

Figure 17.5 Exchange of actin-GFP via a bridging nanotube between two T24 cells. Stable actin–GFP transfected T24 cells were frequently found to be interconnected by TNTs. Occasionally, connections were observed between a high expressing cell and a cell devoid of actin–GFP (cell borders are indicated by a dashed line). The spreading of actin–GFP into the second cell is clearly visible as a cone of fluorescence growing into the GFP-actin negative cell (A). Two nanotubes indicated by arrows connect the shown non-transfected cell with an actin–GFP positive cell outside the imaged area (the imaging pinhole is indicated by a full line) (B). Multiple diffraction-limited spots could be observed at high mobility, indicating the presence of free actin–GFP molecules in the non-transfected cell (see also supplemental material in III and Veranič et al. (2008). Reprinted from *Biophysical Journal*, 95(9), Peter Veranič, Maruša Lokar, Gerhard J. Schütz, Julian Weghuber, Stefan Wieser, Henry Hägerstrand, Veronika Kralj-Iglič, and Aleš Iglič, Different types of cell-to-cell connections mediated by nanotubular structures, pp. 4416–4425, Copyright 2008, with permission from Elsevier.

on type II nanotubes are larger, usually placed in the middle of the tube and do not move along the tube (Veranič et al., 2008). On the other hand, type I nanotubes frequently have vesicular dilatations that move along the tubes in both directions, as seen in Fig. 17.10. Such vesicular dilatations (gondolas) move by 5 to 15 μm in a certain direction with an average speed of 40 n m per second. They sometimes appear in the middle of the nanotube and travel along the nanotube until they fuse with the cell body (Fig. 17.10).

These observed distensions of the nanotubes (gondolas) moving along the bridging nanotubes of type I (Fig. 17.10) may be formed in different ways. In some cases the formation of gondolas, corresponding to transient excited states, may be induced by a sudden tension (caused, e.g., by diverging cells) in the membrane nanotubes

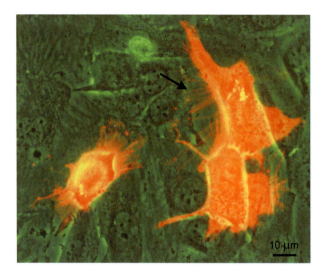

Figure 17.6 Urothelial T24 cells labelled with lipophilic stain DiI were co-cultured with unlabelled T24 cells. The nanotubes (arrow) of stained cells (red) became extended and attached to unstained cells (green) in 3 hours. However, even after 24 h DiI stain did not spread to the connected cells. Reprinted from *Biophysical Journal*, 95(9), Peter Veranič, Maruša Lokar, Gerhard J. Schütz, Julian Weghuber, Stefan Wieser, Henry Hägerstrand, Veronika Kralj-Iglič, and Aleš Iglič, Different types of cell-to-cell connections mediated by nanotubular structures, pp. 4416–4425, Copyright 2008, with permission from Elsevier.

at specific sites where the local membrane constituents of the nanotubes enable and favour the formation of such dilatations. The tension-induced dilatation of the nanotube may appear anywhere along the nanotube and then travel as a wave along the bridging nanotube in the direction that is energetically favourable. Tension could be the most probable origin of gondolas that suddenly appear in the middle of a nanotube. These tension-induced dilatations of the nanotubes, like any other excited state of the membrane, relaxed after a certain time. It was previously reported that slight undulations relax in seconds while sphere-like blebs relax in minutes (Bar-Ziv and Moses, 1994; Bar-Ziv et al., 1999). The distension of the nanotubes may also be formed because of a small organelle inside the nanotube, if the diameter of the organelle is larger than the inner diameter of the nanotube (Gerdes et al.,

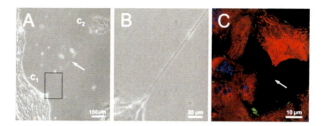

Figure 17.7 In the T24 urothelial line, a long tubular structure connects cells of the two cell clusters C1 and C2 (A). Panel B is a magnified region of the area in the black frame in A. Such long singular tubes of type II contain thin cytokeratin filaments (↑ in C). In C, cytokeratin 7 is labelled in red, actin in green, and the nucleus with DAPI in blue. Reprinted from *Biophysical Journal*, 95(9), Peter Veranič, Maruša Lokar, Gerhard J. Schütz, Julian Weghuber, Stefan Wieser, Henry Hägerstrand, Veronika Kralj-Iglič, and Aleš Iglič, Different types of cell-to-cell connections mediated by nanotubular structures, pp. 4416–4425, Copyright 2008, with permission from Elsevier.

2007). An organelle inside a nanotube my be actively transported by different acto–myosin-dependent mechanisms (Gerdes et al., 2007; Hurtig et al., 2010; Önfelt et al., 2004; Rustom et al., 2004).

The vesicular dilatations of nanotubes observed moving along bridging nanotubes of type I (Figs. 17.9 and 17.10) show a striking similarity to the dilatations of phospholipid nanotubes which move along nanotubes (Fig. 17.2). Therefore, it is also possible that the initiation of gondola formation (Fig. 17.11A) may be based on similar physical mechanisms to those governing the formation of free membrane daughter vesicles, which are created in the processes of budding. In contrast to the latter process, however, in gondolas the connection to the parent membrane from which they originate is not disrupted when the gondola is detached from the parent cell (Fig. 17.11B). From observations in pure lipid systems (Fig. 17.2), it is clear that for the existence of a vesicle, which is a distended integral part of the nanotube membrane (Fig. 17.11), it is not always necessary that the diameter of the enclosed material (e.g., an organelle) be larger than the inner diameter of the nanotube (Gerdes et al., 2007). Transported material (multiple small particles moving synchronously within the distension) may be enclosed within the gondola or may be a part of the gondola membrane

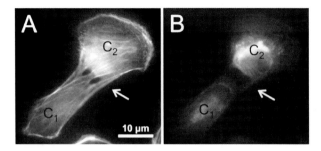

Figure 17.8 Two separating T24 cells (C1 and C2) having actin (A) and cytokeratin (B) filaments present in the forming protrusions. Membranes of the two cells detach at certain sites forming tail-like protrusions between the membranes. The membranes gradually separate as the cells move apart, pulling and dividing their cytoskeletal content. Note that both actin (A) and cytokeratin (B) filaments are still present in the growing tubular connections. Reprinted from *Biophysical Journal*, 95(9), Peter Veranič, Maruša Lokar, Gerhard J. Schütz, Julian Weghuber, Stefan Wieser, Henry Hägerstrand, Veronika Kralj-Iglič, and Aleš Iglič, Different types of cell-to-cell connections mediated by nanotubular structures, pp. 4416–4425, Copyright 2008, with permission from Elsevier.

(Fig. 17.11). Once the gondola is formed, its movement along the nanotube (Fig. 17.11C) requires no additional bending energy. Nevertheless, some process is needed to provide the energy for the gondola to travel along the nanotube. It is possible that gondola movement is driven by the difference in chemical potential between the molecules packed inside the gondola and the molecules in the interior of the target cell, or the difference in chemical potential between the molecules composing the membrane of the gondola and the molecules in the membrane of the target cell. The final event of the transport process is the fusion of the gondola with the target membrane (Iglič et al., 2003; Veranič et al., 2008). In this process, molecules of the gondola's membrane which originate from the parent, a nearly flat membrane, redistribute again in an almost flat target membrane (Fig. 17.11E). This may be energetically favourable and therefore, also part of the driving mechanism to facilitate fusion of the gondola with the membrane. Prior to fusion of the gondola with the target cell membrane, no neck formation is needed (Fig. 17.11D) since the neck is already part of the nanotube

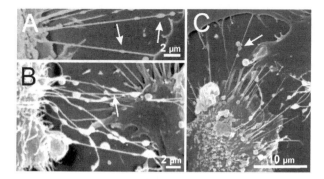

Figure 17.9 Membrane nanotubes with gondolas (white arrows) observed between cells in the human urothelial RT4 cell line (A) and T24 (B and C) by scanning electron microscopy under physiological conditions. Note that the gondolas are an integral part of the tubes. Reprinted from *Biophysical Journal*, 95(9), Peter Veranič, Maruša Lokar, Gerhard J. Schütz, Julian Weghuber, Stefan Wieser, Henry Hägerstrand, Veronika Kralj-Iglič, and Aleš Iglič, Different types of cell-to-cell connections mediated by nanotubular structures, pp. 4416–4425, Copyright 2008, with permission from Elsevier.

connecting the gondola to the membrane of the target cell. This is contrary to the case of a free transport vesicle. It can therefore be concluded that the transport of material in gondolas (or the transport of molecules composing the membrane of gondolas) may be energetically advantageous over free vesicle transport.

Since the bridging nanotubes differ in their structural components, they probably also differ in their functions. Some of the observed bridging nanotubes are certainly TNT (Rustom et al., 2004). The cloud of cytosolic non-polymerized (free) actin–GFP molecules in a cell originally devoid of actin–GFP (Fig. 17.5) clearly shows the transport of free actin–GFP molecules through the bridging nanotubes connecting two neighbouring cells. Nevertheless, further investigations are required to explain in detail what kind of material, signals or information could be exchanged via the observed bridging nanotubes and nanotube-directed gondolas, and in what form or which cytoskeletal components are involved in possible nanotube-mediated communication between neighbouring cells.

It was shown in the previous Chapters 9 and 10 of this book that the lateral distribution of membrane components may

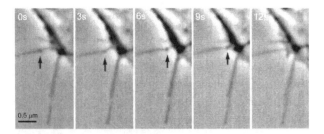

Figure 17.10 Fusion of a gondola (↑) with a cell body is seen from a time-lapse sequence showing directional movement of the gondola along a nanotube. The time sequence in seconds is indicated on the upper left side of each micrograph. Reprinted from *Biophysical Journal*, 95(9), Peter Veranič, Maruša Lokar, Gerhard J. Schütz, Julian Weghuber, Stefan Wieser, Henry Hägerstrand, Veronika Kralj-Iglič, and Aleš Iglič, Different types of cell-to-cell connections mediated by nanotubular structures, pp. 4416–4425, Copyright 2008, with permission from Elsevier.

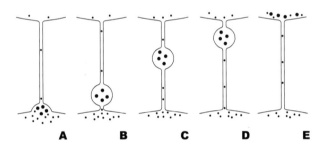

Figure 17.11 Schematic illustration of nanotubule-directed transport of small carrier vesicles (gondolas) transporting granular content and membrane particles. Reprinted from *Biophysical Journal*, 95(9), Peter Veranič, Maruša Lokar, Gerhard J. Schütz, Julian Weghuber, Stefan Wieser, Henry Hägerstrand, Veronika Kralj-Iglič, and Aleš Iglič, Different types of cell-to-cell connections mediated by nanotubular structures, pp. 4416–4425, Copyright 2008, with permission from Elsevier.

strongly depend on their intrinsic shape. Therefore the formation and mechanical stability of intercellular (tunnelling) nanotubes are also determined by the intrinsic shape of membrane components. Fig. 17.12 is an illustrative example showing the theoretically predicted accumulation of an anisotropic membrane component in the membrane tube that connects two spheroidal cells, where the

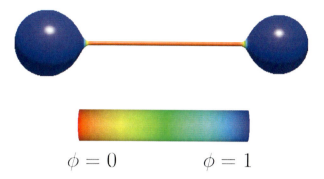

Figure 17.12 The calculated equilibrium membrane shape and lateral distribution of membrane components obtained by miminization of the elastic energy of a two-component membrane composed of an isotropic component (92 percent) and an anisotropic component (8 percent). In the colour map, the hot colours (i.e., red) denote more of the anisotropic component, and the cold colours (i.e., blue) denote more of the isotropic component (Bobrowska et al., 2013; Kabaso et al., 2012a). Reprinted from *Bioelectrochemistry*, 87, Doron Kabaso, Nataliya Bobrovska, Wojciech Góźdź, Ekaterina Gongadze, Veronika Kralj-Iglič, Robert Zorec, Aleš Iglič, The transport along membrane nanotubes driven by the spontaneous curvature of membrane components, pp. 204–210, Copyright 2012, with permission from Elsevier.

isotropic membrane component is predominantly accumulated in the spherical membrane regions. The equilibrium membrane shape and equilibrium lateral distribution of the membrane components presented in Fig. 17.12 were determined in the same minimization procedure (Bobrowska et al., 2013; Kabaso et al., 2012a). In accordance with the results presented in Figs. 9.2–9.4 and 10.8, the energetically favourable accumulation of anisotropic membrane components is indicated to be the main driving force in the formation and stabilisation of the intercellular tube connecting the two spheroidal membrane regions (Kabaso et al., 2012a; Veranič et al., 2008).

Chapter 18

Biological Impact of Membranous Nanostructures

In this book the basic biophysical mechanisms governing biological membrane configurations are considered. The membrane configuration comprises the lateral redistribution of membrane constituents and the related membrane curvature. As membrane constituents are small, the resulting curvatures are large. Membranous nanostructures are formed such as nanovesicles (NVs), nanotubules, and inverted hexagonal stacks. These structures represent an important pool of biological membranes (Kralj-Iglič, 2012). They are composed in a way similar to the mother cell and also enclose a cell interior. Nanotubules explore the surroundings and may become attached to neighbouring cells. NVs are free to move in body fluids and travel with the circulation. They can reach distant cells and interact with them. Nanotubules and NVs transfer matter and information to other cells. Therefore, they can be considered as cell–cell communication systems. By fusing with recipient cells, nanotubules and NVs convey to these cells surface-bound ligands and receptors (Ratajczak et al., 2006a,b), prion proteins (Fevrier et al., 2004; Vella et al., 2008), genetic material including RNA and DNA (Baj-Krzyworzeka et al., 2006; Pisetsky, 2009), and infectious

---

Nanostructures in Biological Systems: Theory and Applications
Aleš Iglič, Veronika Kralj-Iglič, and Damjana Drobne
Copyright © 2015 Pan Stanford Publishing Pte. Ltd.
ISBN 978-981-4267-20-5 (Hardcover), 978-981-4303-43-9 (eBook)
www.panstanford.com

agents (Coltel et al., 2006; Pelchen-Matthews et al., 2004). It has been suggested that NVs are involved in cancer metastasis (Janowska-Wieczorek et al., 2006). Nanotubules and NVs contribute to tumour progression and the spreading of inflammation and infection. It is therefore indicated that basic biophysical mechanisms such as membrane budding and vesiculation play an important role in health and disease. To manipulate these mechanisms it is necessary to describe and understand the processes leading to stable membranous nanostructures.

Methods have been developed to harvest NVs from body fluids. Information on homeostasis can be obtained by harvesting and analysing NVs. For example, the presence of tumours can be detected by characterization of isolated NVs. It was recently demonstrated that RNA profiles, in particular microRNA, are appropriate biomarkers for tumours of various origin (Lu et al., 2005) and various clinical outcome (Calin et al., 2005). MicroRNAs are short (about 18–25 nucleotides long) non-coding RNAs. They are classified as small interfering siRNA, ribosomal rRNA, transfer tRNA, and small nuclear snRNA (Metias et al., 2009). It was reported that over 700 different microRNAs have been identified within the human genome (Patel and Saute, 2011). It is indicated that the microRNA profile is associated with prognosis and development of the disease (Patel and Saute, 2011; White and Yousef, 2010). Furthermore, mutations in microRNA genes are frequent and may have functional importance (Calin et al., 2005); they can either suppress tumours or promote their growth and proliferation (Patel and Saute, 2011). MicroRNA profiling has already been applied to chronic lymphocytic leukemia to distinguish between slowly expanding or aggressive forms of cancer (Lu et al., 2005). Also, the composition of NVs isolated from the blood of patients with early (stage II) colorectal cancer could be distinguished from the composition of those isolated from sex- and age-matched healthy volunteers (Nielsen et al., 2010). Compared to current invasive methods that are used to diagnose most malignancies, the assessment of NVs is advantageous as it only requires a relatively small amount of blood. Assessment of NVs can be used to diagnose the disease, and to follow development and treatment of the disease. Therefore, NVs are considered as potential biomarkers for various diseases, including cancer.

In studying the origin of various diseases and the mechanisms that underlie them, extensive work was performed using chemical and biochemical methods. These methods focus on specific molecules, their binding, reactions, and pathways. Although important progress has been achieved, in many diseases (such as cancer), an essential unifying mechanism or mechanisms has have not yet been revealed. Up to now, the contributions of physics and biophysics cannot match that of chemistry and biochemistry. Apparently, living creatures were so far commonly considered too complex to be adequately described by the physical methods which proved effective in the description of simple systems. However, even in highly complex living creatures, some relevant issues can be exposed to simplify the system. In such cases the methods of theoretical physics can then be applied.

By using the methods of statistical mechanics and thermodynamics it will be demonstrated that the shape of membranous nanostructures is consistent with the ordering of membrane constituents in strongly anisotropically curved membrane regions, an arrangement which is energetically favourable (see Chapters 7, 9 and 10). These theoretical predictions are supported by experimental evidence. Furthermore, orientational ordering of particles with internally distributed charge provides an explanation of the mediated attractive interaction between membranes (see Section 14) which is clinically relevant as a nanovesiculation suppressive mechanism.

The cell membrane is a basic building element of the cell (see Section 18.2). In order to understand the interdependence between processes which take place in cells, it is necessary to understand those features that are relevant for the cell membrane. For this purpose, the cell membrane has been extensively studied. Following a thorough investigation, Singer and Nicolson in 1972 proposed the fluid mosaic model of the membrane. The membrane was described as a lipid bilayer (see Chapter 2) in which proteins and other large molecules are embedded (Singer and Nicolson, 1972). From a physical point of view, the fluid mosaic model expresses the fact that the phospholipid bilayer exhibits the properties of a two-dimensional laterally isotropic liquid. Proteins and other large molecules can more or less freely move laterally within the membrane. Studies (theoretical and experimental) over the last 40 years confirmed that the fluid mosaic model provides a good description of the biological membrane and established it as the standard model.

Twenty-five years later, the fluid mosaic model was complemented by considering lateral inhomogeneities (Brown and London, 1998b; Simons and Ikonen, 1997) (see also Chapters 8–10). According to the modified model, the membrane is described as a two-dimensional liquid with embedded nanodomains (see Chapter 8) of specific composition. These nanodomains are called membrane rafts. Membrane rafts are rather small (10–200 nm) and relatively heterogeneous dynamic structures which exhibit an increased concentration of cholesterol and sphingolipids (Pike, 2006; Simons and Gerl, 2010). From a biochemical point of view, membrane rafts are structures which at low temperatures resist solvation by detergents while from a biophysical point of view, it is considered that increased ordering of membrane constituents takes place in the raft due to interactions between the highly saturated fatty acids of sphingolipids. It was suggested that fatty acids within rafts have limited mobility with respect to the unsaturated fatty acids which are located in other parts of the membrane. Dynamic accumulation of specific membrane constituents in rafts regulates the spatial and temporal dependence of signalization and transport of matter, thereby forming transient but vitally important signalling platforms.

Membrane curvature is determined by the shape of membrane constituents and their interactions (see Chapter 8). By accumulation of a specific type of constituent, an intrinsic curvature of the raft is determined which may be different from the curvature of the surrounding membrane (see also Chapter 8). In other words, lateral sorting of membrane constituents may cause changes in the local membrane curvature (see Chapter 9). Considering this interdependence, the fluid mosaic model was further upgraded as described earlier in this book. Hence, this and previous chapters are devoted to theoretical and experimental evidence showing that membranous nanostructures are a stable pool of cell membranes and that they play a functional role in cellular processes.

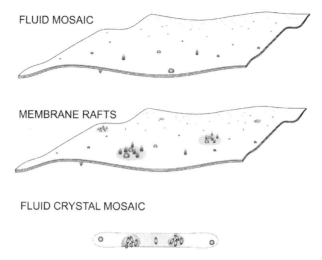

Figure 18.1 A schematic representation of three models of the membrane: the fluid mosaic model (Singer and Nicolson, 1972), the membrane raft model (Brown and London, 1998a,b; Simons and Ikonen, 1997), and the fluid crystal mosaic model (Kralj-Iglič, 2012). Violet colour indicates orientational ordering of lipid molecules on the tubular part. Republished with permission of DOVE Medical Press, from Stability of membranous nanostructures: A possible key mechanism in cancer progression, Kralj-Iglič, V., *Int. J. Nanomed*, 7, copyright 2012; permission conveyed through Copyright Clearance Center, Inc.

To simplify the system, it is considered that one of the membrane extensions (the thickness) is much smaller than the other two extensions, so the membrane may be treated as a two-dimensional surface (see Chapter 5). Also, the membrane is viewed as composed of a large number of particles (building units) which mutually interact (Kralj-Iglič, 2012). Taking into account the above supposition, the membrane layer is described as a surface composed of building units (molecules, groups of molecules, membrane rafts, and nanodomains), which attains a shape corresponding to the minimum of its free energy (see Chapter 9). Orientational ordering of membrane building units on strongly anisotropically curved membrane regions (such as nanotubules, hexagonal stacks, and narrow necks) provides an explanation for the stability of different types of membranous nanostructures (see Chapters 7–10).

Accordingly, the extended model may be referred to as the "fluid crystal mosaic model" expressing that curvature-related lateral and orientational redistribution of membrane constituents takes place.

18.1 Nanovesiculation and Nanovesicles

NVs isolated from blood were first described as an inert platelet dust (Wolf, 1967). Later, it was observed that NVs are shed from the membrane of erythrocytes during storage (Cole et al., 1979; Greenwalt, 2006; Rumsby et al., 1977; Shukla et al., 1978; Simak and Gilderman, 2006), or *in vitro* following the addition of different stimuli to a suspension of erythrocytes (Allan et al., 1976; Araki, 1979; Hägerstrand and Isomaa, 1989, 1992, 1994; Yamaguchi et al., 1991). Nanovesiculation was observed in platelets (George et al., 1982; Hägerstrand et al., 1996; Heijnen et al., 1999), white blood cells (Cerri et al., 2006), endothelial cells (Brogan et al., 2004; Combes et al., 1999; Martinez et al., 2005; Shet et al., 2003), and cancer cells (Black, 1980; Ginestra et al., 1998; Huber et al., 2005; Koga et al., 2005; Kralj-Iglič et al., 1998; Sheddon et al., 2003; Taylor et al., 1983a,b; Valenti et al., 2007; Whiteside, 2005), where it was related to procoagulant activity (Bastida et al., 1983, 1985, 1986; Rauch and Antoniak, 2007).

It is now considered (Diamant et al., 2004; Flaumenhaft, 2006; Greenwalt, 2006; Hugel et al., 2005; Pisetsky, 2009; Ratajczak, 2006; Ratajczak et al., 2006b; Taylor and Black, 1987; Whiteside, 2005) that NVs are sub-micron sized, membrane-enclosed compartments of the cell interior which are released into the surrounding solution in the final stage of the budding process and become free to move with body fluids.

It was found that platelet-derived NVs contain compounds which catalyse formation of blood clots (Berckmans et al., 2002; Bona et al., 1987; del Conde et al., 2005; Furie et al., 2005; Mallat et al., 1999; Müller et al., 2003; Sabatier et al., 2002); moreover, the area-to-volume ratio of platelet-derived NVs is much larger than that of intact platelets, so that nanovesiculation significantly increases the catalytic surface for blood clot formation and is considered to be a procoagulant mechanism. The interplay between these processes takes part especially through NV-mediated interaction among platelets, endothelial cells, and tumour cells; and is reflected in secondary thromboembolic events (e.g., in cancer (del Conde et al., 2007; Furie and Furie, 2006; Hron et al., 2007; Rauch and Antoniak, 2007), autoimmune diseases (Dignat-George et al., 2004; Jy et al., 2007; Kravitz and Shoenfeld, 2005; Pereira et al., 2006; Warkentin et al., 1994)), and in tumour progression (Huber et al., 2005; Janowska-Wieczorek et al., 2005; Valenti et al., 2007).

It would be beneficial to perform diagnosis on samples of peripheral blood instead of on samples obtained by biopsy. It is believed that blood contains circulating NVs (Dey-Hazra et al., 2010; Orozco and Lewis, 2010; Piccin et al., 2007; Sellam et al., 2009) carrying information on clinical status. Also it is believed that these NVs can be harvested by isolation. Isolated NVs can be assessed for concentration and composition. Different protocols for the isolation of NVs can be found in the literature (Biro et al., 2004; Diamant et al., 2002; Dignat-George et al., 2004; Hugel et al., 2004; Nomura, 2004; Shet et al., 2004), usually consisting of centrifugation and washing of the sample and then assessing the NVs by flow cytometry (Dey-Hazra et al., 2010; Huica et al., 2011; Orozco and Lewis, 2010; Robert et al., 2009; Shah et al., 2008). However, a method based on the isolation and assessment of NVs from blood that would be of satisfactory repeatability and accuracy and therefore, suitable for diagnosis and treatment in clinical practice has not yet been established.

It is also interesting to observe the isolates NVs. Due to their size and shape, membrane constituents can induce strong curvature in the membrane, which then forms protrusions and eventually NVs. Due to this potential for strongly curving the membrane, the pinched off NVs are very small and therefore cannot be observed directly under an optical microscope. Other techniques appropriate for observation of biological material are required to reveal their shape, such as imaging with an atomic force microscope (AFM), imaging with a scanning electron microscope (SEM), and imaging with a transmission electron microscope (TEM) (Drobne et al., 2005; Vesel, 2008; Wilson et al., 1995).

Observation by AFM, SEM, and TEM can only be made on a limited number of NVs, whereas flow cytometry is able to record a very large number of NVs and thereby, also give information on the

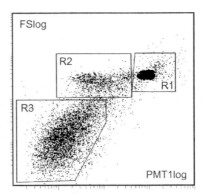

Figure 18.2 A typical dot plot detected by a flow cytometer: FS: forward scattered light, PMT1: side scattered light. The three regions marked comprise R1, microspheres with 10 μm diameter; R2, residual cells; and R3, microvesicles. Reprinted from Šuštar, V., Bedina-Zavec, A., Štukelj, R., Frank, M., Ogorevc, E., Janša, R., Mam, K., Veranič, P., and Kralj-Iglič, V. (2011). Postprandial rise of microvesicles in peripheral blood of healthy human donors. *Lipids Health Dis.*, 10, pp. 47, copyright 2011, permission conveyed through Copyright Clearance Center, Inc.

size distribution. Thus, microscopic imaging and flow cytometry are complementary in gathering information on NVs.

Figure 18.2 shows a dot plot of events detected by flow cytometer. As cells are expected to be found in isolates, we defined three regions: R1, microspheres with a known diameter of 10 μm; R2, residual cells; and R3, NVs.

18.1.1 Nanovesicles Isolated from Blood

To isolate NVs, peripheral blood samples (1.7–20 ml) were taken from human and animal donors. In patients, blood was taken when it was collected for therapeutic reasons, within the same phlebotomy. Similarly in students, blood was taken when it was collected for obligatory check-ups, but for the experiments only, blood was taken from the authors and staff. Mare's blood was used because the large size of the animal allowed collection of a larger volume of blood with minimal discomfort to the animal.

The sampled blood was centrifuged at 1550 g for 20 min. The upper 250 μl of plasma was slowly removed from each tube and transferred to a 1.5 ml Eppendorf tube. The samples were centrifuged at 17570 g for 30 min and The supernatant (225 µl) was discarded and the pellet (25 µl) re-suspended in 225 µl of citrated phosphate buffer saline (PBS). Samples were centrifuged again at 17570 g for 30 min and the supernatant (225 µl) discarded. The pellet (25 µl) was re-suspended in an appropriate quantity of citrated PBS.

For scanning electron imaging of isolates, NVs were suspension-fixed in 1% glutaraldehyde dissolved in PBS/citrate buffer for 60 min at 22°C, post-fixed for 60 min at 22°C in 1% OsO_4 dissolved in 0.9% NaCl, and then dehydrated in a graded series of acetone/water (50%–100%, v/v). The samples were critical-point dried, gold-sputtered, and examined using a SEM.

Figure 18.3 shows a scanning electron micrograph of an isolate, while Fig. 18.4 shows scanning electron micrographs of chosen regions within an isolate from the blood of a healthy human donor. Heparin (Fig. 18.4A–D) and trisodium citrate (Fig. 18.4E,F) were used as the anticoagulants. Many NVs and some residual erythrocytes can be seen in the isolate (Fig. 18.3, Fig. 18.4A, marked with a black arrow). Also activated platelets (Fig. 18.4A, marked with a white arrow) were present in the isolate. NVs had diverse shapes and sizes. Tubular structures of different lengths could be observed (Fig. 18.4B–F), which were more abundant with heparin than with trisodium citrate as the anticoagulant. Peculiar structures (e.g., torus) (Fig. 18.4E, marked with white arrows) and starfish (Fig. 18.4F, marked with a black arrow) were found. The white arrow in Fig. 18.4F points to a cell which formed protrusions with bulbous ends.

Figure18.5 shows some characteristic NP shapes found in an isolate from the blood of a patient with pancreatic cancer (female, 60 years). Some rather large fragments with a low volume:area ratio (A, B), nano-sized discocytes (C), and dumbbell shapes (D) can be seen. Comparison with shapes obtained by minimization of the membrane free energy (E, F) showed good agreement. This indicates that these particles are membrane-enclosed entities without an internal structure and can therefore be described as vesicles.

The shapes shown in Fig. 18.5E and F were calculated theoretically by minimization of the membrane bilayer free energy as

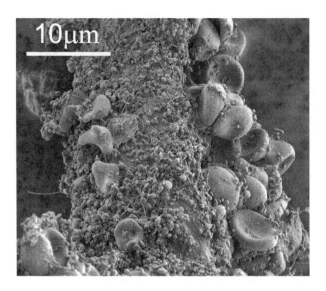

Figure 18.3 Scanning electron micrograph of an isolate from the peripheral blood of a healthy human donor (male, 28 years). A mass of microparticles and numerous residual erythrocytes can be seen. The image was taken using a Quanta TM 250 FEG (FEI, Hillsboro, Oregon, U.S.A.) SEM at FEI Quanta, Eindhoven, The Netherlands, by applying 1.5 kV. Republished with permission of DOVE Medical Press, from Nanoparticles isolated from blood: A reflection of vesiculability of blood cells during the isolation process, Šuštar V, Bedina-Zavec A, Štukelj R, Frank M, Bobojevič G, Janša R, Ogorevc E, Kruljc P, Mam K, Šimunič B, Manček-Keber M, Jerala R, Rozman B, Veranič P, Hägerstrand H, Kralj-Iglič V, *Int J Nanomed*, 6, copyright 2011; permission conveyed through Copyright Clearance Center, Inc.

described in details in Chapter 7 (Kralj-Iglič et al., 2006) (see also Chapters 9 and 10). It was assumed that the vesicle has no internal structure and that its shape was determined by the properties of the membrane. The calculated shapes of minimal elastic energy were characterized by a high degree of symmetry and smooth contours that avoided sharp bending, which is energetically unfavourable. Vesicles undergo fluctuations in shape due to thermal effects, so their instantaneous shapes deviate somewhat from the ideal morphology predicted by theory and calculations. Nevertheless, matching of the appearance of the observed and the calculated shapes of blood-derived NVs is excellent (Figs. 18.5C–F). It can also

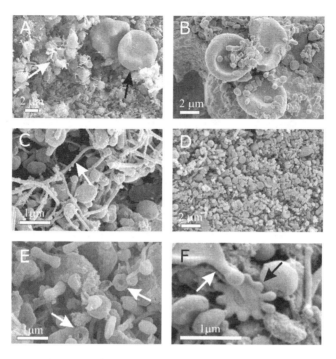

Figure 18.4 Scanning electron micrograph of chosen regions of an isolate from the peripheral blood of a healthy human donor (male, 28 years). In addition to the numerous NVs which are present all the pictures, erythrocytes (A-black arrow, B), activated platelets (A-white arrow), tubules (C), tori (E-white arrows), starfish (F-black arrow), and a deformed erythrocyte exhibiting a protrusion with a bulbous end (F-white arrow) were observed. Images (A-D) were taken using a LEO Gemini 1530 (LEO, Oberkochen, Germany) SEM by applying 8 kV (A,C,D) and 2.7 kV (B) at Åbo Akademi University, Åbo/Turku, Finland. Image E was taken by a Quanta TM 250 FEG (FEI, Hillsboro, Oregon, USA) SEM at FEI Quanta, Eindhoven, The Netherlands, by applying 1.5 kV. Republished with permission of DOVE Medical Press, from Nanoparticles isolated from blood: A reflection of vesiculability of blood cells during the isolation process, Šuštar V, Bedina-Zavec A, Štukelj R, Frank M, Bobojevič G, Janša R, Ogorevc E, Kruljc P, Mam K, Šimunič B, Manček-Keber M, Jerala R, Rozman B, Veranič P, Hägerstrand H, Kralj-Iglič V, *Int J Nanomed*, 6, copyright 2011; permission conveyed through Copyright Clearance Center, Inc.

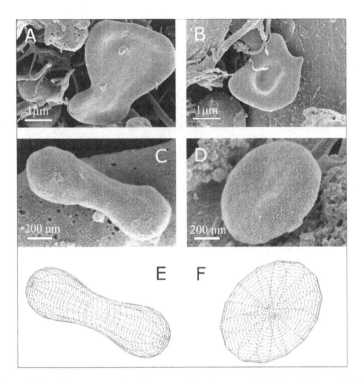

Figure 18.5 Representative characteristic shapes of NVs found in an isolate from the blood of a patient with pancreatic cancer (female, 60 years). Shapes include shizocytes (A,B), a dumbbell (C), a submicron discocyte (D), and the corresponding shapes calculated by minimization of the membrane free energy (E,F). The shape in panel E was obtained for a relative volume $v = 36\pi V^{2/3}/A^{3/2} = 0.65$, where V is the volume of the vesicle, A is the surface area of the vesicle and for the relative average mean curvature $\langle h \rangle = 1/2A \int (C_1 + C_2)\mathrm{d}A = 1.32$, where C_1 and C_2 are the two principal curvatures at a chosen point on the membrane surface and integration is performed over the entire surface of the vesicle A. For the shape in panel F, $v = 0.55$ and $\langle h \rangle = 1.055$ (see also Chapter 7). The intrinsic principal curvatures were equal to 0 for both shapes. The images were taken using a LEO Gemini 1530 (LEO, Oberkochen, Germany) SEM by applying 8 kV at Åbo Akademi University, Åbo/Turku, Finland. Republished with permission of DOVE Medical Press, from Nanoparticles isolated from blood: A reflection of vesiculability of blood cells during the isolation process, Šuštar V, Bedina-Zavec A, Štukelj R, Frank M, Bobojevič G, Janša R, Ogorevc E, Kruljc P, Mam K, Šimunič B, Manček-Keber M, Jerala R, Rozman B, Veranič P, Hägerstrand H, Kralj-Iglič V, *Int J Nanomed*, 6, copyright 2011; permission conveyed through Copyright Clearance Center, Inc.

be seen in Figs. 18.3 and 18.4 that the contours of the NVs are highly symmetrical and smooth, indicating that these shapes correspond to NVs with no internal structure.

Imaging of NVs by AFM in the phase mode gives further information about their properties. In phase mode imaging, the phase shift of the oscillating cantilever relative to the driving signal is measured and correlated with specific properties of the material, which depend on the cantilever tip–sample interaction. Therefore, the phase shift can be used to differentiate areas by friction, adhesion, and viscoelasticity. By operating AFM in the tapping mode, the friction and adhesive force is reduced and imaging of soft biological samples is enabled. Individual NVs can be distinguished by detecting their boundaries (dark parts on the phase images). Figures 18.6 and 18.7 show atomic force micrographs of NV-rich blood plasma of two healthy blood donors (H1 and H2, respectively). The height images and the phase images are presented. The globular structures which differ in elasticity from the surroundings and protrude out of the surface (Fig. 18.6) could correspond to NVs ranging from 100 to 300 nm in width and from 30 to 60 nm in height. Also Fig. 18.7 shows a scanning electron micrograph of NVs isolated from healthy donor H3, revealing globular and tubular structures with shapes characteristic of vesicles (membrane-enclosed entities with no internal structure).

The height of NVs determined by AFM (about 60 nm) is considerably smaller than their diameter (about 150 nm). To some extent this could be attributed to AFM tip broadening (Wilson et al., 1995), but most probably due to the collapse of NVs during the drying process. SEM analysis yields comparable dimensions (Junkar et al., 2009), while the procedure for preparation of samples prevents NVs from collapsing. In analysing samples (NV-rich plasma, isolated plasma NVs) both techniques (AFM and SEM) reveal the presence of globular structures which according to their size and shape can be interpreted as NVs.

18.1.2 *Nanovesicles Isolated from other Body Fluids*

Besides in blood, NVs were also found in other body fluids, that is, the synovial fluid of inflamed joints (Junkar et al., 2009), pleural fluid

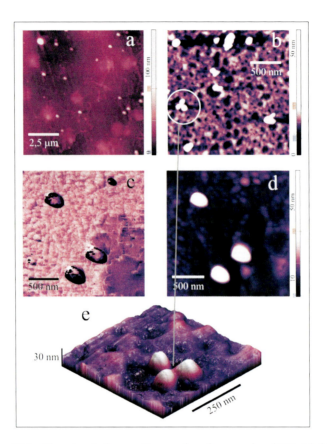

Figure 18.6 The atomic force micrographs of a sample of NV-rich blood plasma of a healthy donor H1. (a,b,d): height images, (b): phase image, (e): enlarged three dimensional representation of the region marked in (b). Reprinted from Junkar, I., Šuštar, V., Frank, M., Janša, V., Bedina-Zavec, A., Rozman, B., Mozetič, M., Hägerstrand, H., and Kralj-Iglič, V. (2009). Blood and synovial microparticles as revealed by atomic force and scanning electron microscope. *Op. Autoimmun. J.*, 1, pp. 50–58, Copyright © 2015 Bentham Open.

(Bard et al., 2004; Mrvar-Brečko et al., 2010), ascites (Mrvar-Brečko et al., 2010) and urine (Pascual et al., 1994).

Figure 18.8 shows material isolated from the chylous fluid (C,D) of a cat, sedimented cells from the same sample (A,B), and material obtained by the isolation protocol from the pleural fluid of a cat.

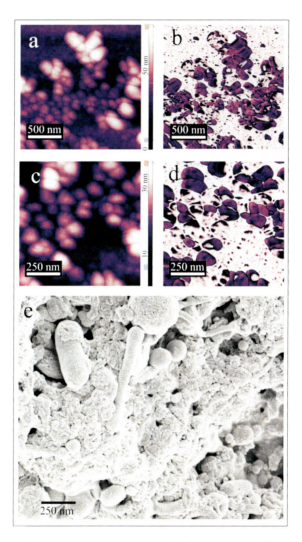

Figure 18.7 An atomic force micrograph of a sample of NV-rich blood plasma from a healthy donor H2. (a,c): phase images, (b,d): height images. (e): scanning electron micrograph of a sample of NVs isolated from the peripheral blood of a healthy donor H3. Reprinted from Junkar, I., Šuštar, V., Frank, M., Janša, V., Bedina-Zavec, A., Rozman, B., Mozetič, M., Hägerstrand, H., and Kralj-Iglič, V. (2009). Blood and synovial microparticles as revealed by atomic force and scanning electron microscope. *Op. Autoimmun. J.*, 1, pp. 50–58, Copyright © 2015 Bentham Open.

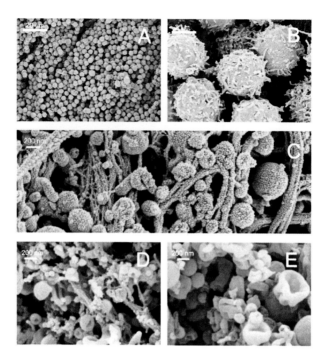

Figure 18.8 Sedimented cells obtained from the chylous fluid of a cat (A,B) and microvesicles isolated from the same sample (C) and from the pleural fluid of a cat (D,E). The sediment of the chylous fluid contains mostly leukocytes (A,B). Reprinted from *Blood Cells, Molecules, and Diseases*, 44(4), Anita Mrvar-Brečko, Vid Šuštar, Vid Janša, Roman Štukelj, Rado Janša, Emir Mujagič, Peter Kruljc, Aleš Iglič, Henry Hägerstrand, and Veronika Kralj-Iglič, Isolated microvesicles from peripheral blood and body fluids as observed by scanning electron microscope, pp. 307–312, Copyright 2010, with permission from Elsevier.

The sediment of the chylous fluid consists mostly of activated leukocytes (A,B), while the isolate from the supernatant is rich in nanostructures which indicate that they derive from leukocytes. The isolate of the cat pleural liquid contains vesicular structures with a low volume-to-area ratio (e.g., stomatocytic shapes). Figure 18.9 shows the sediment and isolate from the postoperative drainage fluid of a human donor. Blood cells (A–C: erythrocytes and B,C: leukocytes) and NVs (A) are present in the sediment, while the supernatant is rich in NVs (C–F).

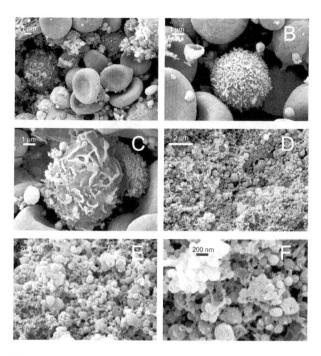

Figure 18.9 Sedimented cells (A–C) and isolated microvesicles (D–F) from human postoperative drainage fluid. The sample was abundant in erythrocytes (A) while leukocytes could also be found (B, C). Numerous microvesicles were found in the supernatant (D–F) as well as in the sediment (A). Reprinted from *Blood Cells, Molecules, and Diseases*, 44(4), Anita Mrvar-Brečko, Vid Šuštar, Vid Janša, Roman Štukelj, Rado Janša, Emir Mujagič, Peter Kruljc, Aleš Iglič, Henry Hägerstrand, and Veronika Kralj-Iglič, Isolated microvesicles from peripheral blood and body fluids as observed by scanning electron microscope, pp. 307–312, Copyright 2010, with permission from Elsevier.

Preparation of samples for scanning electron microscopy yields certain artefacts. Nano-sized grain-like structures can be observed on the globular core of NVs isolated from blood, the chylothorax and ascites (Figs. 18.8C and 18.10B,F). These structures are gold grains formed as a consequence of excessive gold sputtering in sample preparation for SEM. Larger gold grains overshadow the otherwise round core shape of smaller NVs from human pleural fluid (Fig. 18.10F). The stomatocytic form of NVs isolated from

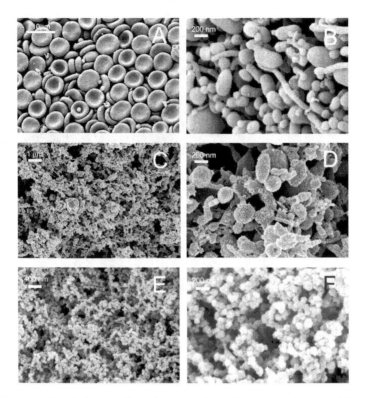

Figure 18.10 Sedimented erythrocytes from human cerebrospinal fluid (A) and NVs isolated from this sample (B). NVs isolated from ascites of a human patient with perforation of ventriculi and diffuse peritonitis (C,D), and from the pleural fluid of a human patient with colon cancer (E,F). Reprinted from *Blood Cells, Molecules, and Diseases*, 44(4), Anita Mrvar-Brečko, Vid Šuštar, Vid Janša, Roman Štukelj, Rado Janša, Emir Mujagič, Peter Kruljc, Aleš Iglič, Henry Hägerstrand, and Veronika Kralj-Iglič, Isolated microvesicles from peripheral blood and body fluids as observed by scanning electron microscope, pp. 307–312, Copyright 2010, with permission from Elsevier.

cat pleural fluid (Fig. 18.10E,F), as well as the holes on NVs isolated from postoperative drainage fluid (Fig. 18.9F) are probably a consequence of improper dehydration in sample preparation for SEM.

Figure 18.11 shows an atomic force micrograph of a sample isolated from the synovial fluid of a patient with psoriatic arthritis

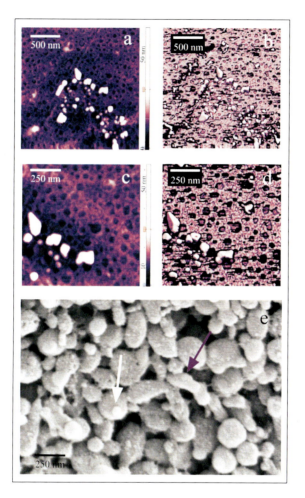

Figure 18.11 An atomic force micrograph of the material isolated from synovial fluid obtained from a patient with psoriatic arthritis P1. (a,c): the phase images, (b,d): the height images. (e): a scanning electron micrograph of the material isolated from synovial fluid of a patient with rheumatoid arthritis P2. Globular and tubular structures with a high degree of symmetry could be NVs (white arrow), while more irregular structures could be protein–lipid assemblies (violet arrow). Reprinted from Junkar, I., Šuštar, V., Frank, M., Janša, V., Bedina-Zavec, A., Rozman, B., Mozetič, M., Hägerstrand, H., and Kralj-Iglič, V. (2009). Blood and synovial microparticles as revealed by atomic force and scanning electron microscope. *Op. Autoimmun. J.*, 1, pp. 50–58, Copyright © 2015 Bentham Open.

(P1) and a scanning electron micrograph of a sample isolated from the synovial fluid of a patient with rheumatoid arthritis (P2). Both, the height images (a,c) and phase images (b,d) are presented. The concentration of NVs isolated from synovial fluid is much higher than the concentration of NVs in the samples obtained by isolation from peripheral blood (Junkar et al., 2009), which is favourable for SEM imaging, but the samples had to be diluted for AFM analysis. The AFM images reveal grain-like structures of different sizes; their height is about 50 nm while their width is between 100 and 150 nm. The SEM image (Fig. 18.11) shows many globular structures with somewhat irregular shape compared to the NVs isolated from blood (Figs. 18.6 and 18.7). AFM images of grains (Fig. 18.11a–d) are smaller in comparison to SEM images (Fig. 18.11e), but the characteristics of the shapes seem alike. Due to the somewhat irregular shapes of these grains which are revealed by the AFM as well as by SEM, we cannot decisively claim that all of these structures are NVs. Grains could also be formed by assembly of proteins and lipids. Further, experiments are needed to reveal the morphology of these grains, such as transmission electron microscopy which could give information on the contents of the grains.

18.2 Isolated Nanovesicles: Clinically Relevant Artefacts

The mechanisms responsible for budding and vesiculation (see Chapters 9 and 10), including processes that occur during the isolation procedure, are poorly understood, thorough solving this problem is a precondition for the reliability and repeatability of the assessment of NVs to be used in clinical studies in which populations are compared quantitatively. The existing method is sensitive to many parameters in the process such as blood uptake, the kind and volume of the anticoagulant used in the tubes for blood collection, centrifugation speed, and temperature, the fraction of blood plasma taken after separation of the cells from plasma, measurement with a flow cytometer, and the time intervals between protocol steps (Junkar et al., 2009). To solve such problems arising from pre-analytical and analytical issues in the analysis of blood NVs, it is not enough to standardize the isolation protocol. The isolation procedure must be better understood otherwise parameters that have important effects on the result may be overlooked.

It is therefore of interest to the study the mechanisms and processes taking place during the isolation of NVs and to reveal the morphology and identity of particles in the isolated material. In particular, it is relevant to determine out whether NVs found in the isolate are present in the sample at uptake, or if they are created from blood cells during the isolation process. In the latter case, clinical results importantly reflect the vesiculability of cells, mostly platelets. For example, due to interaction of native NVs with platelets, platelets are a potential pool of tumour material and also a source of tumour seeding following removal of a tumour from the body. To diminish the probability of metastases spreading, possible simple therapeutic procedures could be suggested based on the removal of a portion of the platelets after tumour resection and their replacement with platelets from a healthy donor. Further, subsequent attempts to optimize platelet number could complement other therapeutic procedures by slowing down or even stopping tumour progression. It is therefore likely that information on the source and identity of NVs could shed light on the interpretation of clinical studies involving determination of NVs in blood. Pursuing a study on the origin and identity of NVs *in vivo*, and examining the effects of blood cell fragmentation during isolation should also improve understanding of the basic mechanisms of cell–cell communication and tumour progression.

To investigate the identity and origin of NVs in blood isolates, a series of experiments and studies was performed. In order to determine whether observation of the isolates by scanning electron microscopy affects the population of NVs in the isolate, samples of NVs isolated from the same (human) blood were divided into two parts; one was imaged at Åbo Akademi University, Åbo/Turku, Finland and the other at FEI Quanta, Eindhoven, Netherlands. The isolation was performed at room temperature (25°C). Drying and gold sputtering/iridium coating were performed in the two laboratories. The effective diameter of NVs measured in the blood isolates by both laboratories was about 300 nm (Table 18.1). The difference between the results of the two laboratories was not statistically significant. As similar results were found in both

Table 18.1 Estimated size of NVs measured from SEM radiographs

Sample	No. of NVs	Diameter ± SD(nm)	p
Human blood (FEI Quanta)	85	321 ± 130	0.28
Human blood (Åbo Akademi)	101	302 ± 131	

Source: Republished with permission of DOVE Medical Press, from Nanoparticles isolated from blood: A reflection of vesiculability of blood cells during the isolation process, Šuštar V, Bedina-Zavec A, Štukelj R, Frank M, Bobojevič G, Janša R, Ogorevc E, Kruljc P, Mam K, Šimunič B, Manček-Keber M, Jerala R, Rozman B, Veranič P, Hägerstrand H, Kralj-Iglič V, *Int J Nanomed*, 6, copyright 2011; permission conveyed through Copyright Clearance Center, Inc.

laboratories, we concluded that scanning electron microscopy is a reliable method for studying the identity and origin of NVs.

Pursuing the origin and mechanisms of NV generation in isolates, different regions of the isolate from mare's blood were inspected. The structures observed in Fig. 18.12A indicate that fragmentation of blood cells occurs during the process. Panel A shows the presence of tubular structures connected to distal bulbous parts (see also Fig. 18.5B). Thin necks were formed (white arrow) which could have been torn by centrifugal shear stress to produce the rather large cell fragments found in the isolates. It is evident that the particles which we considered to be NVs (Figs. 18.3 and 18.4) attained the sizes and shapes indicated in deformed cells (Fig. 18.12A).

The micrograph shown in Fig. 18.12B was taken close to the interface between the isolate and the tube wall where the shear force was expected to be greatest. Numerous elongated shapes, preferentially oriented in a particular direction, can be seen, indicating that shear stress in the centrifuge affects NV shape.

These results indicate that platelet fragmentation in a shear stress field takes place during isolation. The question is whether these fragments represent a marginal or a substantial subpopulation of the NVs found in isolates.

18.2.1 *The Effect of Temperature on Isolates from Blood*

The process of NV isolation was studied at different temperatures that were kept constant throughout the isolation process using a water-bath and a temperature-regulated centrifuge (Šuštar et al., 2011a). For this series of experiments on the effect of temperature,

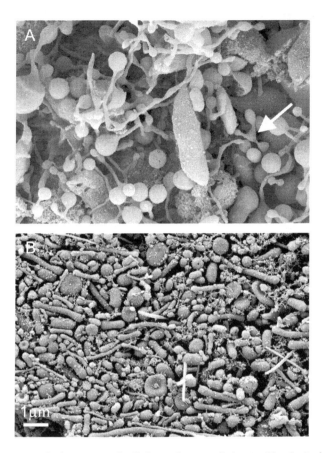

Figure 18.12 Deformation of cell-derived material obtained by the isolation procedure. Deformed cells from the blood of a healthy mare (aged 5 years) exhibit protrusions connected by thin necks, which were torn, eventually yielding membrane-enclosed cell fragments (A). Close to the tube wall the shear forces in the centrifuge are high and therefore the cell fragments in the isolate from the blood of a healthy human donor (male, 28 years) are elongated and exhibit preferential orientation (B). The images were taken using a LEO Gemini 1530 (LEO, Oberkochen, Germany) SEM applying 8 kV at Åbo Akademi University, Åbo/Turku, Finland. Republished with permission of DOVE Medical Press, from Nanoparticles isolated from blood: A reflection of vesiculability of blood cells during the isolation process, Šuštar V, Bedina-Zavec A, Štukelj R, Frank M, Bobojevič G, Janša R, Ogorevc E, Kruljc P, Mam K, Šimunič B, Manček-Keber M, Jerala R, Rozman B, Veranič P, Hägerstrand H, Kralj-Iglič V, *Int J Nanomed*, 6, copyright 2011; permission conveyed through Copyright Clearance Center, Inc.

Table 18.2 Concentration of NVs obtained by isolating NVs from the blood of 42 donors with no record of disease, at different temperatures

T (°C)	Number of subjects	NPs/spheres $\pm$ SD	p vs. 37°C (P)	p vs. 40°C (P)
30	12	2.90 $\pm$ 1.85	0.01 (0.64)	0.001 (0.82)
37	17	1.31 $\pm$ 1.45	1	0.31 (0.16)
40	13	0.87 $\pm$ 0.45	1	

Source: Republished with permission of DOVE Medical Press, from Nanoparticles isolated from blood: A reflection of vesiculability of blood cells during the isolation process, Šuštar V, Bedina-Zavec A, Štukelj R, Frank M, Bobojevič G, Janša R, Ogorevc E, Kruljc P, Mam K, Šimunič B, Manček-Keber M, Jerala R, Rozman B, Veranič P, Hägerstrand H, Kralj-Iglič V, *Int J Nanomed*, 6, copyright 2011; permission conveyed through Copyright Clearance Center, Inc.
Note: The statistical significance of differences (p) and the corresponding statistical power (P) are shown. NP indicates nanoparticles and T indicates temperature.

blood samples were collected from 56 subjects (students and staff) with no record of disease, after a 12 hour overnight fast. Up to eight samples were processed within a single experiment. The chosen temperature was kept constant during the isolation procedure. The NVs in fresh isolates were counted by flow cytometry immediately after isolation. The final analysis comprised samples obtained from 42 subjects with no record of disease (29 females and 13 males). It can be seen in Table 18.2 that the concentration of NVs decreased with increase in temperature.

As the accuracy of flow cytometry in determining NV concentration is rather poor, a further study was designed to obtain a more decisive result. In a second set of experiments, blood was collected from 7 subjects with no record of disease (4 females and 3 males) after a 12 hour fast. Isolation was first performed at 37°C and then a second blood sample was collected from the same subjects in the same consecutive order and the isolation performed at 20°C. The procedure was then again repeated at 4°C. The volunteers, consisting of hospital staff and the authors, did not eat or drink during the period of blood sampling and were requested to refrain from physical activity. Blood was acquired by free flow to minimize activation of platelets in the needle which could represent an additional source of difference between the samples. The isolation procedures were performed at the three different temperatures in a single day so that fresh isolates could be assessed using the same setting of the flow cytometer.

Table 18.3 Concentration of NVs isolated from the blood of healthy donors at different temperatures

Subject	NVs (4°C)	Time (4°C)	NVs (20°C)	Time (20°C)	NVs (37°C)	Time (37°C)
1	0.54	64	0.58*	110*	0.35	68
2	0.29	55	0.22	57	0.29*	40*
3	1.21	104	0.78*	114*	0.21	90
4	0.34*	72*	0.23*	163*	0.42	55
5	0.58	76	0.32	81	0.17	86
6	0.26*	108*	0.55	82	0.28	84
7	0.90*	64*	0.38	81	0.23	80
Average	0.59	78	0.43	98	0.29	72
Average*	0.65	75	0.38	75	0.28	77

Source: Republished with permission of DOVE Medical Press, from Nanoparticles isolated from blood: A reflection of vesiculability of blood cells during the isolation process, Šuštar V, Bedina-Zavec A, Štukelj R, Frank M, Bobojevič G, Janša R, Ogorevc E, Kruljc P, Mam K, Šimunič B, Manček-Keber M, Jerala R, Rozman B, Veranič P, Hägerstrand H, Kralj-Iglič V, *Int J Nanomed*, 6, copyright 2011; permission conveyed through Copyright Clearance Center, Inc.
Note: Average * denotes the average values calculated without the data marked by asterisks.

The results of this second study confirmed the results of the first study in that the concentrations of NVs in the isolates were higher at lower isolation temperatures (Table 18.3). However, it was observed that the time needed to acquire the required volume of blood by free flow differed markedly between subjects and also in repetitive acquisitions from the same subject, indicating corresponding differences in shear stress. Because this could be a source of the considerable difference in the NV concentrations in isolates, another analysis of the results was performed using only data on blood samples that differed in collection time by less than 15 s for a given subject. The data which was omitted is marked with asterisks in Table 18.3. In subject 4, all three collection times differed by more than 15 s, so only one result was retained. These results show that in all subjects the concentration of NVs in the isolates decreased gradually with increase in temperature during isolation (Table 18.3).

Platelets are affected by shear stress in the needle during blood sampling. Assuming laminar stationary flow of a Newtonian viscous fluid and the validity of the Poiseuille–Hagen law, the velocity in the

Table 18.4 Size of nanoparticles isolated from mare's blood at different temperatures, that is, diameter measured from SEM images

T (°C)	NPs	Diameter (SD) (nm)	p vs 30 °C (P)	p vs 37 °C (P)
20	44	273 (82)	0.33 (0.166)	0.00 (0.99)
30	51	291 (101)		0.00 (0.95)
37	67	362 (100)	1	

Source: Republished with permission of DOVE Medical Press, from Nanoparticles isolated from blood: A reflection of vesiculability of blood cells during the isolation process, Šuštar V, Bedina-Zavec A, Štukelj R, Frank M, Bobojevič G, Janša R, Ogorevc E, Kruljc P, Mam K, Šimunič B, Manček-Keber M, Jerala R, Rozman B, Veranič P, Hägerstrand H, Kralj-Iglič V, *Int J Nanomed*, 6, copyright 2011; permission conveyed through Copyright Clearance Center, Inc.
Abbreviations: NP, nanoparticles; SD, standard deviation.

direction of flow is subject to a parabolic profile that is dependent on the distance from the centre of the needle. During free flow, the flow rate is determined by the difference between the pressure in the vein and atmospheric pressure, resulting in the rather slow dripping of blood. The gradient of velocity determines the shear force which is greatest near the inner wall of the needle. The variation in time that reflects the speed of blood in the needle may be the cause of the poor accuracy when determining the concentration of NVs. The lower pressure in evacuated tubes used for blood sampling results in faster flow and therefore, shorter times to acquire the same volume of blood, with a correspondingly larger velocity of blood and shear stresses in the needle.

Scanning electron micrographs indicated that the NVs were rather large (the average size was around 300 nm) and their size depended on the temperature during isolation; they were larger if the isolation was performed at higher temperatures (Table 18.4). The differences between the size of NVs isolated from mare's blood at 20°C and 37°C and at 30°C and 37°C were considerable (29% and 22%, respectively). These differences were statistically significant ($p \leq 0.00$) and of sufficient power (P values at $\alpha = 0.05$ were 0.99 and 0.95, respectively) (Table 18.4). All the differences between the mean size of NVs isolated from human blood at 4, 20, and 37°C

Table 18.5 Mean of the parameter representing flow cytometric measurement of light scattering in the forward direction (size of NVs in relative units) at different temperatures

Subject	Mean FS ($T = 4°C$)	Mean FS ($T = 20°C$)	Mean FS ($T = 37°C$)
1	1.2	2.1	2.1
2	1.4	1.7	2.7
3	0.9	1.3	2.3
4	0.9	1.8	2.0
5	1.5	2.1	2.4
6	1.7	1.9	2.4
7	1.3	1.8	1.9
Average	1.3	1.8	2.3

Source: Republished with permission of DOVE Medical Press, from Nanoparticles isolated from blood: A reflection of vesiculability of blood cells during the isolation process, Šuštar V, Bedina-Zavec A, Štukelj R, Frank M, Bobojevič G, Janša R, Ogorevc E, Kruljc P, Mam K, Šimunič B, Manček-Keber M, Jerala R, Rozman B, Veranič P, Hägerstrand H, Kralj-Iglič V, *Int J Nanomed*, 6, copyright 2011; permission conveyed through Copyright Clearance Center, Inc.
Abbreviation: FS, forward scatter.

and measured by flow cytometry were shown to be statistically significant (Table 18.5).

Measurements with a flow cytometer showed that the increase in size with increase in temperature was gradual in all subjects (Table 18.5).

18.2.2 Origin of Micro- and Nanovesicles in Blood Isolates

Studies of the origin of NVs isolated from peripheral blood showed that the largest pool of NVs in isolates derives from platelets (around 80%), followed by erythrocytes (around 10%) and other cells (T-helper cells, T-suppressor cells, monocytes, B-lymphocytes, granulocytes, and endothelial cells) (Diamant et al., 2002). Cancer cells are prone to shed NVs, but a significant increase of the number of NVs found in peripheral blood of patients with certain types of cancer are ascribed to platelets (Janowska-Wieczorek et al., 2006) which can be activated by NVs from neoplastic cells. In such experiment, NVs were labelled with antibodies which interact with endothelial, platelet and erythrocyte surface molecules (CD31/CD42b and CD235). Staining with antibodies for platelet origin (anti-CD42bPE and anti-CD31FITC positive events) showed that the majority (70%) of NVs contain receptors derived from platelets (Šuštar et al., 2011a). This finding agrees with previous reports (Diamant et al., 2002). In labelling with anti-CD31-FITC and anti-CD42b-PE, about 30% of events corresponded to unlabelled particles. Out of these, about 15% could be ascribed to anti-CD235-FITC-labelled particles and about 9% to the background. This left around 6% of unlabelled particles in the isolates (Šuštar et al., 2011a).

Because budding and vesiculation are common processes in all cells, it could be expected that NVs created *in vivo* would also be present in blood and could be detected by isolation. However, it seemed unclear how particles sized 300 nm or greater that were mainly quasi-globular shaped could be obtained by budding of activated platelets which are sized about 1.5 μm. For example, filopodia of activated platelets are thinner (Figs. 18.13A–F), so if these were pinched off from the mother cell, the NVs produced would be evidently smaller and/or tubular. Further, despite considerable evidence that platelets are the main origin of NVs in blood isolates using the described protocol for isolation no correlation between the concentration of platelets in blood and the concentration of NVs in blood isolates was found in blood isolates (Šuštar et al., 2011a). Such a relationship should be expected if the NVs found in isolates were predominantly present in blood *in vivo*. Therefore, the following questions may be posed: (1) Are the NVs found in isolates present in blood *in vivo*? (2) What are the processes leading to the formation of NVs in isolates? (3) What is the content of the isolates? (4) What is the identity of NVs in isolates with respect to the mother cell(s)?

It was suggested above that the isolation procedure depends on external parameters. These parameters cannot be kept constant with the existing equipment and protocol which explains the poor repeatability and accuracy of NV isolation in different experiments and certainly adds to the lack of correlation between the concentration of NV in isolates and the concentration of platelets in blood. Namely, it is indicated that the majority of NVs are created during and after blood sampling, and accordingly the results reflect the properties and composition of blood cells and plasma. For example,

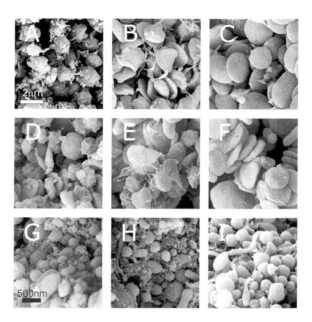

Figure 18.13 Platelets and NVs at different temperatures. NVs were isolated from platelet-rich plasma of a healthy human donor (female, 28 years) at different temperatures (A: 4°C, B: 20°C, C: 37°C), platelets from platelet-rich plasma of a mare (D: 4°C, E: 20°C, F: 37°C), and NVs isolated from blood of the mare (G: 4°C, H: 20°C, I: 37°C). The images were taken using a LEO Gemini 1530 (LEO, Oberkochen, Germany) SEM applying 8 kV at Åbo Akademi University, Åbo/Turku, Finland. Republished with permission of DOVE Medical Press, from Nanoparticles isolated from blood: A reflection of vesiculability of blood cells during the isolation process, Šuštar V, Bedina-Zavec A, Štukelj R, Frank M, Bobojevič G, Janša R, Ogorevc E, Kruljc P, Mam K, Šimunič B, Manček-Keber M, Jerala R, Rozman B, Veranič P, Hägerstrand H, Kralj-Iglič V, *Int J Nanomed*, 6, copyright 2011; permission conveyed through Copyright Clearance Center, Inc.

membrane and plasma constituents may affect the membrane curvature (Kabaso et al., 2011a,c; Pavlič et al., 2010) which is the basic mechanism underlying the budding and vesiculation of membranes.

It was suggested that platelets had different properties at different temperatures as regards their fragmentation during isolation. Platelets in platelet-rich plasma were visualized at different temperatures in a healthy human donor (Figs. 18.4A–C)

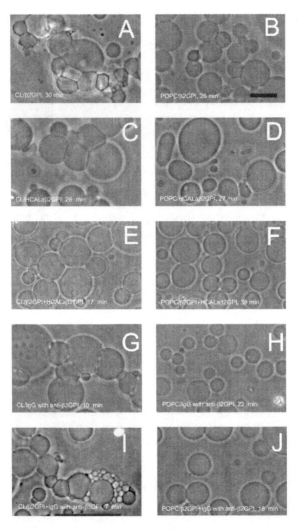

Figure 18.14 Effect of β_2GPI and anti-β_2GPI aPL antibodies (anti-β_2GPIs) on giant phospholipid vesicles. Left side (A,C,E,G,I): negatively charged cardiolipin-containing vesicles; right side (B,D,F,H,J): neutral POPC vesicles. Bar = 10 μm. Reprinted from *Autoimmune Reviews*, 6(1), Ambrožič, A., Čučnik, S., Tomšič, N., Urbanija, J., Lokar, M., Babnik, B., Rozman, B., Iglič, A., and Kralj-Iglič, V., Interaction of giant phospholipid vesicles containing cardiolipin and cholesterol with b_2-glycoprotein-I and anti-b_2-glycoprotein-I antibodies, pp. 10–15, Copyright 2006, with permission from Elsevier.

and a healthy mare (Figs. 18.4D–F). The respective NVs isolated from these samples are shown in Figs. 18.13G–I. At temperatures below room temperature, platelet shapes exhibited filopodia and distortion compared to the resting disc-like shape in the human subject and the mare (Figs. 18.13B,E).

In order to understand the dependence of the concentration and size of NVs in isolates on temperature, the laws of hydromechanics must be taken into account. The following equation taking into account centrifugal force, buoyancy, and Stokes law governs the sedimentation velocity of a spherical particle,

$$v = \frac{9\Delta\rho a d^2}{8\eta}, \qquad (18.1)$$

where $\Delta\rho$ is the difference in densities of the NVs and the medium (plasma), d is the effective diameter of the NV, a is the acceleration of the centrifugal force created in the centrifuge rotor and η is the viscosity of the medium. It follows from Eq. (18.1) that both, native NVs possibly present in blood and NVs possibly created after sampling would sediment more slowly at lower temperatures due to the higher viscosity of plasma at these temperatures. Therefore, clearance of cells from the upper part of the tube that is used to isolate NVs during the first centrifugation is less effective. Cells remaining in this compartment may shed NVs into the sample during centrifugation. Platelets become activated below room temperature and increasingly deform with decreasing temperature (Fig. 18.13) causing changes in the integrity of their cytoskeleton and rendering the cells prone to fragmentation, thereby contributing to an increased number of NVs in the isolates at lower temperatures. All the above explains the fact that a lower concentration of NVs was observed in isolates prepared at higher temperature (Tables 18.2, 18.3). Because the effects on NV concentration of factors that determine the sedimentation speed of existing NVs and the creation of new NVs during the first step of isolation are synergistic, we could not distinguish between their respective contributions to the overall effect. However, the mean size of NVs was also different at different isolation temperatures. If isolation primarily yields the NVs that were present in blood *in vivo*, the average size of NVs present in the upper compartment of plasma after the first centrifugation should be smaller at higher temperatures according to Eq. (18.1), and the clearance of larger NVs would be more effective. Assuming that the second and the third centrifugation collects NVs in the pellet, the average size of NVs in isolates was expected to be smaller at higher temperatures. In contrast, it was observed that NVs are larger when isolated at higher temperatures.

The dependence of their properties on temperature, the large size of NVs in the isolates, the shapes of the intermediate structures leading to isolated material, and the sensitivity of the concentration and mean size of NVs to external parameters all indicate that a large pool of NVs are created after blood sampling. NVs which are shed after sampling blood, especially from temperature or shear-activated platelets (Maurer-Spurej et al., 2001), are detected in the isolated material. The properties of blood cells and plasma may therefore have an important influence on the state of the isolate. One can interpret the alteration of blood cells in cancer patients by the presumable integration of native tumour cell-derived NVs into their membranes. Blood cells, especially platelets, may convey tumour cell material to distal cells and render it functional by inducing processes in these cells (Baj-Krzyworzeka et al., 2006; Holmes et al., 2009; Janowska-Wieczorek et al., 2006). It has been suggested that metastases are seeded by tumour cells and that the probability of this happening is greater when microemboli composed of tumour cells and platelets travel slowly in capillaries, thereby enhancing the probability of tumour cells entering the tissues through the endothelium. Platelets are known to stick to tumour cells and shield them from attack by leukocytes (Gay and Felding-Habermann, 2011). Indeed, there is evidence that platelets support tumour metastasis (Gay and Felding-Habermann, 2011) and platelet counts are related to prognosis in cancer patients (Arslan and Coskun, 2005; Gasic et al., 1968). Because tumour cells are unlikely to be found *in vivo* in patients, the above hypothesis is based on cancer induction by injection of tumour cells directly into the blood of animals. On the other hand, it appears likely that native NVs shed by cancer cells are the origin of metastases, either as vehicles or as mediators of transport by mobile cells, most probably platelets. It has been reported that NVs shed from cells interact with other cells (Boilard et al., 2010; Pap et al., 2009; Prokopi et al., 2009; Szajnik et al., 2010) so it is possible that material shed from blood cells is exchanged constantly between cells via native NVs. Because platelets are prone to vesiculate, the material shed during this process is likely to be found in other cells, such as erythrocytes, leukocytes and endothelial cells. The NV-mediated exchange of material between cells may explain the intriguing data of Boilard et al (2010), who found platelet-derived material, but no platelets, in the synovial fluid of patients with rheumatoid arthritis.

The isolate is composed of cell fragments, which were most likely formed as a result of mechanical stress during centrifugation and also of thermal stress during isolation. The concentration, size, and identity of NVs in the isolates appear to depend on the properties of blood cells and the surrounding medium, which may be altered by disease. The isolated NVs, therefore, represent a clinically relevant parameter, even though they may have been created after blood sampling.

As regards characterization of samples, controlled manipulation of the size of the cell fragments (NVs) could be advantageous. Avoiding production of fragments of the size of immune complexes (mean diameter 50 nm) may avoid problems with artefacts when measuring the NV concentration by flow cytometry (György et al., 2011).

18.3 Post-Prandial Increase in Concentration of Nanovesicles in Isolates from Blood

Studies involving NVs in a healthy human population revealed a post-prandial increase of endothelial-derived (Ferreira et al., 2004; Tushuizen et al., 2007) and plasma total NVs (Michelson et al., 2009; Šuštar et al., 2011b; Tushuizen et al., 2006) in isolates from peripheral blood, while studies on lipoprotein and glucose metabolism reported changes in blood cholesterol and glucose levels (Alssema et al., 2010; Cohn et al., 1988; DeRosa et al., 2010; Ferreira et al., 2004; Michelson et al., 2009; Tushuizen et al., 2007, 2006). In the *in vitro* study, it was found that the cholesterol concentration in the surrounding medium and in the membrane considerably affects the nanovesiculation of membranes of epithelial cells (Marzesco et al., 2009) which is also supported by findings that membrane rafts (which are enriched in cholesterol) are precursors of NVs (Hägerstrand et al., 2006). It was hypothesized (Šuštar et al., 2011b) that NVs are an important pool of blood cholesterol, so it is of interest to focus on the correlations of the total number of NVs with concentrations of blood cholesterol post-fasting and postprandial. The total number of NVs is supposed to be relevant since all NVs contain cholesterol. It was indicated that cholesterol plays an important role in budding and vesiculation, especially due to partitioning into cholesterol-enriched membrane rafts (Brown and London, 1998a; Simons and Ikonen, 1997) which favour strongly curved membrane regions (Biro et al., 2005). Due to a self-consistent minimization of the free energy and lateral distribution of membrane constituents, a highly curved local membrane shape with increased content of constituents that favour such a curvature is attained, and budding of the membrane is promoted (Aeffner et al., 2009; Dubnickova et al., 2000; Hägerstrand et al., 2001, 2006; Marzesco et al., 2009; Tenchov et al., 2006).

The post-prandial increase of NVs was studied in relation to blood cholesterol and blood glucose in a population of 33 donors with no record of disease, 18 female, and 15 male (Šuštar et al., 2011b). The experiment was performed in two days. The first day, blood uptake started at 7 a.m., after a 15-hour fast. After the test, donors were encouraged to eat food rich in cholesterol, fat and carbohydrates all day. They were advised not to be extremely physically active. The second day, they consumed a breakfast at 7 a.m. consisting of two eggs, bread and a dairy product and another meal consisting of a dairy product at 10 a.m. On the second day, blood uptake, from the medial cubital vein on the other arm started at 12 p.m.

The final analysis included 21 subjects, 10 female (average age 29 years $\pm$ standard deviation 13 years), and 11 male (31 years $\pm$ 10 years). Starting with 33 subjects, one male subject was excluded from the study since it was found that he underwent an 8 hour plane flight a day before taking the first blood test. Three subjects (1 male and 2 female) were excluded because it was found that they had not fasted for the prescribed 15 hours before the first blood test. Five subjects were excluded as their post-fasting levels of triglycerides were increased. Three subjects were excluded due to statin therapy. One subject received beta blocking and anti-hypertensive therapy, while 20 were medication-free. Data for two subjects on cholesterol and glucose was lost, but data on NVs of these two subjects were included in the analysis.

In most subjects the glucose concentration decreased post-prandially with a concomitant increase of triglycerides, HDL cholesterol and NVs, and a slight decrease in LDL cholesterol. However, in five subjects (two male and three female) trigylcerides decreased. In one subject, all the considered parameters decreased post-prandially.

Averaged over post-fasting and the post-prandial results, NVs were more abundant in the female population (0.90 ± 0.71) than in the male population (0.53 ± 0.30). The male population had slightly higher concentrations of total cholesterol (5.09 ± 0.96) mmol/l, glucose (4.97 ± 0.29) mmol/l triglycerides (1.03 ± 0.35) mmol/l and LDL-C (2.97 ± 0.89) mmol/l than the female population, where the concentration of total cholesterol was (4.80 ± 0.73) mmol/l, of glucose (4.76 ± 0.57) mmol/l, of triglycerides (0.98 ± 0.26) mmol/l and of LDL-C (2.64 ± 0.65) mmol/l. The concentration of HDL-C was higher in the female population (1.62 ± 0.22) mmol/l than in the male population (1.52 ± 0.15) mmol/l. The two populations differed statistically significantly only in the number of NVs ($p = 0.03$), while differences in all other parameters were statistically insignificant. None of these parameters measured post-fasting differed statistically significantly between women and men, while the number of NVs was the only parameter that differed statistically significantly between women and men in the postprandial state.

The average number of NVs was considerably (52%) and statistically significantly higher ($p = 0.01$) in the post-prandial than in the fasting state with the power $P = 0.67$ at $\alpha = 0.05$. The number of NVs increased in 16 and decreased in 5 subjects; the greatest increase was by 135% and the greatest decrease by 52% which is taken to be considerable. Concentrations of total cholesterol, LDL-C and HDL-C remained on average within 2% of the initial (post-fasting) values. We found a 11% increase in triglyceride concentration ($p = 0.12$). Also we found a 6% decrease in the blood glucose concentration ($p \leq 0.01$) with power $P = 0.76$ at $\alpha = 0.05$.

Considering all the data (from both the first and the second day), a statistically significant negative correlation between the number of NVs and the LDL-C concentration ($r = -0.29$, $p = 0.04$) was obtained. Although the average values of parameters, especially of total cholesterol, LDL-C and HDL-C, were only moderately affected by food consumption, there were large variations of the respective parameters within the population, as was already outlined before (Cohn et al., 1988). Measured at a given time interval, it can therefore not be concluded that a post-prandial increase or decrease in any of the parameters is an indicator of a normal or a pathological process at the level of the individual. Further, based on the existing evidence it could not be concluded that any particular mechanism is the one which keeps the average values of parameters relatively constant through fasting and post-prandial states (Šuštar et al., 2011b).

The post-prandial number of NVs negatively correlated with fasting total cholesterol concentration ($r = -0.46$, $p = 0.035$), while the difference in NVs between the postprandial and post-fasting states (in per cent) correlated positively with the respective differences in total cholesterol concentration ($r = 0.17$, $p = 0.00$), HDL-C concentration ($r = 0.37$, $p = 0.00$), LDL-C concentration ($r = 0.20$, $p = 0.00$), and triglyceride concentration ($r = 0.23$, $p = 0.00$). The correlation between the difference in NVs and glucose concentration was negative ($r = -0.39$, $p = 0.00$).

Men and women were considered in the same group as there were no decisive reasons why the process of membrane vesiculation should essentially differ in men and women. So it was assumed that the postprandial effect on NVs would be the same in men and women, that is, the number of NVs would increase after meals. If the effects differed in magnitude between the sexes, considering both groups together would only increase the noise in the statistical analysis. This means that it would be possible to obtain a lower or no statistical significance of the effect in the combined group due to larger scattering of data. Analysis, however, shows no correlation between total post-fasting blood cholesterol and the post-prandial number of NVs in men, while there is a considerable and statistically significant effect in women which also prevails in the effect of the combined group.

It should be taken into consideration that circadian rhythm has an effect on the level of blood constituents. Since the first day blood was taken at 7 a.m. and on the second day it was taken at 12 p.m., the concentrations of blood cholesterol and glucose would differ. Based on the reported dependencies of blood cholesterol and triglyceride concentrations on time of day (Bremner et al., 2000; Ogita et al., 2007), it was estimated that due to the circadian rhythm effect, on the average the concentration of total cholesterol would increase by about 3%, the concentration of triglycerides by 7%, the concentration of LDL-C by 2%, while the concentration of HDL-C would be unchanged. If these results are taken into account, the observed effect on total cholesterol, LDL cholesterol and HDL cholesterol could be ascribed to circadian rhythm, while the effect on triglycerides is somewhat larger (by 4%). However, the subjects considered in the circadian rhythm study received regular meals (Bremner et al., 2000; Ogita et al., 2007).

18.4 Mediated Interaction between Membranes

The manipulation of nanovesiculation can be considered as a possibility to control homeostasis. It was found that membrane buds can adhere to the mother membrane, subject to mutual attraction mediated by constituents of the solution (Urbanija et al., 2007). Thereby, buds cannot become free NVs. It was suggested that orientational ordering of the mediating particles with internally distributed charge is a possible mechanism of suppression of nanovesiculation. In body fluids, probable candidates for mediating molecules are proteins. In blood, antibodies are likely to contribute to this effect due to their dimeric structure.

Antiphospholipid (aPL) antibodies are present in the blood of patients with anti-phospholipid syndrome (APS). Besides the presence of antibodies, APS is defined by thromboembolic disorders and recurrent premature termination of pregnancy in female patients (Levine et al., 2002; Roubey, 1996). Interestingly, it was found that the concentration of NVs was elevated in patients with APS (Dignat-George et al., 2004). It is therefore relevant to explore how the aPL antibodies affect the vesiculation of membranes.

aPL antibodies are assessed by ELISA tests. Antibodies are captured by the negatively charged phospholipid cardiolipin in the presence of the plasma protein beta 2 glycoprotein I (β_2GPI). Namely, it was found (Galli et al., 1996; Matsuura et al., 1990; McNeil et al., 1990) that aPL antibodies are directed to β_2GPI–cardiolipin complexes and that β_2GPI is an absolute requirement for an antibody–phospholipid interaction (McNeil et al., 1990). β_2GPI is considered to exhibit a variety of physiological roles, among them in the process of blood clot formation. It was found that it affects the metabolism of triacylglycerol-rich lipoproteins, the function of platelets, and the activation of endothelial cells (Bevers et al., 2005). Moreover, β_2GPI inhibits the transformation of prothrombin into thrombin (Nimpf et al., 1986). It binds to structures which contain negatively charged phospholipid molecules such as platelets (Schousboe, 1980), platelet-derived microvesicles, apoptotic cells (Price et al., 1996) and serum lipoproteins (Kobayashi et al., 2003; Polz and Kostner, 1979). Further, it mediates cellular recognition of negatively charged phospholipid-exposing microparticles (Balasubramanian et al., 1997; Moestrup et al., 1998; Thiagarajan et al., 1999), thereby indicating its anticoagulant role in the clearance of procoagulant negatively charged microvesicles from the circulation (Aupeix et al., 1996; Choon et al., 1995; Zwaal, 1978; Zwaal et al., 1997). aPL antibodies were indicated to inhibit protein C activation (Hasselaar et al., 1989), while the binding of aPL antibody-β_2GPI complexes to cell surfaces was found to promote activation of platelets (Khamashta et al., 1988), as well as endothelial cells *in vitro* (Del Papa et al., 1995; Simantov et al., 1995) and *in vivo* (Pierangeli et al., 1999).

In spite of the considerable knowledge gathered on the role of the complex interactions between phospholipids, β_2GPI and aPL antibodies in thrombosis and haemostasis, the underlying mechanisms are not yet completely understood. However, these interactions also can also be studied in relatively simple model systems such as an aqueous solution of giant phospholipid vesicles (GPVs) with exogeneously added β_2GPI and/or aPL antibodies. In observing collective effects, the coalescence of negatively charged cardiolipin-containing vesicles and neutral palmitoyloleoylphosphatidylcholine (POPC) vesicles was found to be induced by a patient's IgG (the most abundant immunoglobulin in plasma) fractions containing aPL antibodies and/or β_2GPI (Ambrožič et al., 2006; Urbanija et al., 2007).

β_2GPI causes coalescence of cardiolipin-containing vesicles (Fig. 18.14A, as well as of POPC vesicles (Fig. 18.14B). It was found (Urbanija et al., 2007) that adhesion to the bottom of the observation chamber occurred simultaneously. Formation of sticky complexes was also observed in samples which contain both kinds of vesicles. This indicates that β_2GPI mediates the interaction between charged–charged, charged–neutral, and neutral–neutral pairs of membranes.

Addition of HCALaβ_2GPI (monoclonal HCAL anti-β_2GPI antibodies-chimeric IgG monoclonal anti-β_2GPI antibodies, consisting of constant human and variable mouse regions), dissolved in PBS, to a GPV solution caused coalescence of charged cardiolipin vesicles and their adhesion to the bottom of the observation chamber (Fig. 18.14C), while neutral POPC vesicles did not coalesce nor adhere to the bottom of the observation chamber (Fig. 18.14D). Addition of HCALaβ_2GPI dissolved in PBS to the mixture of charged and neutral vesicles yielded two coexisting populations: one forming sticky complexes that adhere to the bottom of the observation chamber, and the other consisting of separate fluctuating vesicles. When β_2GPI and HCALaβ_2GPI were well-mixed and incubated for 10 min before addition to the solution containing vesicles, coalescence of cardiolipin-containing vesicles (Fig. 18.14E), but not of POPC vesicles (Fig. 18.14F) took place.

Addition of the APS patient's IgG fraction which contained anti-β_2GPI antibodies caused coalescence of the charged vesicles and their adhesion to the bottom of the observation chamber, while these effects were absent in neutral vesicles (Figs. 18.14G and H, respectively). Addition of the pre-incubated mixture of β_2GPI and IgG caused coalescence of charged vesicles and of neutral vesicles (Fig. 18.14I); however, in neutral vesicles, the effect was very weak (Fig. 18.14J).

Binding of β_2GPI to negatively charged phospholipids has been considered to mediate the interaction between phospholipid assemblies and macrophages (Thiagarajan et al., 1999). The complex of anionic phospholipid vesicles and β_2GPI was found to be a specific requirement for anionic phospholipids to be

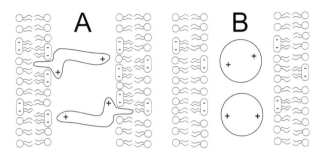

Figure 18.15 Schemes of the β_2GPI-mediated (A) and antibody-mediated (B) interactions between negatively charged phospholipid bilayers. Reprinted from *Chemistry and Physics of Lipids*, 150(1), Jasna Urbanija, Nejc Tomšič, Maruša Lokar, Aleš Ambrožič, Saša Čučnik, Blaž Rozman, Maša Kandušer, Aleš Iglič, and Veronika Kralj-Iglič, Coalescence of phospholipid membranes as a possible origin of anticoagulant effect of serum proteins, pp. 49–57, Copyright 2007, with permission from Elsevier.

recognized by a putative cell surface receptor on macrophages. However, the above experiments indicated that β_2GPI may also directly mediate attractive interactions between charged–charged (Fig. 18.14A), charged–neutral and neutral–neutral phospholipid membranes (Fig. 18.14B) (Urbanija et al., 2007). Even when added alone, HCALaβ_2GPI and patient's anti-β_2GPIs were observed to act similarly to β_2GPI in mediating the attractive interaction between negatively charged surfaces (Fig. 18.14C,G), but these antibodies alone or previously mixed with β_2GPI failed to mediate the attractive interaction between neutral POPC membranes (Fig. 18.14D,H and F,J, respectively) (Urbanija et al., 2007).

The mediating effect of solution constituents (Fig. 18.15) is quantitatively assessed by the average angle of contact between the adhered GPVs (Frank et al., 2008) (Fig. 18.16).

The above experiments show an attraction between membranes of negatively charged GPVs and adhesion between them which cannot be explained by the classical theory of the electric double layer (Verwey and Overbeek, 1948), but the affinity of β_2GPI for apoptotic membrane blebs that contain phospholipids with negatively charged headgroups can be explained by their opposite charges. Namely, some β_2GPI domains are highly positively charged (Bouma et al., 1999; Kertesz et al., 1995). It was found that

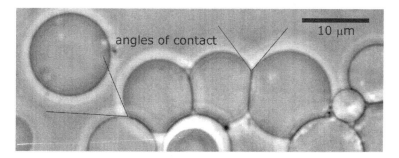

Figure 18.16 Adhesion of GPVs after the addition of plasma to a suspension of GPVs, with angles of contact between GPVs indicated. Reprinted from *Autoimmunity Reviews*, 7(3), Mojca Frank, Mateja Manček-Keberb, Mojca Kržan, Snežna Sodin-Šemrl, Roman Jerala, Aleš Iglič, Blaž Rozman, and Veronika Kralj-Iglič, Prevention of microvesiculation by adhesion of buds to the mother cell membrane: A possible anticoagulant effect of healthy donor plasma, pp. 240–245, Copyright 2008, with permission from Elsevier.

besides electrostatic interactions, β_2GPI also binds to phospholipid layers by hydrophobic interaction (Wang et al., 1998). Therefore, a β_2GPI molecule can intercalate in the membrane of GPV with its hydrophobic part and is simultaneously attracted to the membrane of another GPV with its poly-lysine segment on the I-st domain, thereby forming a bridge between the membranes of the vesicles (Fig. 18.15A). Such a configuration is favourable with respect to the electrostatic energy of the electric double layer. The antibodies, being composed of two heavy and two light polypeptide chains, form a dimeric structure with a particular internal distribution of charge. Within a simple model such a structure can be represented by a dimeric ion consisting of two equal point charges separated by a fixed distance. Orientational ordering of dimeric ions in the gradient of the local electric field (Fig. 18.15B) gives rise to an attractive force between the two electric double layers (see Chapter 14). The above mechanisms are suggested to prevail in the observed attractive interactions between charged membranes involving β_2GPI and anti-β_2GPIs (Fig. 18.14A,C,E,G,I), although there may be other contributions to the interaction such as van der Waals attraction, suppression of fluctuations (Helfrich, 1995) and water ordering near the interfaces (Israelachvili, 1997).

Furthermore, the adhesion between negatively charged GPVs in the presence of β_2GPI depends on the concentration of β_2GPI. Specifically, the average effective angles of contact between GPVs are larger for higher concentrations of β_2GPI. No adhesion was observed between negatively charged GPVs at β_2GPI concentrations lower than 4.6 mg/l, while a rather high contact angle (93°) was reached within the physiological range of β_2GPI concentrations (200 mg/l) (Frank et al., 2008). IgG antibodies (IgG antibodies from a healthy donor, polyclonal anti-β_2GPI IgG antibodies from a patient with APS, and monoclonal β_2GPI-dependent anti-cardiolipin IgG antibody HCAL) did not induce adhesion between negatively charged GPVs (as shown by zero values of the average effective angles of contact between GPVs in Table 18.6). Also, no adhesion between negatively charged GPVs could be observed when PBS/sugar solution alone was added to the GPV suspension. (Table 18.6). However, when negatively charged GPVs were incubated with higher concentrations ($\geq$1 mg/l) of an IgG antibody fraction from a patient with APS, containing high titres of both anti-β_2GPI and anti-cardiolipin antibodies, a dose-dependent increase in the average effective angles of contact between the negatively charged GPVs was observed (Frank et al., 2008). The average effective angles of contact increased from 0° at an IgG antibody concentration of 77 mg/ml to 107° at an IgG antibody concentration of 5.2 mg/ml, which is approximately half the IgG antibody concentration in human plasma.

In the presence of IgG antibodies from a healthy donor, a statistically significant increase in β_2GPI-induced adhesion between negatively charged GPVs was observed (Table 18.6) already at a β_2GPI concentration as small as 10.5 μg/ml. However, there was no further increase in membrane adhesion when the antibody concentration was increased to 33.6 μg/ml. Polyclonal anti-β_2GPI IgG antibodies from an APS patient, the IgG fraction from another APS patient (containing high titres of anti-β_2GPI and anti-cardiolipin antibodies) and the monoclonal β_2GPI-dependent antibody HCAL (but not IgG antibodies from a healthy donor) significantly reduced the β_2GPI-induced adhesion between negatively charged GPVs in a concentration-dependent manner. Also, pre-incubation of β_2GPI and healthy donor IgG antibodies with high avidity polyclonal anti-β_2GPI

Table 18.6 Effect of a therapeutic concentration of nadroparin (1.2 IU anti-Xa/ml) on the effective angle of contact between negatively charged (POPS-containing) GPVs (Y) in the presence of β_2GPI, IgG antibodies of a healthy donor, anti-β_2GPI antibodies from a patient with aPL syndrome, and β_2GPI (55 μg/ml)

	Y1 (°)	Y2 (°)	Y3 (°)
β_2GPI	105 ± 20	93 ± 19	94 ± 16
β_2GPI + healthy donor IgG	110 ± 17	100 ± 24	91 ± 17
β_2GPI + anti β_2GPI IgG	47 ± 11	64 ± 23	69 ± 23
Nadroparin	0	0	0
β_2GPI + nadroparin	93 ± 27	n.d.	n.d.
β_2GPI + healthy donor IgG + nadroparin	n.d.	104 ± 30	95 ± 28
Healthy donor IgG	0	0	0
Anti β_2GPI IgG	0	0	0
Healthy donor IgG + nadroparin	n.d.	0	0
Anti β_2GPI IgG + nadroparin	n.d.	0	0
Background control (PBS/sugar)	0	0	0

Source: Reprinted from *Autoimmunity Reviews*, 7(3), Mojca Frank, Mateja Manček-Keberb, Mojca Kržan, Snežna Sodin-Šemrl, Roman Jerala, Aleš Iglič, Blaž Rozman, and Veronika Kralj-Iglič, Prevention of microvesiculation by adhesion of buds to the mother cell membrane: A possible anticoagulant effect of healthy donor plasma, pp. 240–245, Copyright 2008, with permission from Elsevier.

Note: Experiments were done on three different batches of electroformation yielding GPVs (n.d. = experiment not done).

IgG antibodies induced a large and statistically significant reduction in the adhesion of negatively charged GPVs.

18.5 Mediated Interaction between Membranes as a Vesiculation-Suppression Mechanism

Mediated interaction between membranes may have important consequences as regards vesiculation of membranes. Namely, if the bud were attracted to the mother membrane it would not become a free vesicle. In this regard, mediated interaction represents a mechanism that suppresses vesiculation. To show this possibility, experiments with GPVs were made in which the expected process can be directly observed in real time. The budding of the vesicle was

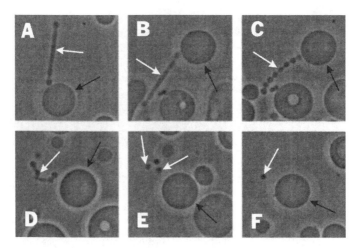

Figure 18.17 The effect of phosphate buffer saline (PBS) on a budding vesicle. The bead-like bud (marked by a white arrow) detached from the mother vesicle (marked by a black arrow) and disintegrated into spherical microvesicles (marked by white arrows) on the time-scale of minute. Bar = 10 μm. Reprinted from *Chemistry and Physics of Lipids*, 150(1), Jasna Urbanija, Nejc Tomšič, Maruša Lokar, Aleš Ambrožič, Saša Čučnik, Blaž Rozman, Maša Kandušer, Aleš Iglič, and Veronika Kralj-Iglič, Coalescence of phospholipid membranes as a possible origin of anticoagulant effect of serum proteins, pp. 49–57, Copyright 2007, with permission from Elsevier.

induced by increasing the temperature of the sample above room temperature. As a result, the bud elongated and appeared tube-like. When the tube was of a sufficient length the temperature was kept constant (typically 35°C) and the substance under investigation was added to the observation chamber (β_2GPI dissolved in PBS or PBS alone as a control). Figure 18.17 shows the effect of PBS of higher osmolarity (283 mosm/l) than the suspension of GPVs (205 mosm/l). The presence of PBS in the outer solution caused the bud to attain a bead-like shape (Fig. 18.17B). The bud detached from the mother vesicle (Fig. 18.17C) and decomposed into separate spherical vesicles (D,E), which were free to migrate away from the mother vesicle (F). When β_2GPI was present in the solution, the bud (Fig. 18.18A–C) coalesced with the mother vesicle before it could detach from it (Fig. 18.18D–F). Figure 18.18G shows a sticky complex formed by a vesicle with a long, initially tubular protrusion.

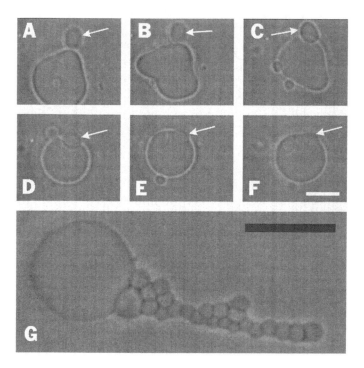

Figure 18.18 The effect of β_2GPI dissolved in PBS on a budding vesicle (A–F). The bud (marked by a white arrow) coalesced with the mother vesicle and remained attached to it. A sticky complex formed by coalescence of a bead-like protrusion and a mother vesicle (G). Bars = 10 μm. Reprinted from *Chemistry and Physics of Lipids*, 150(1), Jasna Urbanija, Nejc Tomšič, Maruša Lokar, Aleš Ambrožič, Saša Čučnik, Blaž Rozman, Maša Kandušer, Aleš Iglič, and Veronika Kralj-Iglič, Coalescence of phospholipid membranes as a possible origin of anticoagulant effect of serum proteins, pp. 49–57, Copyright 2007, with permission from Elsevier.

In contrast to the case presented in Fig. 18.18, the beads reunited with the mother vesicle.

Figure 18.20 shows budding of membranes and adhesion of buds to the mother membrane in blood cells. Adding an ionophore to the suspension of erythrocytes caused a discocyte–echinocyte transformation (Fig. 18.20A). Budding of the membrane took place at the tips of the echinocyte spicules (Fig. 18.20A). Some buds prolonged into tubular protrusions (Fig. 18.20A, white arrow)

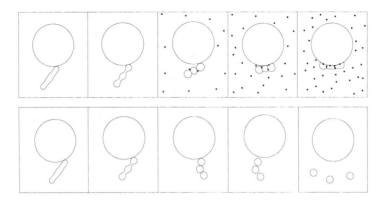

Figure 18.19 Scheme of the budding and vesiculation of a membrane in the presence (upper) and in the absence (lower) of adhesion mediators. If adhesion mediators are present, the buds adhere to the membrane, while if adhesion mediators are absent, the buds pinch off from the mother membrane and become NVs. Reprinted from *Chemistry and Physics of Lipids*, 150(1), Jasna Urbanija, Nejc Tomšič, Maruša Lokar, Aleš Ambrožič, Saša Čučnik, Blaž Rozman, Maša Kandušer, Aleš Iglič, and Veronika Kralj-Iglič, Coalescence of phospholipid membranes as a possible origin of anticoagulant effect of serum proteins, pp. 49–57, Copyright 2007, with permission from Elsevier.

while others appeared to be composed of a series of globular units. Figure 18.20B shows the adhesion of such units to each other (Fig. 18.20B, white arrows and black arrow). Adhesion of a bud to the mother membrane and to the membrane of the adjacent cell was also observed in platelets (Fig. 18.20C, white arrows) and in GPVs (Fig. 18.20D, white arrow), while adhering NVs were found in leukocytes (Fig. 18.20E) and erythrocytes (Fig. 18.20F). Spherical NVs may have adhered to the erythrocyte membrane (Fig. 18.20F, black arrow) while contact between the two erythrocytes was made through NVs adhering at their tips (Fig. 18.20E, gray arrow). The transmission electron microscopy image shows that the nanostructures are lighter (Fig. 18.20E), indicating that they do not contain haemoglobin. Either the membrane of these structures was permeable to haemoglobin while the connection with the mother cells (the necks) did not allow effective exchange of this protein between them and the respective mother cells, or the adhering NVs did not derive from the cell to which they

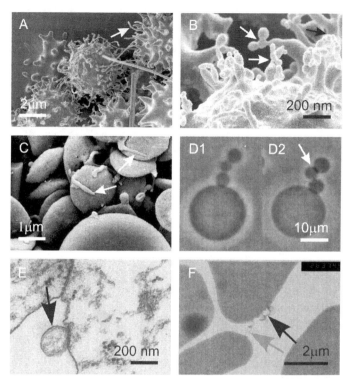

Figure 18.20 Budding of biological membranes and adhesion of buds to the mother membrane. A SEM image of echinocytes with tubular protrusions induced by the calcium ionophore A21387 (A), a SEM image of the adhesion of beads on protrusions (B), an SEM image of the adhesion of a tubular platelet protrusion to the mother platelet and to the adjacent platelet (C), a phase contrast microscope image of a giant phospholipid vesicle in a suspension with added PBS-dissolved beta 2 glycoprotein I 10 min after the addition of the sample (D1) and 20 min after the addition of the sample (D2), a TEM image of a bud adhering to the leukocyte membrane (E) and a TEM image of vesicles adhering to an erythrocyte membrane (F). Arrows in panels A–C point to buds, the arrow in panel D points to the area of adhesion between membrane parts connected by a thin neck, the black arrows in E and F point to globular membranous nanostructures adhering to the plasma membrane and the grey arrow in F points to a connection between cells formed by adhering nano-sized protrusions. (Štukelj, 2013).

adhered, but from another cell. As the adhering nanostructures were lighter, the mother cell was most probably not an erythrocyte.

In cells there may be different mechanisms that promote budding from those in GPVs, such as redistribution of membrane constituents (Hägerstrand et al., 2006), increase in the area of the outer layer with respect to the area of the inner layer (Sheetz and Singer, 1974) and increase in the temperature (Käs and Sackmann, 1991; Lipowsky, 1991). Regardless of the mechanism which induces budding, by causing adhesion of buds to the mother cell (Fig. 18.18) the presence of certain proteins could suppress the release of cell membrane exovesicles. The mechanism of NV-suppression in question is a physical mechanism that is common in all membranes, regardless of accompanying chemical processes which finally lead, for example, to blood clot formation or to protein synthesis. As a similar process may also take place in cells, a possible anticoagulant, anti cancer-progression and anti-inflammation effect of plasma constituents was suggested (Šuštar et al., 2009; Urbanija et al., 2007). According to the hypothesis, natural or artificial suppressors of nanovesiculation would act simultaneously as anticoagulants, cancer invasive potential decelerators, and inflammation suppressors. The proposed hypothesis is supported by the facts that a decrease of the level of plasma β_2GPI (Brighton, 1996) and an increase of the level of prothrombogenic NVs (Dignat-George et al., 2004; Morel et al., 2004) was observed in isolates from the blood of patients with disseminated intravascular coagulation.

Adhesion of the membrane bud to the mother membrane due to attractive-mediated interaction is a possible mechanism that could underlie the anticoagulant and anti-metastatic role of molecules in the solution in contact with the cell. Our results indicated that suppression of nanovesiculation (which was observed in erythrocytes, leukocytes, and platelets) involves development of a stable (energetically favourable) neck and adhesion of the membranes of the bud and of the mother membrane to each other.

As the mechanism of vesiculation suppression by mediated attractive interaction between membranes is non-specific, it could involve many kinds of plasma constituents which give an overall mediating effect. Further, the dissolved compounds not only enter into chemical reactions with membrane-bound receptors, but also

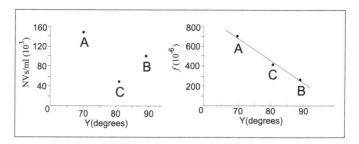

Figure 18.21 Left: The dependence of plasma NV concentration on the adhesion angle (Y) measured 25 min after the addition of plasma from subjects A, B, and C. Right: The dependence of the ratio $f =$ NV concentration/platelet concentration (indicating the ability of the membrane pool to shed NVs) on the adhesion angle (Y) measured 25 min after the addition of plasma from subjects A, B and C. Reprinted from *Autoimmunity Reviews*, 7(3), Mojca Frank, Mateja Mančan-Keberb, Mojca Kržan, Snežna Sodin-Šemrl, Roman Jerala, Aleš Iglič, Blaž Rozman, and Veronika Kralj-Iglič, Prevention of microvesiculation by adhesion of buds to the mother cell membrane: A possible anticoagulant effect of healthy donor plasma, pp. 240–245, Copyright 2008, with permission from Elsevier.

may affect the budding and vesiculation process by physical mechanisms (Brighton, 1996; Evans, 1974; Sheetz and Singer, 1974).

The addition of human plasma to a suspension of GPVs induced the adhesion of GPVs (Fig. 18.21) in a timescale of minutes. The mediating effect of human plasma can be quantitatively assessed by the average angle of contact between the adhering GPVs (Fig. 18.16), while the ability of the membrane to release NVs is assessed by the ratio $f =$ MV concentration/platelet concentration. Figure 18.21a shows measurement of the angles of contact between adhered GPVs. The adhesion angle Y is the average of all clearly visible angles measured from all the micrographs taken at a defined time. The concentration of NVs and the parameters Y and f reflect hemostasis and can therefore be used as biomarkers. For example, the adhesion angles of subjects A and B were compared at 6, 10, 15, 20, and 25 min after the addition of the subject's plasma to the GPVs. At all defined times Y in subject B was found to be significantly larger than Y in subject A ($p < 0.05$) (Frank et al., 2008), so the method can be considered sensitive enough to distinguish between subjects.

In a study considering the effect of human plasma on the adhesion of GPVs, the concentration of NVs in blood isolates of three healthy subjects was related to the adhesion angle Y (Fig. 18.21b). It can be seen roughly that a higher NV concentration indicates a weaker adhesion between membranes (smaller Y) since subject A, in whom the concentration of NVs was the highest, had the smallest Y. In subjects B and C, however, a larger Y did not correspond to a lower NV concentration (Fig. 18.21b). However, the three subjects differed considerably in platelet concentrations, which were $214 \times 10^9/l$, $394 \times 10^9/l$, and $120 \times 10^9/l$ in subjects A, B, and C, respectively. Figure 18.21c shows an excellent correspondence between the ability of the membrane to shed vesicles (f) and the adhesion angle Y. A negative relationship can be observed: f is smaller if Y is larger. (Fig. 18.21c). It was therefore concluded that the parameter f could be an efficient indicator of the ability of the membrane pool to shed NVs.

Heparin is a highly sulfated glycosaminoglycan stored within the secretory granules of mast cells and released into the vasculature at sites of tissue injury. Its role is still unclear, but it was found that it has anticoagulant and anti-inflammatory effects and that it decelerates the spread of metastases in cancer (Šuštar et al., 2009; Young, 2008). In order to explain the anti-tumour progression effect of heparin, various mechanisms were suggested. An acknowledged mechanism of metastatic potential is based on the scenario where after intravasation, a metastatic cancer cell passes into the bloodstream where it forms a micro-embolus composed of the metastatic cell, platelets, and leukocytes. The micro-embolus travels to the vessel of the target organ where the cell interacts with the endothelium of the blood vessel and passes to the organ, where it can form a metastasis. It was suggested that heparin affects the interaction of a free malignant cell with platelets, rendering it more accessible to leukocytes and diminishing its probability of adhering to the endothelium (Borsig, 2003; Stevenson et al., 2005). The underlying mechanism was suggested to be based on blocking of selectins by heparin. Another proposed mechanism based on the fibrinolytic activity of heparin. It was suggested (O'Meara and Jackson, 1958) that the fibrin mesh may serve as a support for metastatic cells which is in line with the results of experiments indicating that fibrinolytic agents are effective in the reduction of metastases (Borsig, 2003; Linhardt, 2004). Furthermore, it was reported (Berry et al., 2004) that heparin uptake into cancer cells can be promoted by conjugation to poly β-amino esters. Detailed studies (Chen et al., 2008) suggest that poly β-amino ester–heparin complexes affect cellular processes, including the induction of transcription factor and caspase activation. Internalized heparin is considered cytotoxic, causing cancer cell death by inducing apoptosis (Chen et al., 2008). However, none of the hitherto proposed mechanisms explain the anticoagulant, anti-tumour progression and anti-inflammation effects by a single underlying mechanism.

All three effects of heparin can be explained by suppression of nanovesiculation which, according to the above hypothesis, can be induced by mediating attractive interaction between membranes of the bud and of the mother cell. It was found that the addition of heparin to plasma increases the ability of plasma to mediate attractive interaction between membranes (Frank et al., 2008; Šuštar et al., 2009). The effect was found in all plasma samples considered: in healthy subjects and in patients (with rheumatoid arthritis and with gastrointestinal cancer) (Šuštar et al., 2009). Heparin in sugar solution exhibits the same effect, albeit too weak to have an impact in therapeutic concentrations (Šuštar et al., 2009).

In studying the effect of heparin *in vivo*, it was found (Frank et al., 2008) that the adhesion between GPVs mediated by β_2GPI was considerably decreased in the presence of serum IgG antibody fraction, containing autoimmune polyclonal antibodies against β_2GPI (isolated from the serum of a patient with APS and thrombosis), while a therapeutic concentration of nadroparin restored this adhesion (Frank et al., 2008). This is in favour of the hypothesis of the non-specific anticoagulant and anti-metastatic effect of plasma constituents is based on suppression of membrane vesiculation.

Nadroparin most probably interferes with anti-β_2GPI antibody binding to membrane-bound β_2GPI, thereby enabling domain I of β_2GPI to interact freely with the negatively charged membrane. This is consistent with the inhibition of *in vitro* binding of aPL antibodies on phospholipid-coated microplates in cofactor (β_2GPI)-dependent phosphatidylserine and cardiolipin ELISAs in the presence of low molecular weight heparin or unfractionated heparin (Ermel et al., 1995; Franklin and Kutteh, 2003; Wagenknecht and McIntyre, 1992). Also, affinity chromatography with low molecular weight heparin and unfractionated heparin columns adsorbed a significant proportion of aPL antibodies from the sera of women with recurrent pregnancy loss due to APS (Ermel et al., 1995). Heparin and proteins interact due to the binding of positively charged amino acids on the protein to negatively charged sulpho- and carboxyl groups on heparin (Capila and Linhardt, 2002). Hydrogen bonds are also important, at least in some cases of protein–heparin interaction (Capila and Linhardt, 2002). Somatic mutations leading to accumulation of positively charged amino acids (arginine, asparagine and lysine) within complementary determining regions of the paratope are a distinguishing feature of IgG aPL antibodies (Giles et al., 2003). Arginine residues were also shown to be implicated in binding of human monoclonal aPL antibodies derived from a patient with APS to β_2GPI (Giles, 2006). Based on these observations it could be inferred that nadroparin might potentially bind positively charged amino acids within the paratope of aPL antibodies and prevent their interaction with β_2GPI.

18.6 The Role of the Stability of Narrow Necks in Suppression of Membrane Vesiculation

The attractive interaction between membranes mediated by molecules in solution is of a short range (of the order of nanometers or even smaller) and therefore, applies to structures which are already very close together. For a bud, these conditions are fulfilled when it is connected to the mother vesicle by a short and thin but stable neck. The adhesion of the bud to the mother membrane, would however take place only if the neck were an energetically favourable structure. The stability of the membrane neck(s) (Bobrowska et al., 2013; Jesenek et al., 2012, 2013; Jorgačevski et al., 2010; Kralj-Iglič et al., 1999, 2006; Urbanija et al., 2008a) (see also Chapter 10) can be studied indirectly, by following the development of thermal fluctuations of a mother giant phospholipid vesicle while the necks are formed in a process of integration of a myelin-like protrusion into the mother GPV. It was suggested (Kralj-Iglič et al., 2001a) that the myelin-like protrusion serves as a reservoir for the membrane area of the mother globule and for the volume of the mother globule. However, the first contribution is more significant than the second one, so that with integration of the protrusion into the mother vesicle, the globular part becomes more and more flaccid, thereby allowing an increase in fluctuations of shape.

In cells, the glycaneous coat prevents adjacent membranes approaching each other to a distance they could be subject to attractive-mediated interaction (see also Chapter 14). We suggest that self-adhesion of nano-sized buds could occur if the membrane around the neck becomes depleted or nude with respect to the glycaneous coat and if appropriate mediating molecules are present in the solution. A favourable composition of the membrane in the neck is attained by curvature-sorting of the membrane constituents (Bobrowska et al., 2013; Gozdz and Gompper, 1999; Jorgačevski et al., 2010; Kralj-Iglič and Veranič, 2007; Shlomovitz et al., 2011; Yaghmur et al., 2007). Glycolipids with extensive parts protruding from the outer membrane layer are not likely to accumulate in the strongly negatively and anisotropically curved region of the neck, which enables the suggested process to take place. It can be suggested that the particular curvature of the neck provides the field for such sorting of membrane constituents in the neck. Theoretically it was predicted that a shape with a thin neck corresponds to a global minimum of the membrane free energy and is therefore stable (Kralj-Iglič et al., 2006).

In GPVs and in cells, tube-like protrusions are commonly observed. The existence of a network of nanotubes was indicated in an experiment (Mathivet et al., 1996) which showed rapid transport of a fluorescent label within the membrane between giant phospholipid vesicles prepared by electroformation (Angelova et al., 1992). Rinsing GPVs from the electroformation chamber tears the network, but its remnants remain attached to the GPVs.

The existence of the nanotubular network (Fig. 12.2) was then proved by an experiment in which the remnants of the network in the form of tubular protrusions (which are attached to the mother globule) became visible under a phase contrast microscope after undergoing a slow spontaneous shape transformation in which the average mean curvature of the vesicle decreased causing the protrusion to become shorter and thicker (Kralj-Iglič et al., 2001a) (see also Chapter 6). As as a results of a spontaneous process the average mean curvature of the GPVs decreases with time (Božič et al., 2002; Kralj-Iglič et al., 2001a). The reason for the transformation is not known, but presumably, phospholipid molecules are slowly removed from the outer membrane layer due to equalization of the chemical potential in the solution and in the membrane, degradation of the lipid and lipid flip flop (Kralj-Iglič et al., 2001a). Immediately after electroformation the vesicles appear spherical, protrusions are not visible and fluctuations of the globular part cannot be observed. A vesicle is chosen and followed for several hours. Some time (on the timescale of half an hour) after the solution containing vesicles is placed in the observation chamber, a tubular protrusion attached to the globular mother vesicle becomes visible (Kralj-Iglič et al., 2001a; Kralj-Iglič, 2002) (see also Section 6.4). The protrusion (Fig. 18.22A) shortens and thickens (Fig. 18.22B–D) and eventually exhibits a bead-like bud (Fig. 18.22E) which further transforms by reduction of the number of beads (Fig. 18.22E-I) (Božič et al., 2002; Kralj-Iglič et al., 2001a). Such shapes are observed in the last stage of the spontaneous process in which myelin-like protrusions are integrated into the mother vesicle (Fig. 18.22); Finally, the neck connecting the protrusion to the mother vesicle opens and the protrusion is integrated into the mother vesicle.

To study the effect of neck formation on the stability of the shape, thermal fluctuations of the mother GPV shape during this process were observed. The solution containing vesicles was placed in the observation chamber immediately after the electroformation of vesicles. A vesicle was chosen and followed during the above described process. The microscope was focused on the chosen vesicle, in particular on the globular part, while an attached video camera recorded it until the protrusion became completely integrated into the mother vesicle. The images of the globular part were digitized at the rate of about one per second. From the binary images the vesicle contour was determined by tracing the inner boundary of the white halo, surrounding the vesicle (Usenik et al., 2011). The coordinates of the contours were calculated relative to

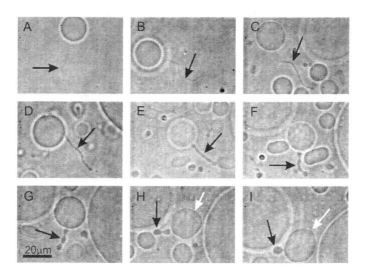

Figure 18.22 Time course of the spontaneous slow shortening of a myelin protrusion from a giant phospholipid vesicle made of POPC in sugar solution. Black arrows point to the protrusion, while white arrows point to the mother vesicle.

the contour centres. An example of a processed vesicle image and the contour obtained are shown in Fig. 18.23.

The shape of a nearly spherical vesicle can be expressed using the expansion into spherical harmonics

$$R(\theta, \varphi) = R_s (1 + \sum_{\ell=0}^{\ell_{max}} \sum_{m=-\ell}^{m=\ell} u_{\ell m} Y_{\ell m}(\theta, \varphi)), \qquad (18.2)$$

where $R(\theta, \varphi)$ is the distance from the contour centre to the membrane, R_s is the effective radius of the mother globule, $u_{\ell m}$ are Fourier coefficients and $Y_{\ell m}$ are the normalized spherical harmonics (Abramowitz and Stegun, 1970):

$$Y_{\ell m}(\theta, \varphi) = N_{\ell m} P_{\ell m}(\cos\theta) e^{im\varphi}, \qquad (18.3)$$

$P_{\ell m}(\cos\theta)$ are the associated Legendre functions and $N_{\ell m}$ are the normalization factors:

$$N_{\ell m} = \sqrt{\frac{(2\ell + 1)}{4\pi} \frac{(\ell - |m|)!}{(\ell + |m|)!}}. \qquad (18.4)$$

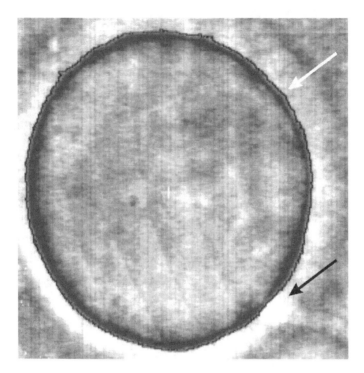

Figure 18.23 A processed image of a phospholipid vesicle and the vesicle contour. The microscope was focused on the globule (white arrow). A part of the protrusion can be seen at the bottom right (black arrow). The white cross marks the centre of the contour. The diameter of the vesicle was about 15 μm. (Štukelj, 2013).

The effective radius R_s is introduced in such a way that all the Fourier coefficients $u_{\ell m}$ are small.

The shape of the cross section of the vesicle which is obtained from Eq. (18.2) by taking $\theta = \pi/2$ is

$$R(\theta = \pi/2, \varphi) = R_s\left(1 + \sum_{m=-\ell_{max}}^{m=\ell_{max}} e^{im\varphi} u_m\right). \quad (18.5)$$

The corresponding Fourier coefficients are

$$u_{\ell m} = \sum_{\ell=|m|}^{\ell=\ell_{max}} u_{\ell m} N_{\ell m} P_{\ell m}(0), \quad (18.6)$$

where

$$P_{\ell m}(0) = 2^{|m|} \frac{1}{\sqrt{\pi}} \cos\left(\frac{\pi}{2}(\ell+m)\right) \frac{\Gamma(\ell/2+|m|/2+1/2)}{\Gamma(\ell/2-|m|/2+1)}.$$
(18.7)

The Fourier coefficients and the contour centre were obtained by least squares fitting of expression (18.5) to the experimentally obtained contour.

Figure 18.24 shows the time dependence of the averaged square of the Fourier coefficients normalized by the square of the effective radius (A) and of the effective radius of the mother vesicle R_s corresponding to the last stages of the slow spontaneous shortening of the myelin protrusion and its integration with the mother vesicle. The effective radius of the mother vesicle R_s and the Fourier coefficients increase on the average. The contribution of the Fourier coefficients with ($m = 2$) was the largest, but also coefficients with higher m can be noted. However, the increase of R_s is not monotonous. Rather, a peculiar stepwise pattern of R_s time-dependence can be observed.

The abrupt increase in the effective radius of the mother globule and of the Fourier coefficients are in step (Figs. 18.24A and B) which is in agreement with previous observations of the width of the protrusion necks (Božič et al., 2002). The duration of the steps increased so that a protrusion with three beads is less persistent than a protrusion with two beads, and the latter is less persistent than a protrusion with one bead. The necks connecting four beads were wider than the necks connecting three beads and these were wider than the neck that connects a single bead to the mother vesicle (Božič et al., 2002). The narrower the neck, the longer the persistence of the given number of beads (Fig. 18.24B). The abrupt increase in the effective radius is especially pronounced when the last bead is integrated into the globular part. It was concluded (Štukelj, 2013) that the narrow neck tends to stabilize the shape. This effect is not limited to the neck that connects the protrusion to the mother globule, but is also present in shapes having protrusions with two or three (wider) necks, although it is not so strong.

Within the last two steps (time between 650 s and 800 s and 800 s and 1300 s in Fig. 18.24), the effective radius of the mother globule decreased (Fig. 18.24B). However, the effective radius

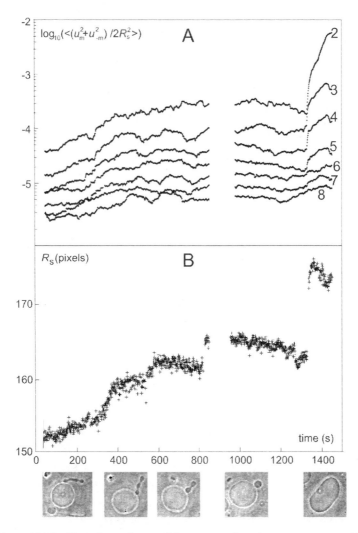

Figure 18.24 Time dependence of the average (moving averages over 100 points) square of the Fourier coefficients normalized by the square of the effective radius $\langle (u_m + u_{-m})^2 / 2R_s^2 \rangle$ for $m = 2$ to 8 as indicated in panel A; the scale on the ordinate is logarithmic (A). Time dependence of the effective radius of the mother globule R_s along the same sequence where the shortened and undulating protrusion integrates with the globular part (B). Each point corresponds to one image. (Štukelj, 2013).

decreased after the protrusion was completely incorporated into the mother globule (times larger than 1300s). It can be expected that the fluctuations immediately after integration of a larger amount of material into the globular part would not be spherically symmetric as the inflow appeared at a certain place where the protrusion was joined to the globular part. After some time the spherically symmetric mode was more or less restored. There may be other reasons for the decrease of R_s such as flow of the membrane and of the contents to and from the protrusion, rearrangement of the phospholipid molecules within the membrane, etc. At this point the observed decrease of R_s within a step remains unexplained.

The shape transformation of SOPC vesicles undergoing a budding transition due to heating was analysed (Döbereiner et al., 1995). It was found that the vesicles change abruptly as temperature T is raised, from a prolate ellipsoidal shape to a shape composed of a spherical mother vesicle and a spherical daughter vesicle connected by a narrow neck (such as in Fig. 18.22F). A similar process was observed in DMPC vesicles (Käs and Sackmann, 1991). It was also observed that in the reverse process in which the vesicles were cooled the neck opened at lower temperature indicating hysteresis (Käs and Sackmann, 1991). The acknowledged theory of membrane isotropic elasticity (Miao et al., 1994) does not offer an explanation for this feature (Döbereiner et al., 1995), but the budding transition was described as a first order transition (Käs and Sackmann, 1991) preceeded by large thermal shape fluctuations and quasi-critical slowing down that was interpreted as fluctuations of a metastable state near its spinodal instability (Döbereiner et al., 1995).

To explain the stability of the neck in a pure phospholipid system, the following mechanism was suggested (Štukelj, 2013). For various reasons (e.g., equilibration of the osmotic pressure, the presence in solution of molecules with particular properties, preferential intercalation of molecules into one of the two layers), the shape of the GPV may change. This change can be such that in some area(s) (e.g., necks) the curvature may become stronger and anisotropic. In order to constitute the membrane at that region, a phospholipid molecule may undergo a conformational change so that that the shape of the molecule becomes strongly anisotropic (in the sense that not all in-plane orientations are energetically equivalent). Such a molecule may be considered as a seed for an anisotropic inclusion. If the curvature relaxes, the conformational change relaxes too. We may say that such an inclusion is transient. However, if the vesicle fluctuates around the shape with an anisotropic region (e.g., a neck), the phospholipid molecule spends more time in a highly anisotropic state. Due to interaction between the phospholipid molecules, clusters of highly anisotropic membrane inclusions may be formed. The interaction of such an inclusion with the curvature field stabilizes the inclusion, which in turn favours regions with a large difference between the two main curvatures (the neck). Inclusions become orientationally ordered while the formation of the neck is promoted. The observed critical fluctuations may therefore, indicate the vicinity of a phase transition in which a pool of phospholipid molecules that are strongly anisotropic and orientationally ordered is localized around the narrow but finite neck. The change of average mean curvature (presumably due to the change in the number of molecules in the outer membrane layer) is however important in driving the shape over the prolate-pear transition where the probability of the proposed mechanism becomes high.

18.7 Clinical Validation of the Hypothesis of Nanovesiculation Suppression

In clinical studies involving populations of blood donors, it is of interest to determine the strength of the mediating effect of different plasma constituents on the interaction between GPVs, to test for a possible correlation with the amount of native NVs isolated from plasma, and to interpret the results in the light of clinical status.

Platelets represent the major pool of vesiculating cell membranes in healthy subjects (Diamant et al., 2002) as well as in many pathological disorders (Horstman et al., 2004; Jy et al., 1992; Martinez et al., 2005; Warkentin et al., 1994). Because NVs are derived from the budding of platelet membranes, in healthy subjects, a lower platelet concentration would imply a lower plasma NV concentration and relatively uniform values of f within the population. In contrast, an increased number of platelet-derived NVs in the presence of thrombocytopenia was found in different disorders, such as heparin-induced thrombocytopenia (HIT) (Hughes et al., 2000; Kravitz and Shoenfeld, 2005; Warkentin et al., 1994) and idiopathic thrombocytopenic purpura (Jy et al., 1992). Similarly, a low concentration of red blood cells and a high concentration of red blood cell-derived NVs were found in a hemolytic anaemias, such as thalassemia (Pattanapanyasat et al., 2004) and sickle-cell anaemia (Shet et al., 2003). In some of these disorders, such as idiopathic thrombocytopenic purpura (Horstman et al., 1994) and thalassemia (Pattanapanyasat et al., 2004), a strong budding process leading to cell lysis occurs. In these cases, a high NV concentration would be associated with a low number of vesiculating cells. High values of the parameter f could therefore be a convenient indicator of enhanced cell destruction in cytopenic states due to its enhanced sensitivity: the denominator (NV concentration) is increased and the numerator (vesiculating cell concentration) is decreased, both contributing to the increase of f.

The parameter f could be an indicator of enhanced platelet activation and destruction in which shedding of NVs in thrombocytopenic states is associated with hypercoagulability and thrombosis. It is known that HIT patients with severe thrombocytopenia are at increased risk of thrombosis (Lewis et al., 2006) and an increased number of potentially procoagulant platelet-derived NVs were reported in acute HIT patients (Warkentin et al., 1994). Also, the presence of aPL antibodies was correlated with an increased risk of thrombosis in aPL-associated thrombocytopenia patients (Atsumi et al., 2005). As aPL were shown to be involved in platelet activation (Nojima et al., 1999), which could be accompanied by enhanced platelet microvesiculation (Solum, 1999), platelet-derived NVs could be potentially increased in aPL-associated thrombocytopenia. In contrast, thrombocytopenia was not found to be related to the increased risk of thrombosis in APS patients (Krause et al., 2005). It was suggested that circulating NVs isolated from APS patients are mainly endothelium-derived (Combes et al., 1999; Dignat-George et al., 2004).

The ratio f is a measure of the ability of the platelet membrane to vesiculate, and is smaller, if the mediating effect of plasma, represented by the adhesion angle (Y) is larger. This is in favour of the hypothesis that plasma-mediated attractive interaction between membranes could represent a NV-suppression mechanism by preventing the release of NVs from cells. However, in order to obtain a decisive answer, the microvesiculation suppression hypothesis should be tested on different populations involving a larger number of subjects.

18.8 Concentration of Nanovesicles in Isolates from Blood of Patients with Gastrointestinal Diseases

Study of a population of subjects with various gastrointestinal diseases (Janša et al., 2008) brought further evidence in favour of the hypothesis of mediated interaction as a microvesiclulation suppression mechanism. To compare patients with diagnosed gastrointestinal cancer with other patients, two groups were formed. The group of patients diagnosed with cancer consisted of 5 patients and the group of patients with other gastrointestinal diseases consisted of 16 patients (for analysis of NVs) or 14 patients (for analysis of the average effective angles of contact between GPVs).

A negative, statistically significant correlation (Pearson coefficient $= -0.50$, $p = 0.031$) was found between the number of NVs in peripheral blood and the ability of plasma to induce coalescence between membranes represented by the average effective angle of contact between adhering GPVs (Y). The statistical significance of the correlation was even higher if the number of NVs was calculated with respect to the number of platelets (Pearson coefficient $= -0.64$, $p = 0.003$).

By comparing patients diagnosed with cancer with patients having other gastrointestinal diseases, a large (140%) and statistically significant ($p = 0.03$) difference between groups A and B regarding the number of NVs in peripheral blood was found, while the difference between the two groups regarding the average effective angles of contact between GPVs was smaller than the difference in NVs, but still considerable (20%) and statistically significant ($p = 0.01$). Further, statistical analysis yielded a power of 100% for NVs at $\alpha = 0.05$ while for the average effective angles of contact, the power at $\alpha = 0.05$ was 90%, which is excellent considering that there were only 5 subjects in group A. On the basis of these results we can conclude that considerable and statistically significant differences in the number of NVs and in the ability of plasma to cause adhesion of membranes are indicated between the two groups. Four out of five patients from group A form a separate group in Fig. 18.25 at large numbers of NVs and small average angles of contact between GPVs. In these patients the disease was well advanced. One patient died two weeks after the blood sample was taken, due to cardiac arrest following coma. The another patient with cancer who had a small number of NVs and a large average effective angle of contact (and with respect to these parameters was indistinguishable from patients from group B), the tumour was smaller and the stage of the disease was described as initial. The large difference in the number of NVs between the group of patients with gastric cancer and the group of patients with other intestinal diseases could therefore be ascribed to the advanced stage of cancer in four out of five patients with cancer. This is in agreement with the results of other authors who found an increased number of NVs in the peripheral blood of patients with gastric cancer with respect to normal controls (Kim, et al., 2003).

The Pearson coefficient representing the strength of the correlation was higher for the parameter f (Fig. 18.25B) than for the NV number (Fig. 18.25A), mostly on account of the patients with diagnosed cancer. In line with the above hypothesis, this indicates that also in these patients platelets represent an important vesiculating pool. Indeed, it was found that an increased number of tissue factor bearing NVs, presumably derived from platelets, were found in the blood of patients with Duke's D colorectal cancer (Hron et al., 2007).

It has been suggested that tissue factor might be transported to the platelet membrane from monocytes and macrophages by means of NVs (Müller et al., 2003). The tissue factor, an integral membrane protein of the vessel wall and the principal initiator of blood coagulation, was found on circulating NVs (del Conde et al., 2005, 2007; Hron et al., 2007; Müller et al., 2003; Rauch and Antoniak, 2007). It was reported that the tissue factor-bearing NVs originate from lipid rafts of the monocyte or macrophage membrane. The rafts are enriched in tissue factor and cholesterol (del Conde et al., 2005) which indicates the importance of redistribution of membrane

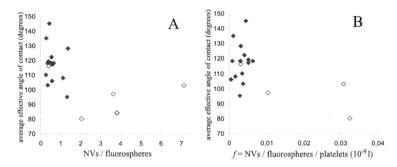

Figure 18.25 Correlation between the number of NVs isolated from blood and the average angle of contact (Y) between GPVs adhering after the addition of plasma from the same blood (a) and the correlation between the number of NVs per number of platelets (parameter f) and the average angle of contact (Y) for the population of patients with gastrointestinal diseases. Reprinted from *Blood Cells, Molecules, and Diseases*, 41(1), Rado Janša, Vid Šuštar, Mojca Frank, Petra Sušanj, Janez Bešter, Mateja Manček-Keber, Mojca Kržan, Aleš Iglič, Number of microvesicles in peripheral blood and ability of plasma to induce adhesion between phospholipid membranes in 19 patients with gastrointestinal diseases, pp. 124–132, Copyright 2008, with permission from Elsevier.

constituents (Kralj-Iglič et al., 1999, 1998) and interactions between membrane constituents (Kralj-Iglič and Veranič, 2007) in the budding process (Hägerstrand et al., 2006).

18.9 Perspectives in the Biophysics of Membranous Nanostructures

Membranous nanostructures were long overlooked due to their small size and fragility. It has now become evident that they play an important role in vital cell processes. They create a communication system that integrates the whole organism and connects it with its surroundings. They underlie epigenetic processes and determine the expression of information contained within genetic material. Revealing the functioning of membranous nanostructures will provide a key to different disorders and help in their prevention and therapy. Theoretical biophysics supported by an experimental approach represents an effective tool in efforts to reach this goal.

Bibliography

Abidor, I. G., Arakelyan, V. B., Chernomordik, L. V., Chizmadzhev, Y. A., Pastushenko, V. F., and Tarasevich, M. R. (1979). Electric Breakdown of Bilayer Lipid-Membranes 1. Main Experimental Facts and their Qualitative Discussion. *Bioelectrochem. Bioener.*, 6, pp. 37–52.

Abramowitz, M., and Stegun, I. A. (1970). *Handbook of Mathematical Functions*, 9th edn. (Dover Publications Inc., New York).

Adams, D. J. (1981). Theory of the Dielectric Constant of Ice. *Nature*, 293, 5832, pp. 447–449.

Aeffner, S., Reusch, T., Weinhausen, B., and Salditt, T. (2009). Membrane Fusion Intermediates and the Effect of Cholesterol: An In-House X-Ray Scattering Study. *Eur. Phys. J.*, 30, pp. 205–214.

Alberts, B., Johnson, A., Lewis, J., Raff, M., Roberts, K., and Walter, P. (2008). *Mol. Biol. Cell*, 5th edn. (Garland Science, New York).

Allain, J. M., and Ben Amar, M. (2004). Biphasic Vesicle: Instability Induced by Adsorption of Proteins. *Physica A*, 337, pp. 531–545.

Allan, D., Billah, M. M., Finean, J. B., and Michell, R. H. (1976). Release of Diacylglycerol-Enriched Vesicles from Erythrocytes with Increased Intracellular (Ca^{2+}). *Nature (London)*, 261, pp. 58–60.

Alssema, M., El-Harchaoui, K., Schindhelm, R. K., Diamant, M., Nijpels, G., Kostense, P. J., Teerlink, T., Heine, R. J., Dallinga-Thie, G. M., Kuivenhoven, J. A., Dekker, J. M., and Scheffer, P. G. (2010). Fasting Cholesteryl Ester Transfer Protein Concentration is Independently Associated with the Postprandial Decrease in High-Density Lipoprotein Cholesterol Concentration after Fat-Rich Meals: The Hoorn Prandial Study. *Metabolism*, 59, pp. 854–860.

Alvarez, O., Brodwick, M., Latorre, R., Mclaughlin, A., Mclaughlin, S., and Szabo, G. (1983). Large Divalent Cations and Electrostatic Potentials Adjacent to Membranes. *Biophys. J.*, 44, pp. 333–342.

Ambrožič, A., Čučnik, S., Tomšič, N., Urbanija, J., Lokar, M., Babnik, B., Rozman, B., Iglič, A., and Kralj-Iglič, V. (2006). Interaction of Giant

Phospholipid Vesicles Containing Cardiolipin and Cholesterol with β_2-Glycoprotein-I and Anti-β_2-Glycoprotein-I Antibodies. *Autoimmun. Rev.*, 6, pp. 10–15.

Andelman, D. (1995). Electrostatic Properties of Membranes: The Poisson-Boltzmann Theory, in R. Lipowsky and E. Sackmann (eds.), *Structure and Dynamics of Membranes* (Elsevier, Amsterdam), pp. 603–642.

Angelini, T. E., Liang, H., Wriggers, W., and Wong, G. C. L. (2003). Like-Charge Attraction between Polyelectrolytes Induced by Counterion Charge Density Waves. *Proc. Natl. Acad. Sci. USA*, 100, 15, pp. 8634–8637.

Angelova, M. I., Soléau, S., Méléard, Ph., Faucon, J. F., and Bothorel, P. (1992). Preparation of Giant Vesicles by External AC Electric Field: Kinetics and Application. *Prog. Colloid Polym. Sci.*, 89, pp. 127–131.

Araki, T. (1979). Release of Cholesterol-Enriched Microvesicles from Human Erythrocytes Caused by Hypertonic Saline at Low-Temperatures. *FEBS Lett.*, 97, pp. 237–240.

Aranda-Espinoza, H., Berman, A., Dan, N., Pincus, P., and Safran, S. (1996). Interaction between Inclusions Embedded in Membranes. *Biophys. J.*, 71, pp. 648–656.

Arfken, G. B., and Weber, H. J. (1995). *Mathematical Methods for Physicists* (Academic Press, San Diego, CA).

Arslan, C., and Coskun, H. S. (2005). Thrombocytosis in Solid Tumors: Review of the Literature. *Turk. J. Haematol.*, 22, pp. 59–64.

Atsumi, T., Furukawa, S., Amengual, O., and Koike, T. (2005). Antiphospholipid Antibody Associated Thrombocytopenia and the Paradoxical Risk of Thrombosis. *Lupus*, 14, pp. 499–504.

Attard, G. S., Glyde, J. C., and Goltner, C. G. (1995). Liquid Crystalline Phases as Templates for the Synthesis of Mesoporous Silica. *Nature*, 378, pp. 366–368.

Aupeix, K., Toti, F., Satta, N., Bischoff, P., and Freyssinet, J. M. (1996). Oxysterols Induce Membrane Procoagulant Activity in Monocytic THP-1 Cells. *Biochem. J.*, 314, pp. 1027–1033.

Bacquet, R., and Rossky, P. J. (1983). Corrections to the HNC Equation for Associating Electrolytes. *J. Chem. Phys.*, 79, pp. 1419–1426.

Bacquet, R., and Rossky, P. J. (1984). Ionic Atmosphere of Rod-Like Polyelectrolytes. A Hypernetted Chain Study. *J. Phys. Chem.*, 88, pp. 2660–2669.

Baj-Krzyworzeka, M., Szatanek, R., Weglarczyk, K., Baran, J., Urbanowicz, B., Brański, P., Ratajczak, M. Z., and Zembala, M. (2006). Tumour-Derived Microvesicles Carry Several Surface Determinants and mRNA of

Tumour Cells and Transfer Some of these Determinants to Monocytes. *Cancer Immunol. Immun.*, 55, pp. 808–818.

Balasubramanian, K., Chandra, J., and Schroit, A. J. (1997). Immune Clearance of Phosphatidylserine: Expressing Cells by Phagocytes. The Role of Beta2-Glycoprotein I in Macrophage Recognition. *J. Biol. Chem.*, 272, pp. 31113–31117.

Balasubramanian, K., and Scroit, A. J. (1998). Characterization of Phosphatidylserine Dependent β_2-Glycoprotein I Macrophage Interactions. Implications for Apoptotic Cell Clearance by Phagocytes. *J. Biol. Chem.*, 273, pp. 29272–29277.

Baptista, G. R. (ed.) (2013). *An Integrated View of the Molecular Recognition and Toxinology: From Analytical Procedures to Biomedical Applications*, (InTech). DOI: 10.5772/3429.

Barbero, G., Evangelista, L. R., and Olivero, D. (2000). Asymmetric Ionic Adsorption and Cell Polarization in Liquid Crystals. *J. Appl. Phys.*, 87, 5, pp. 2646–2648.

Bard, M. P., Hegmans, J. P., Hemmes, A, Luider, T. M., Kleijmeer, M. J., Prins, J. B., Zitvogel, L., Burgers, S. A., Hoogsteden, H. C., and Lambrecht, B. N. (2004). Proteomic Analysis of Exosomes Isolated from Human Malignant Pleural Effusions. *Am. J. Respir. Cell Mol. Biol.*, 31, pp. 114–121.

Bar-Ziv, R., and Moses, E. (1994). Instability and "Pearling" States Produced in Tubular Membranes by Competition of Curvature and Tension. *Phys. Rev. Lett.*, 73, pp. 1392–1395.

Bar-Ziv, R., Tlusty, E., Moses, E., Safran, S. A., and Bershadsky, A. (1999). Pearling in Cells: A Clue to Understanding Cell Shape. *Proc. Natl. Acad. Asci. USA*, 96, pp. 10140–10145.

Bastida, E., Ordinas, A., and Jamieson, G. A. (1983). Identity of Procoagulant and Platelet Aggregating Activities in Microvesicles from Human Glioblastoma Cells. *Thromb. Haemostasis.*, 50, pp. 218–218.

Bastida, E., Escolar, G., Ordinas, A., and Jamieson, G. A. (1985). Identical Thrombogenic Effects of Human-Tumor Cells and Shed Microvesicles with Different Mechanisms of Platelet Activation. *Thromb. Haemost.*, 54, pp. 264–264.

Bastida, E., Escolar, G., Ordinas, A., and Jamieson, G. A. (1986). Morphometric Evaluation of Thrombogenesis by Microvesicles from Human-Tumor Cell-Lines with Thrombin-Dependent (u87mg) and Adenosine-Diphosphate Dependent (sknmc) Platelet-Activating Mechanisms. *J. Lab. Clin. Med.*, 108, pp. 622–627.

Baumgart, T., Hess, S. T., and Webb, W. W. (2003). Imaging Coexisting Fluid Domains in Biomembrane Models Coupling Curvature and Line Tension. *Nature*, 425, 6960, pp. 821–824. DOI: 10.1038/nature02013.

Bazant, M., Kilic, M., Storey, B., and Ajdari, A. (2009). Towards an Understanding of Induced-Charge Electrokinetics at Large Applied Voltages in Concentrated Solutions. *Adv. Colloid Interf. Sci.*, 152, 1–2, pp. 48–88.

Ben-Shaul, A. (1995). Molecular Theory of Chain Packing, Elasticity and Lipid-Protein Interactions in Lipid Bilayers, in R. Lipowsky and E. Sackmann (eds.), *Structure and Dynamics of Membranes* (Elsevier, Amsterdam), pp. 382.

Berckmans, R. J., Nieuwland, R., Tak, P. P., Boing, A. N., Romijn, F. P., Kraan, M. C., Breedveld, F. C., Hack, C. E., and Sturk, A. (2002). Cell-Derived Microparticles in Synovial Fluid from Inflamed Arthritic Joints Support Coagulation Exclusively via a Factor VII-Dependent Mechanism. *Arthritis Rheum.*, 46, pp. 2857–2866.

Berg, J. M., Tymoczko, J. L., and Stryer, L. (2002). *Biochemistry*, 5th edn. (W. H. Freeman, New York).

Berkowitz, M. L., Bostick, D. L., and Pandit, S. (2006). Aqueous Solutions Next to Phospholipid Membrane Surfaces: Insights from Simulations. *Chem. Rev.*, 106, pp. 1527–1539.

Berry, D., Lynn, D. M., Sasisekharan, R., and Langer, R. (2004). Poly(Beta-amino Ester)s Promote Cellular Uptake of Heparin and Cancer Cell Death. *Chem. Biol.*, 11, pp. 487–498.

Bessis, M. (1973). *Living Blood Cells and their Ultrastructure* (Springer, New York).

Betterton, M. D., and Brenner, M. P. (1999). Electrostatic Edge Instability of Lipid Membranes. *Phys. Rev. Lett.*, 82, pp. 1598–1601.

Bevers, E. M., Janssen, M. O., Comfurius, P., Balasubramanian, K., Schroit, A. J., Zwaal, R. F., and Willems, G. M. (2005). Quantitative Determination of the Binding of β_2-Glycoprotein I and Prothrombin to Phosphatidylserine-Exposing Blood Platelets. *Biochem. J.*, 386, pp. 271–279.

Bhuiyan, L. B., and Outhwaite, C. W. (2009). Comparison of Exclusion Volume Corrections to the Poisson-Boltzmann Equation for Inhomogeneous Electrolytes. *J. Coll. Int. Sci.*, 331, pp. 543–547.

Bhuiyan, L. B., Outhwaite, C. W., and Bratko, D. (1992). Structure and Thermodynamics of Micellar Solutions in the Modified Poisson-Boltzmann Theory. *Chem. Phys. Lett.*, 193, pp. 203–210.

Bibi, S., Kaur, R., Henriksen-Lacey, M., McNeil, S. E., Wilkhu, J., Lattmann, E., Christensen, D., Mohammed, A. R., and Perrie, Y. (2011). Microscopy Imaging of Liposomes: From Coverslips to Environmental SEM. *Int. J. Pharm.*, 417, 1–2, pp. 138–150. DOI: 10.1016/j.ijpharm.2010.12.021.

Biesheuvel, P. M., and van Soestbergen, M. (2007). Counterion Volume Effects in Mixed Electrical Double Layers. *J. Coll. Int. Sci.*, 316, pp. 490–499.

Bikerman, J. J. (1942). Structure and Capacity of the Electrical Double Layer. *Phil. Mag.*, 33, pp. 384–397.

Biro, E., Akkerman, J. W. N., Hoek, F. J., Gorter, G., Pronk, L. M., Sturk, A., and Nieuwland, R. (2005). The Phospholipid Composition and Cholesterol Content of Platelet-Derived Microparticles: A Comparison with Platelet Membrane Fractions. *J. Thromb. Haemostas.*, 3, pp. 2754–2763.

Biro, E., Nieuwland, R., and Sturk, A. (2004). Measuring Circulating Cell-Derived Microparticles. *J. Thromb. Haemost.*, 2, pp. 1843–344.

Bivas, I., and Ermakov, Y. A. (2007). Elasticity and Electrostatics of Amphiphilic Layers, in A. Leitmannova Liu (ed.), *Advances in Planar Lipid Bilayers and Liposomes* (Elsevier, Amsterdam), 5, pp. 313–343.

Black, P. H. (1980). Shedding from Normal and Cancer-Cell Surfaces. *New Engl. J. Med.*, 303, pp. 1415–1416.

Bloomfield, V. (1996). DNA Condensation, *Curr. Opin. Struct. Biol.*, 6, pp. 334–341.

Božič, B., Gomišček, G., Kralj-Iglič, V., Svetina, S., and Zeks, B. (2002). Shapes of Phospholipid Vesicles with Bead-Like Protrusions. *Eur. Biophys. J.*, 31, pp. 487–496.

Božič, B., Kralj-Iglič, V., and Svetina, S. (2006). Coupling between Vesicle Shape and Lateral Distribution of Mobile Membrane Inclusions. *Phys. Rev. E*, 73, pp. 041915.

Boal, D. (2002). *Mechanics of the Cell* (Cambridge University Press, Cambridge, UK).

Bobrowska-Hägerstand, M., Kralj-Iglič, V., Iglič, A., Bialkowska, K., Isomaa, B., and Hägerstrand, H. (1999). Torocyte Membrane Endovesicles Induced by Octaethyleneglycol Dodecylether in Human Erythrocytes. *Biophys. J.*, 77, pp. 3356–3362.

Bobrowska, N., Góźdź, W., Kralj-Iglič, V., and Iglič, A. (2013). On the Role of Anisotropy of Membrane Components in Formation and Stabilization of Tubular Structures in Multi-Component Membranes. *Plos. One*, 8, e73941.

Bobyn, J. D., Pilliar, R. M., Cameron, H. U., Weatherly, G. C., and Kent, G. M. (1980). The Effect of Porous Surface Configuration on the Tensile Strength of Fixation of Implants by Bone Ingrowth. *Clin. Orthop. Relat. Res.*, 149, pp. 291–298.

Bobyn, J. D., Wilson, G. J., MacGregor, D. C., Pilliar, R. M., and Weatherly, G. C. (1982). Effect of Pore Size on the Peel Strength of Attachment of Fibrous Tissue to Porous-Surfaced Implants. *J. Biomed. Mater. Res.*, 16, pp. 571–584.

Bohinc, K., Gimsa, J., Kralj-Iglič, V., Slivnik, T., and Iglič, A. (2005). Excluded Volume Driven Counterion Condensation Inside Nanotubes in a Concave Electrical Double Layer Model. *Bioelectrochemistry*, 67, pp. 91–99.

Bohinc, K., Iglič, A., and May, S. (2004). Interaction between Macroions Mediated by Divalent Rod-Like Ions. *Europhys. Lett.*, 68, 4, pp. 494–500.

Bohinc, K., Kralj-Iglič, V., and Iglič, A. (2001). Thickness of Electrical Double Layer. Effect of Ion Size. *Electrochim. Acta.*, 46, pp. 3033–3040.

Boilard, E., Nigrovic, P. A., Larabee, K., Watts, G. F., Coblyn, J. S., Weinblatt, M. E., Massarotti, E. M., Remold-O'Donnell, E., Farndale, R. W., Ware, J., and Lee, D. M. (2010). Platelets Amplify Inflammation in Arthritis via Collagen-Dependent Microparticle Production. *Science*, 327, 5965, pp. 580–583. (PMC free article) (PubMed).

Bona, R., Lee, E., and Rickles, F. (1987). Tissue Factor Apoprotein: Intracellular-Transport and Expression in Shed Membrane-Vesicles. *Thromb. Res.*, 48, pp. 487–500.

Booth, F. (1951). The Dielectric Constant of Water and the Saturation Effect. *J. Chem. Phys.*, 19, pp. 391–394.

Borsig, L. (2003). Selectins Facilitate Carcinom Metastasis and Heparin can Prevent them. *News Physiol. Sci.*, 19, pp. 16–21.

Borukhov, I. (2004). Charge Renormalization of Cylinders and Spheres: Ion Size Effect. *J. Pol. Sci. B, Pol. Phys.*, 42, pp. 3598.

Borukhov, I., Andelman, D., and Orland, H. (1997). Steric Effects in Electrolytes: A Modified Poisson Boltzmann Equation. *Phys. Rev. Lett.*, 79, pp. 435–438.

Bouafsoun, A., Helali, S., Mebarek, S., Zeiller, C., Prigent, A. F., Othmane, A., Kerkeni, A., Jaffrézic-Renault, N., and Ponsonnet, L. (2007). Electrical Probing of Endothelial Cell Behaviour on a Fibronectin/Polystyrene/Thiol/Gold Electrode by Faradaic Electrochemical Impedance Spectroscopy (EIS). *Bioelectrochemitry*, 70, pp. 401–407.

Boulbitch, A. A. (1998). Deflection of a Cell Membrane under Application of Local Force. *Phys. Rev. E*, 57, pp. 1–5.

Bouma, B., de Groot, P. G., van den Elsen, J. M. H., Ravelli, R. B. G., Schouten, A., Simmelink, J. A., Derksen, M. J. A., Kroon, J., and Gros, P. (1999). Adhesion Mechanism of Human β_2-Glycoprotein I to Phospholipids Based on its Crystal Structure. *EMBO J.*, 18, pp. 5166–5174.

Boya, P., and Kroemer, G. (2008). Lysosomal Membrane Permeabilization in Cell Death. *Oncogene*, 27, 50, pp. 6434–6451. DOI: 10.1038/onc.2008.310.

Bratko, D. (1990). Hypernetted Chain Approximation for Ion Distribution in Reverse Micelles. *Chem. Phys. Lett.*, 169, pp. 555–560.

Bratko, D., and Vlachy, V. (1982). Distribution of Counterions in the Double Layer around a Cylindrical Polyion. *J. Phys. Chem.*, 90, pp. 434–438.

Bremner, W. F., Sothern, R. B., Kanabrocki, E. L., Ryan, M., McCormick, J. B., Dawson, S., Connors, E. S., Rothschild, R., Third, J. L. H. C., Vahed, S., Nemchausky, B. M., Shirazi, P., and Olwin, J. H. (2000). Relation between Circadian Patterns in Levels of Circulating Lipoprotein(a), Fibrinogen, Platelets, and Related Lipid Variables in Men. *Am. Heart J.*, 139, pp. 164–173.

Brighton, T. A., Hogg, P. J., Dai, Y. P., Murray, B. H., Chong, B. H., and Chesterman, C. N. (1996). Beta2-Glycoprotein I in Thrombosis: Evidence for a Role as a Natural Anticoagulant. *Br. J. Haematol.*, 93, pp. 185–194.

Brogan, P. A., Shah, V., Brachet, C., Harnden, A., Mant, D., Klein, N., and Dillon, M. J. (2004). Endothelial and Platelet Microparticles in Vasculitis of the Young. *Arthritis Rheum.*, 50, pp. 927–936.

Brown, D. A., and London, E. J. (1998a). Function of Lipid Rafts in Biological Membranes. *Annu. Rev. Cell Biol.*, 14, pp. 111–136.

Brown, D. A., and London, E. J. (1998b). Structure and Origin of Ordered Lipid Domains in Biological Membranes. *J. Membr. Biol.*, 164, pp. 103–114.

Butler, J. C., Angelini, T., Tang, J. X., and Wong, G. C. L. (2003). Ion Multivalence and Like-Charge Polyelectrolyte Attraction. *Phys. Rev. Lett.*, 91, 2, pp. 028301-4.

Butt, H. J., Graf, K., and Kappl, M. (2003). *Physics and Chemistry of Interfaces* (Wiley-VCH, Weinheim).

Calin, G. A., Ferracin, M., Cimmino, A. Di Leva, G., Shimizu, M., Wojcik, S. E., Iorio, M. V., Visone, R., Sever, N. I., Fabbri, M., Iuliano, R., Palumbo, T., Pichiorri, F., Roldo, C., Garzon, R., Sevignani, C., Rassenti, L., Alder, H.,

Volinia, S., Liu, C. G., Kipps, T. J., Negrini, M., and Croce, C. M. (2005). A microRNA Signature Associated with Prognosis and Progression in Chronic Lymphocytic Leukemia. *New Engl. J. Med.*, 353, pp. 1793–1801.

Cammack, R., Attwood, T., Campbell, P., Parish, H., Smith, A., Vella, F., and Stirling, J. (2006). *Oxford Dictionary of Biochemistry and Molecular Biology*, 2nd edn. (Oxford University Press, USA).

Canham, P. B. (1970). The Minimum Energy of Bending as a Possible Explanation of the Biconcave Shape of the Human Red Blood Cell. *J. Theor. Biol.*, 26, pp. 61–81.

Capila, I., and Linhardt, R. J. (2002). Heparin-Protein Interactions. *Angew. Chem. Int. Ed. Engl.*, 41, pp. 390–412.

Carnie, S. L., Chan, D. Y. C., and Stankovich, J. (1994). Computation of Forces between Spherical Colloidal Particles-Nonlinear Poisson-Boltzmann Theory. *J. Colloid Interf. Sci.*, 165, pp. 116–128.

Carnie, S., and McLaughlin, S. (1983). Large Divalent Cations and Electrostatic Potentials Adjacent to Membranes. A Theoretical Calculation. *Biophys. J.*, 44, pp. 325–332.

Causeret, M., Taulet, N., Comunale, F., Favard, C., and Gauthier-Rouvire, C. (2005). N-cadherin Association with Lipid Rafts Regulates its Dynamic Assembly at Cell-Cell Junctions in C_2C_{12} Myoblasts. *Mol. Biol. Cell.*, 16, pp. 2168–2180.

Ceccarelli, B., Hurlbut, W., and Mauro, A. (1973). Turnover of Transmitter and Synaptic Vesicles at the Frog Neuromuscular Junction. *J. Cell. Biol.*, 57, pp. 499–524.

Cerri, C., Chimenti, D., Conti, I., Neri, T., Paggiaro, P., and Celi, A. Monocyte/Macrophage-Derived Microparticles Up-Regulate Inflammatory Mediator Synthesis by Human Airway Epithelial Cells. *J. Immunol.*, 177, pp. 1975–1980.

Cevc, G. (1990). Membrane Electrostatics. *Biochim. Biophys. Acta.*, 1031, 3, pp. 311–382.

Cevc, G., and Marsh, D. (1987). *Phospholipid Bilayers. Physical Principles and Models.* (Wiley-Interscience, New York).

Chakraborty, H., Mondal, S., Sarkar, M. (2008). Membrane Fusion: A New Function of Non Steroidal Anti-Inflammatory Drugs. *Biophys. Chem.*, 137, 1, pp. 28–34. DOI: 10.1016/j.bpc.2008.06.007.

Chan, Y. H. M., and Boxer, S. G. (2007). Model Membrane Systems and their Applications. *Curr. Opin. Chem. Bio.*, 11, 6, pp. 581–587. DOI: 10.1016/j.cbpa.2007.09.020.

Chandler, D. (2002). Hydrophobicity: Two Faces of Water. *Nature*, 417, pp. 491.

Chandler, D. (2005). Interfaces and the Driving Force of Hydrophobic Assembly. *Nature*, 437, pp. 640–647.

Chanturiya, A., Yang, J., Scaria, P., Stanek, J., Frei, J., Mett, H., and Woodle, M. (2003). New Cationic Lipids form Channel-Like Pores in Phospholipid Bilayers. *Biophys. J.*, 84, pp. 1750–1755.

Chapman, D. L. (1913). A Contribution to the Theory of Electrocapillarity. *Philos. Mag.*, 25, pp. 475–481.

Chen, X., Xiao, W., Qu, X., and Zhou, S. (2008). The Effect of Dalteparin, a Kind of Low Molecular Weight Heparin, on Lung Adenocarcinoma A549 Cell Line in Vitro. *Cancer Inv.*, 26, pp. 718–724.

Chen, Z., and Rand, R. (1997). The Influence of Cholesterol on Phospholipid Membrane Curvature and Bending Elasticity. *Biophys. J.*, 73, pp. 267–276.

Chernomordik, L. V., and Kozlov, M. M. (2008). Mechanics of Membrane Fusion. *Nat. Struct. and Mol. Bio.*, 15, pp. 675–683.

Chernomordik, L. V., Kozlov, M. M., Melikyan, G. B., Abidor, I. G., Markin, V. S., and Chizmadzhev, Y. A. (1985). The Shape of Lipid Molecules and Monolayer Membrane-Fusion. *Biochim. Biophys. Acta*, 812, pp. 643–655.

Chinnery, H. R., Peralman, E., and McMenamin, P. G. (2008). Cutting Edge: Membrane Nanotubes In Vivo: A Feature of MHC Class II+ Cells in Mouse Cornea. *J. Immunol.*, 180, pp. 5779–5783.

Chonn, A., Semple, S. C., and Cullis, P. R. (1995). β_2-Glycoprotein I is a Major Protein Associated with Very Rapidly Cleared Liposomes in Vivo, Suggesting Significant Role in the Immune Clearance of Non-Self Particles. *J. Biol. Chem.*, 270, pp. 25845–25849.

Chou, T. (2007). Stochastic Entry of Enveloped Viruses: Fusion Versus Endocytosis. *Biophys. J.*, 93, pp. 1116–1123.

Churchward, M., Rogasevskaia, T., Brandman, D., Khosravani, H., Nava, P., Atkinson, J., and Coorssen, J. (2008). Specific Lipids Supply Critical Negative Spontaneous Curvature: An Essential Component of Native Ca^{2+}-Triggered Membrane Fusion. *Biophys. J.*, 94, pp. 3976–3986.

Cliffton, E. E., and Agostino, D. (1964). Effect of Inhibitors of Fibrinolytic Enzymes on Development of Pulmonary Metastases. *J. Natl. Cancer Inst.*, 33, pp. 753–763.

Cohn, J. S., McNamara, J. R., Cohn, D., Ordovas, J. M., and Schaefer, E. J. (1988). Postprandial Plasma Lipoprotein Changes in Human Subjects of Different Ages. *J. Lip. Res.*, 29, pp. 469–478.

Cole, W. F., Rumsby, M. G., Longster, G. H., and Tovey, L. A. D. (1979). Changes in the Inhibition of Specific Agglutination by Plasma Due to Microvesicles Released from Human Red-Cells during Storage for Transfusion. *Vox Sang.*, 37, pp. 73–77.

Coltel, N., Combes, V., Wassmer, S. C. Chimini, G., and Grau, G. E. (2006). Cell Vesiculation and Immunopathology: Implications in Cerebral Malaria. *Microbes Infect.*, 8, pp. 2305–2316.

Combes, V., Simon, A. C., Grau, G. E., Arnoux, D., Camoin, L., Sabatier, F., Mutin, M., Sanmarco, M., Sampol, J., and Dignat-George, F. (1999). In Vitro Generation of Endothelial Microparticles and Possible Prothrombotic Activity in Patients with Lupus Anticoagulant. *J. Clin. Invest.*, 104, pp. 93–102.

Cooper, A., Paran, N., and Shaul, Y. (2003). The Earliest Steps in Hepatitis B Virus Infection. *Biochim. Biophys. Acta*, 1614, pp. 89–96.

Cooper, G. M. (2000). *Cell: A Molecular Approach*, 2nd edn. (ASM Press, Sunderland MA).

Corbeil, D., Röper, K., Fargeas, C. A., Joester, A., and Huttner, W. B. (2001). Prominin: A Story of Cholesterol, Plasma Membrane Protrusions and Human Pathology. *Traffic*, 2, pp. 82–91.

Corless, J. M., and Costello, M. J. (1981). Paracrystalline Inclusions Associated with the Disk Membranes of Frog Retinal Rod Outer Segments. *Exp. Eye Res.*, 32, pp. 217–228.

Crowley, J. M. (1973). Electrical Breakdown of Biomolecular Lipid-Membranes as an Electromechanical Instability. *Biophys. J.*, 13, pp. 711–724.

Cullis, P. R., Hope, M. J., and Tilcock, C. P. S. (1986). Lipid Polymorphism and the Roles of Lipids in Membranes. *Chem. Phys. Lipids*, 40, pp. 127–144.

Döbereiner, H. G., Evans, E., Seifert U., and Wortis, M. (1995). Spinodal Fluctuations of Budding Vesicles. *Phys. Rev. Lett.*, 75, pp. 3360.

Dan, N., and Safran, S. A. (1998). Effect of Lipid Characteristics on the Structure of Transmembrane Proteins. *Biophys. J.*, 75, pp. 1410–1414.

Dan, N., Berman, A., Pincus, P., and Safran, S. A. (1994). Membrane-Induced Interactions between Inclusions. *J. Phys. II (France)*, 4, pp. 1713–1725.

Dan, N., Pincus, P., and Safran, S. A. (1993). Membrane-Induced Interactions Between Inclusions. *Langmuir*, 9, pp. 2768–2771.

Das, T., Bratko, D., Bhuiyan, L. B., and Outhwaite, C. W. (1995). Modified Poisson-Boltzmann Theory Applied to Linear Polyelectrolyte Solutions. *J. Phys. Chem.*, 99, pp. 410–418.

Das, T., Bratko, D., Bhuiyan, L. B., and Outhwaite, C. W. (1997). Polyelectrolyte Solutions Containing Mixed Valency Ions in the Cell Model: A Simulation and Modified Poisson-Boltzmann Theory. *J. Phys. Chem.*, 107, pp. 9197–9207.

Davis, D. M., and Sowinski, S. (2008). Membrane Nanotubes: Dynamic Long-Distance Connections between Animal Cells. *Nat. Rev. Mol. Cell Biol.*, 6, pp. 431–436.

del Conde, I., Shrimpton, C. N., Thiagarajan, P., and Lopez, J. A. (2005). Tissue Factor-Bearing Microvesicles Arise from Lipid Rafts and Fuse with Activated Platelets to Initiate Coagulation. *Blood*, 106, pp. 1604–1611.

del Conde, I., Bharwani, L. D., Dietzen, D. J., Pendurthi, U., Thaigarajan, P., and Lopez, J. A. (2007). Microvesicle-Associated Tissue Factor and Trousseau's Syndrome. *J. Thromb. Haemost.*, 5, pp. 70–74.

del Papa, N., Guidali, L., Spatola, L., Bonara, P., Borghi, M. O., Tincani, A., Balestrieri, G., and Meroni, P. L. (1995). Relationship between Anti-Phospholipid and Anti-Endothelial Cell Antibodies III: 2 Glycoprotein I Mediates the Antibody Binding to Endothelial Membranes and Induces the Expression of Adhesion Molecules. *Clin. Exp. Rheumatol.*, 13, pp. 179–185.

Delacroix, H., Gulik-Krzywicki, T., and Seddon, M. (1996). Freeze Fracture Electron Microscopy of Lyotropic Lipid Systems: Quantitative Analysis of the Inverse Micellar Cubic Phase of Space Group Fd3m ($Q^2 27$). *J. Mol. Biol.*, 258, pp. 88–103.

Derényi, I., Jülicher, F., and Prost, J. (2002). Formation and Interaction of Membrane Tubes. *Phys. Rev. Lett.*, 88, pp. 238101.

DeRosa, G., Ferrari, I., D'Angelo, A., Salvadeo, S. A. T., Fogari, E., Gravina, A., Mereu, R., Palumbo, I., Maffioli, P., Randazzo, S., and Cicero, A. F. G. (2010). Effects of a Standardized Oral Fat Load on Vascular Remodeling Markers in Healthy Subjects. *Microvasc. Res.*, 80, pp. 110–115.

Deserno, M. (2004a). Elastic Deformation of a Fluid Membrane upon Colloid Binding. *Phys. Rev. E*, 69, pp. 031903.

Deserno, M. (2004b). When Do Fluid Membranes Engulf Sticky Colloids? *J. Phys. Cond. Mat.*, 16, pp. S2061–S2070.

Deserno, M. (2009). Mesoscopic Membrane Physics: Concepts, Simulations, and Selected Applications. *Macromol. Rapid Comm.*, 30, 9–10, pp. 752–771. DOI:10.1002/marc.200900090.

Deserno, M., and Bickel, T. (2003). Wrapping of a Spherical Colloid by a Fluid Membrane. *Europhys. Lett.*, 62, pp. 767–773.

Deuling, H. J., and Helfrich, W. (1976). Curvature Elasticity of Fluid Membranes: Catalog of Vesicle Shapes. *J. Phys. (France)*, 37, pp. 1335–1345.

Dey-Hazra, E., Hertel, B., Kirsch, T., Woywodt, A., Lovric, S., Haller, H., Haubitz, M., and Erdbruegger, U. (2010). Detection of Circulating Microparticles by Flow Cytometry: Influence of Centrifugation, Filtration of Buffer, and Freezing. *Vasc. Health Risk Manag.*, 6, pp. 1125–1133 (PMC free article) (PubMed).

Di Scipio, R. G. (1992). Ultrastructures and Interactions of Complement Factors H and I. *J. Immunol.*, 149, pp. 2592–2599.

Diamant, M., Nieuwland, R., Pablo, R. F., Sturk, A., Smit, J. W., and Radder, J. K. (2002). Elevated Numbers of Tissue-Factor Exposing Microparticles Correlate with Components of the Metabolic Syndrome in Uncomplicated Type 2 Diabetes Mellitus. *Circulation*, 106, pp. 2442–2447.

Diamant, M., Tushuizen, M. E., Sturk, A., and Nieuwland, R. (2004). Cellular Microparticles: New Players in the Field of Vascular Disease? *Eur. J. Clin. Invest.*, 34, pp. 392–401.

Dignat-George, F., Camoin-Jau, L., Sabatier, F., Arnoux, D., Anfosso, F., Bardin, N., Veit, V., Combes, V., Gentile, S., Moal, S., Sanmarco, M., and Sampol, J. (2004). Endothelial Microparticles: A Potential Contribution to the Thrombotic Complications of the Antiphospholipid Syndrome. *Thromb. Haemost.*, 91, pp. 667–673.

Diguet, A., Yanagisawa, M., Liu, Y. J., Brun, E., Abadie, S., Rudiuk, S., and Baigl, D. (2012). UV-Induced Bursting of Cell-Sized Multicomponent Lipid Vesicles in a Photosensitive Surfactant Solution. *J. Am. Chem. Soc.*, 134, 10, pp. 4898–4904. DOI: 10.1021/ja211664f.

Dill, K., and Bromberg, S. (2003). *Molecular Driving Forces: Statistical Thermodynamics in Chemistry and Biology* (Garland Science, USA).

Ding, H. M., and Ma, Y. Q. (2012). Role of Physicochemical Properties of Coating Ligands in Receptor-Mediated Endocytosis of Nanoparticles. *Biomaterials*, 33, 23, pp. 5798–5802. DOI: 10.1016/j.biomaterials.2012.04.055.

Discher, D. E. N., and Mohandas, N. (1996). Kinematics of Red Cell Aspiration by Fluorescence-Imaged Microdeformation. *Biophys. J.*, 71, pp. 1680–1694.

Discher, D. E. N., Mohandas, N., and Evans, E. A. (1994). Molecular Maps of Red Cell Deformability: Hidden Elasticity and In Situ Connectivity. *Science*, 266, pp. 1032–1035.

Dommersnes, P. G., and Fournier, J. B. (1999). N-Body Study of Anisotropic Membrane Inclusions: Membrane Mediated Interactions and Ordered Aggregation. *Eur. Phys. J. B*, pp. 9–12.

Dommersnes, P. G., and Fournier, J. B. (2002). The Many-Body Problem for Anisotropic Membrane Inclusions and the Self-Assembly of "Saddle" Defects into an "Egg Carton". *Biophys. J.*, 83, pp. 2898–2905.

Drobne, D. (2013). 3D Imaging of Cells and Tissues by Focused Ion Beam/Scanning Electron Microscopy (FIB/SEM), in A. A. Sousa and M. J. Kruhlak (eds.), *Nanoimaging: Methods and Protocols* (Humana Press, New York), 950, pp. 275–292. DOI: 10.1007/978-1-62703-137-0_16.

Drobne, D., Milani, M., Leser, V., Tatti, F., Zrimec, A., Znidarsic, N., Kostanjsek, R., and Strus, J. (2008). Imaging of Intracellular Spherical Lamellar Structures and Tissue Gross Morphology by a Focused Ion Beam/Scanning Electron Microscope (FIB/SEM). *Ultramicroscopy*, 108, 7, pp. 663–670. DIO: 10.1016/j.ultramic.2007.10.010.

Drobne, D., Milani, M., Zrimec, A., Zrimec, M. B., Tatti, F., and Draslar, K. (2005). Focused Ion Beam/Scanning Electron Microscopy Studies of Porcellio Scaber (Isopoda, Crustacea) Digestive Gland Epithelium Cells. *Scanning*, 27, pp. 30–34.

Dubnickova, M., Bobrowska-Hägerstrand, M., Soderstrom, T., Iglič, A., and Hägerstrand, H. (2000). Gemini (Dimeric) Surfactant Perturbation of the Human Erythrocyte. *Acta Biochim. Polonica*, 47, pp. 651–660.

Duesing, P. M., Templer, R. H., and Seddon, J. M. (1997). Quantifying Packing Frustration Energy in Inverse Lytropic Mesophases. *Langmuir*, 13, pp. 251–359.

Duman, J., and Forte, J. (2003). What is the Role of SNARE Proteins in Membrane Fusion? *Am. J. Physiol. Cell. Physiol.*, 285, pp. C237–C249.

Dutta, M., and Sengupta, M. (1954). A Theory of Strong Electrolytes in Solution Based on New Statistics. *Proc. Natl. Inst. Scif. India*, 20, pp. 1–11.

Duwe, H. P., Käs, J., and Sackmann, E. (1990). Bending Elastic Moduli of Lipid Bilayers: Modulations of Solutes. *J. Phys. (France)*, 51, pp. 945–962.

Eigen, M., and Wicke, E. (1954). The Thermodynamics of Electrolytes at Higher Concentrations. *J. Phys. Chem.*, 58, 9, pp. 702–714.

Elsgolc, L. E. (1961). *Calculus of Variations* (Pergamon Press, Oxford).

Ermel, L. D., Marshburn, P. B., and Kutteh, W. H. (1995). Interaction of Heparin with Antiphospholipid Antibody (APA) from the Sera of Women with Recurrent Pregnancy Loss (RPL). *Am. J. Reprod. Immunol.*, 33, pp. 14–20.

Evans, E. (1974). Bending Resistance and Chemically Induced Moments in Membrane Bilayers. *Biophys. J.*, 14, pp. 923–931.

Evans, E. A., and Skalak, R. (1980). *Mechanics and Thermodynamics of Biomembranes* (CRC Press, Boca Raton).

Evans, D. F., and Wennerström, H. (1999). *The Colloidal Domain: Where Physics, Chemistry, Biology, and Technology Meet*, 2nd edn. (Wiley-VCH, New York).

Ewald, P. P. (1921). Evaluation of Optical and Electrostatics Lattice Potentials. *Ann. Phys. (Leipzig)*, 64, pp. 253–287.

Fang, Q., Berberian, K., Gong, L., Hafez, I., Sörensen, J., and Lindau, M. (2008). The Role of the C Terminus of the SNARE Protein SNAP-25 in Fusion Neck Opening and a Model for Fusion Neck Mechanics. *Proc. Natl. Acad. Sci. USA*, 105, pp. 15388–15392.

Farsad, K., and De Camilli, P. (2003). Mechanisms of Membrane Deformation. *Curr. Opin. Cell Biol.*, 15, pp. 372–381.

Faucon, J. F., Mitov, M., Meleard, P., Bivas, I., and Bothorel, P. (1989). Bending Elasticity and Thermal Fluctuations of Lipid Membranes. Theoretical and Experimental Requirements. *J. Physique*, 50, pp. 2389–2414.

Fedorov, M. V., and Kornyshev, A. A. (2008). Towards Understanding the Structure and Capacitance of Electrical Double Layer in Ionic Liquids. *Electrochim. Acta*, 53, pp. 6835–6840.

Fedorov, M. V., Georgi, N., and Kornyshev, A. A. (2010). Double Layer in Ionic Liquids: The Nature of the Camel Shape of Capacitance. *Electrochem. Commun.*, 12, pp. 296–299.

Fernfindez-Nieves, A., Richter, C., and de las Nieves, F. J. (1998). Point of Zero Charge Estimation for a TiO_2/Water Interface. *Prog. Colloid. Polym. Sci.*, 110, pp. 21–24.

Ferreira, A. C., Peter, A. A., Mendez, A. J., Jimenez, J. J., Mauro, L. M., Chirinos, J. A., Ghany, R., Virani, S., Garcia, S., Horstman, L. L., Purow, J., Jy, W., Ahn, Y. S., and de Marchena, E. (2004). Postprandial Hypertriglyceridemia Increases Circulating Levels of Endothelial Cell Microparticles. *Circulation*, 110, pp. 3599–3603.

Fevrier, B., Vilette, D., Archer, F., Loew, D., Faigle, W., Vidal, M., Laude, H., and Raposo, G. (2004). Cells Release Prions in Association with Exosomes. *Proc. Natl. Acad. Sci. USA.*, 101, pp. 9683–9688.

Fischer, T. (1992). Bending Stiffness of Lipid Bilayers. 3. Gaussian Curvature. *J. Phys. II (France)*, 2, pp. 337–343.

Fischer, T. (1993). Bending Stiffness of Lipid Bilayers. V. Comparison of Two Formulations. *J. Phys. II (France)*, 3, pp. 1795–1805.

Flaumenhaft, R. (2006). Formation and Fate of Platelet Microparticles. *Blood Cells Mol. Dis.*, 36, pp. 182–187.

Fleck, C. C., and Netz, R. R. (2004). Electrostatic Colloid-Membrane Binding. *Europhys. Lett.*, 67, pp. 314–320.

Fošnarič, M., Bohinc, K., Gauger, D. R., Iglič, A., Kralj-Iglič, V., and May, S. (2005). The Influence of Anisotropic Membrane Inclusions on Curvature Elastic Properties of Lipid Membranes. *J. Chem. Inf. Mod.*, 45, pp. 1652–1661.

Fošnarič, M., Iglič, A., and May, S. (2006). Influence of Rigid Inclusions on the Bending Elasticity of a Lipid Membrane. *Phys. Rev. E*, 174, pp. 051503.

Fošnarič, M., Iglič, A., Kroll, D. M., and May, S. (2009). Monte Carlo Simulations of Complex Formation between a Mixed Fluid Vesicle and a Charged Colloid. *J. Chem. Phys.*, 131, pp. 105103.

Fošnarič, M., Kralj-Iglič, V., Bohinc, K., Iglič, A., and May, S. (2003). Stabilization of Pores in Lipid Bilayers by Anisotropic Inclusions. *J. Phys. Chem. B.*, 107, pp. 12519–12526.

Fošnarič, M., Nemec, M., Kralj-Iglič, V., Hägerstrand, H., Schara, M., and Iglič, A. (2002). Possible Role of Anisotropic Membrane Inclusions in Stability of Torocyte Red Blood Cell Daughter Vesicles. *Colloid. Surf. B.*, 26, pp. 243–253.

Fournier, J. B. (1996). Nontopological Saddle-Splay and Curvature Instabilities from Anisotropic Membrane Inclusions. *Phys. Rev. Lett.*, 76, pp. 4436–4439.

Fournier, J. B. (1998). Coupling between Membrane Tilt-Difference and Dilation: A New "Ripple" Instability and Multiple Crystalline Inclusions Phases. *Europhys. Lett.*, 43, pp. 725–730.

Fournier, J. B. (1999). Microscopic Membrane Elasticity and Interactions among Membrane Inclusions: Interplay between the Shape, Dilation, Tilt and Tilt-Difference Modes. *Eur. Phys. J. B*, 11, pp. 261–272.

Fournier, J. B., and Galatola, P. (1998). Bilayer Membranes with 2-D Nematic Order of the Surfactant Polar Heads. *Braz. J. Phys.*, 28, pp. 329–338.

Fröhlich, H. (1964). *Theory of Dielectrics* (Clarendon Press).

Frank, M., Manček-Keber, M., Kržan, M., Sodin-Šemrl, S., Jerala, R., Iglič, A., Rozman, B., and Kralj-Iglič, V. (2008). Prevention of Microvesiculation by Adhesion of Buds to the Mother Cell Membrane: A Possible

Anticoagulant Effect of Healthy Donor Plasma. *Autoimmun. Rev.*, 7, pp. 240–245.

Frank, M., Sodin-Šemrl, S., Rozman, B., Potočnik M., and Kralj-Iglič, V. (2009). Effects of Low-Molecular-Weight Heparin on Adhesion and Vesiculation of Phospholipid Membranes: A Possible Mechanism for the Treatment of Hypercoagulability in Antiphospholipid Syndrome. *Ann. NY Acad. Sci.*, 1173, pp. 874–886.

Franklin, R. D., and Kutteh W. H. (2003). Effects of Unfractionated and Low Molecular Weight Heparin on Antiphospholipid Antibody Binding in Vitro. *Obstet. Gynecol.*, 101, pp. 455–462.

Franks, F. (1972). *Water. A Comprehensive Treatise* (Plenum Press, New York).

Freise, V. (1952). Zur Theorie der Diffusendoppeltsch Icht. *Z. Elektrochem.*, 56, pp. 822–827.

Frenkel, D., and Smith, B. (1996). *Understanding Molecular Simulation* (Academic Press, San Diego).

Furie, B., Furie, B. C. (2006). Cancer-Associated Thrombosis. *Blood Cells Mol. Dis.*, 36, pp. 177–181.

Furie, B., Zwicker, J., LaRocca, T., Kos, C., Bauer, B., and Furie, B. C. (2005). Tissue Factor-Bearing Microparticles and Cancer-Associated Thrombosis. *Haematol. Rep.*, 1, 9, pp. 5–8.

Galkina, S. I., Molotkovsky, J. G., Ullrich, V., and Sudina, G. F. (2005). Scanning Electron Microscopy Study of Neutrophil Membrane Tubulovesicular Extensions (Cytonemes) and their Role in Anchoring, Aggregation and Phagocytosis. The Effect of Nitric Oxide. *Exp. Cell Res.*, 304, pp. 620–629.

Galli, M., Grassi, A., and Barbui, T. (1996). Platelet-Derived Microvesicles in Thrombotic Thrombocytopenic Purpura and Hemolytic Uremic Syndrome. *Thromb. Haemost.*, 75, pp. 427–431.

Gamsjaeger, R., Johs, A., Gries, A., Gruber, H. J., Romanin, C., Prassl, R., and Hinterdorfer, P. (2005). Membrane Binding of β_2-Glycoprotein I Can be described by a Two-State Reaction Model: An Atomic Froce Microscopy and Surface Plasmon Resonance Study. *Biochem. J.*, 389, pp. 665–673.

Gao, H. J., Shi, W. D., and Freund, L. B. (2005). Mechanics of Receptor-Mediated Endocytosis, *Proc. Nat. Acad. Sci. USA*, 102, pp. 9469–9474.

Gasic, G. J., Gasic, T. B., and Stewart, C. C. (1968). Antimetastatic Effects Associated with Platelet Reduction, *Proc. Natl. Acad. Sci. USA*, 61, 1, pp. 46–52. (PMC free article) (PubMed).

Gay, L. J., and Felding-Habermann, B. (2011). Contribution of Platelets to Tumor Metastasis. *Nat. Rev. Cancer*, 11, 2, pp. 123–134.

Gelbart, W. M., Bruinsma, R., Pincus, P. A., and Parsegian, V. A. (2000). DNA-Inspired Electrostatics. Not Just the Repository of our Genetic Information, DNA is Also a Fascinating, Shape-Shifting Molecule whose Behavior in Solution Counters our Intuition and Challenges our Physical Understanding. *Phy. Today*, 53, pp. 38–44.

George, J. N., Thoi, L. L., McManus, L. M., and Reimann, T. A. (1982). Isolation of Human Platelet Membrane Microparticles from Plasma and Serum. *Blood.*, 60, pp. 834–840.

Gerdes, H. H., Bukoreshtiev, N. V., and Barroso, J. F. V. (2007). Tunneling Nanotubes: A New Route for the Exchange of Components between Animal Cells. *FEBS Lett.*, 581, pp. 2194–2201.

Gerdes, H. H., and Carvalho, R. N. (2008). Intercellular Transfer Mediated by Tunneling Nanotubes. *Curr. Opin. Cell Biol.*, 20, pp. 470–475.

Giles, I. P., Haley, J. D., Nagl, S., Isenberg, D. A., Latchman, D. S., and Rahman, A. (2003). A Systematic Analysis of Sequences of Human Antiphospho-Lipid and Anti-β_2-Glycoprotein I Antibodies: The Importance of Somatic Mutations and Certain Sequence Motifs. *Semin. Arthritis Rheum.*, 32, pp. 246–265.

Giles, I., Lambrianides, N., Pattni, N., Faulkes, D., Latchman, D., Chen, P. J., Pierangeli, S., Isenberg, D., and Rahman, A. (2006). Arginine Residues are Important in Determining the Binding of Human Monoclonal Antiphospholipid Antibodies to Clinically Relevant Antigens. *J. Immunol.*, 177, pp. 1729–1736.

Gimsa, U., Iglič, A., Fiedler, S., Zwanzig, M., Kralj-Iglič, V., Jonas, L., and Gimsa, J. (2007). Actin is Not Required for Nanotubular Protrusions of Primary Astrocytes Grown on Metal Nano-Lawn. *Mol. Membr. Biol.*, 24, pp. 243–255.

Ginestra, A., La Placa, M. D., Saladino, F., Cassara, D., Nagase, H., and Vittorelli, M. L. (1998). The Amount and Proteolytic Content of Vesicles Shed by Human Cancer Cell Lines Correlates with their in Vitro Invasiveness. *Anticancer Res.*, 18, pp. 3433–3437.

Gompper, G., and Kroll, D. M. (1997). Network Models of Fluid, Hexatic and Polymerized Membranes. *J. Phys. Cond. Mat.*, 9, pp. 8795–8834.

Gompper, G., and Kroll, D. M. (2004). Triangulated-Surface Models of Fluctuating Membranes, in D. Nelson, T. Piran, S. Weinberg (eds.), *Statistical Mechanics of Membranes and Surfaces*, 2nd edn. (World Scientific, Singapore), pp. 359–426.

Gongadze, E. (2011). *Influence of the Surface Structure of a Biomaterial on the Field Distribution in the Neighbouring Biosystem*, Ph.D. thesis, University of Rostock.

Gongadze, E., Bohinc, K., van Rienen, U., Kralj-Iglič, V., and Iglič, A. (2010). Spatial Variation of Permittivity near a Charged Membrane in Contact with Electrolyte Solution, in Iglič, A. (ed.), *Advances in Planar Lipid Bilayers and Liposomes* (Elsevier, Amsterdam), 11, pp. 101–126.

Gongadze, E., and Iglič, A. (2012a). Decrease of Permittivity of an Electrolyte Solution near a Charged Surface Due to Saturation and Excluded Volume Effects. *Bioelectrochemistry*, 87, pp. 199–203.

Gongadze, E., and Iglič, A. (2012b). Physical Properties of Water near a Charged Metal Surface Due to Saturation and Excluded Volume Effect. *Bulg. J. Phys.*, 39, pp. 12–28.

Gongadze, E., and Iglič, A. (2013). Excluded Volume Effect of Counterions and Water Dipoles near a Highly Charged Surface. *Gen. Phys. Biophys.*, 32, pp. 143–145.

Gongadze, E., Kabaso, D., Bauer, S., Slivnik, T., Schmuki, P., van Rienen, U., and Iglič, A. (2011a). Adhesion of Osteoblasts to a Nanorough Titanium Implant Surface. *Int. J. Nanomed.*, 6, pp. 1801–1816.

Gongadze, E., van Rienen, U., and Iglič, A. (2011b). Generalized Stern Models of an Electric Double Layer Considering the Spatial Variation of Permittivity and Finite Size of Ions in Saturation Regime. *Cell. Mol. Biol. Lett.*, 16, pp. 576–594.

Gongadze, E., van Rienen, U., Kralj-Iglič, V., and Iglič, A. (2011c). Langevin Poisson-Boltzmann Equation: Point-Like Ions and Water Dipoles near Charged Membrane Surface. *Gen. Physiol. Biophys.* 30, 130–137.

Gongadze, E., Kabaso, D., Bauer, S., Park, J., Schmuki, P., and Iglič, A. (2012). Adhesion of Osteoblast to a Vertically Aligned TiO_2 Nanotube Surface. *Mini-Reviews in Medicinal Chemistry.* 13, 194–200.

Gongadze, E., van Rienen, U., Kralj-Iglič, V., and Iglič, A. (2013). Spatial Variation of Permittivity of an Electrolyte Solution in Contact with a Charged Metal Surface: A Mini Review. *Comput. Meth. Biomech. Biomed. Eng.*, 16, pp. 463–480.

Gongadze, E., Velikonja, A., Perutková, Š., Kramar, P., Maček-Lebar, A., Kralj-Iglič, V., and Iglič, A. (2014). Ions and Water Molecules in an Electrolyte Solution in Contact with Charged and Dipolar Surfaces. *Electrochimica Acta* (in press).

Goniakowski, J., and Gillan, M. (1996). The Adsorption of H_2O on TiO_2 and SnO_2(110) Studied by First-Principles Calculations. *Surf. Sci.*, 350, pp. 145–158.

Gonzalez-Tovar, E., Lozada-Cassou, M., and Henderson, D. (1985). Hypernetted Chain Approximation for the Distribution of Ions around a Cylindrical Electrode: II. Numerical Solution for a Model Cylindrical Polyelectrolyte. *J. Chem. Phys.*, 83, pp. 361–372.

Goracci, L., Ceccarelli, M., Bonelli, D., and Cruciani, G. (2013). Modeling Phospholipidosis Induction: Reliability and Warnings. *J. Chem. Inf. Model.*, 53, 6, pp. 1436–1446. DOI: 10.1021/ci400113t

Gorter, E., and Grendel, F. (1925). On Bimolecular Layers of Lipoids on the Chromocytes of the Blood. *J. Exp. Med.*, 41, 4, pp. 439–443. DOI: 10.1084/jem.41.4.439

Gouy, M. G. (1910). Sur la Constitution Dela Charge Electrique ala Surface d'un Electrolyte. *J. Physique (France)*, 9, pp. 457–468.

Gozdz, W. T., and Gompper, G. (1999). Shapes and Shape Transformations of Two-Component Membranes of Complex Topology. *Phys. Rev. E.*, 59, 4, pp. 4305–4316.

Greenwalt, T. J. (2006). The How and Why of Exocytic Vesicles. *Transfusion*, 46, pp. 143–152.

Grimley, T. B. (1950). The Contact between a Solid and a Liquid Electrolyte, in *Proc. R. Soc. Lond. Ser. A*, 201, pp. 40–61.

Grimley, T. B., and Mott, N. F. (1947). The Contact between a Solid and a Liquid Electrolyte. *Discuss. Faraday Soc.*, 1, pp. 3–11.

Grosberg, A. Y., Nguyen, T. T., and Shklovskii, B. I. (2002). The Physics of Charge Inversion in Chemical and Biological Systems, *Mod. Rev. Phys.* 74, pp. 329–345.

Gruen, D. W. R., and Marčelja, S. (1983). Spatially Varying Polarization in Water. *J. Chem. Soc. Faraday Trans. II*, 79, 2, pp. 225–242.

Gruler, H. (1975). Chemoelastic Effect of Membranes. *Z. Naturforsch.*, 30c, pp. 608–614.

Guldbrand, L., Jönsson, B., Wennerström, H., and Linse, P. (1984). Electrical Double Layer Forces. A Monte-Carlo Study. *J. Chem. Phys.*, 80, 5, pp. 2221–2228.

György, B., Módos, K., Pállinger, E., Pálóczi, K., Pásztói, M., Misják, P., Deli, M. A., Sipos, A., Szalai, A., Voszka, I., Polgár, A., Tóth, K., Csete, M., Nagy, G., Gay, S., Falus, A., Kittel, A., and Buzás, E.I. (2011). Detection and Isolation of Cell-Derived Microparticles are Compromised by Protein Complexes Due to Shared Biophysical Parameters. *Blood.*, 117, 4, pp. e39–e48.

Hägerstrand, H., Bobrowska-Hagerstrand, M., Lillsunde, I., and Isomaa, B. (1996). Vesiculation Induced by Amphiphiles and Ionophore A23187 in Porcine Platelets: A Transmission Electron Microscopic Study. *Chem. Biol. Interact.*, 101, pp. 115–126.

Hägerstrand, H., Danieluk, M., Bobrowska-Hägerstrand, M., Iglič, A., Wróbel, A., Isomaa, B., and Nikinmaa, M. (2000). Influence of Band 3 Protein Absence and Skeletal Structures on Amphiphile and Ca^{2+} Induced Shape Alteration in Erythrocytes: A Study with Lamprey (*Lampetra fluviatilis*), Trout (*Onchorhynchus mykiss*) and Human Erythrocytes. *Biochim. Biophys. Acta*, 1466, pp. 125–138.

Hägerstrand, H., Danieluk, M., Bobrowska-Hägerstrand, M., Pector, V., Ruysschaert, J. M., Kralj-Iglič, V., and Iglič, A. (1999). Liposomes Composed of a Double-Chain Cationic Amphiphile (Vectamidine) Induce their Own Encapsulation into Human Erythrocytes. *Biochim. Biophys. Acta*, 1421, pp. 125–130.

Hägerstrand, H., Iglič, A., Bobrowska-Hägerstrand, M., Lindqvist, C., Isomaa, B., and Eber, S. (2001). Amphiphile-Induced Vesiculation in Aged Hereditary Spherocytosis Erythrocytes Indicates Normal Membrane Stability Properties Under Non-Starving Conditions. *Mol. Membr. Biol.*, 18, pp. 221–227.

Hägerstrand, H., and Isomaa, B. (1989). Vesiculation Induced by Amphiphiles in Erythrocytes. *Biochem. Biophys. Acta.*, 982, pp. 179–186.

Hägerstrand, H., and Isomaa, B. (1992). Morphological Characterization of Exovesicles and Endovesicles Released in Human Erythrocytes Following Treatment with Amphiphiles. *Biochim. Biophys. Acta*, 1109, pp. 117–126.

Hägerstrand, H., and Isomaa, B. (1994). Lipid and Protein Composition of Exovesicles Released from Human Erythrocytes Following Treatment with Amphiphiles. *Biochim. Biophys. Acta.*, 1190, pp. 409–415.

Hägerstrand, H., Kralj-Iglič, V., Bobrowska-Hägerstrand, M., and Iglič, A. (1999). Membrane Skeleton Detachment in Spherical and Cylindrical Microexovesicles. *Bull. Math. Biol.*, 61, pp. 1019–1030.

Hägerstrand, H., Kralj-Iglič, V., Fošnarič, M., Bobrovska-Hägerstrand, M., Mrowczynska, L., Söderström, T., and Iglič, A. (2004). Endovesicle Formation and Membrane Perturbation Induced by Polyoxyethyleneglycolalkylethers in Human Erythrocytes. *Biochim. Biophys. Acta*, 1665, pp. 191–200.

Hägerstrand, H., and Mrowczynska, L. (2008). Patching of gangliosideM1 in Human Erythrocytes: Distribution of CD47 and CD59 in Patched and Curved Membrane. *Mol. Membr. Biol.*, 25, pp. 258–265.

Hägerstrand, H., Mrowczynska, L., Salzer, U., Prohaska, R., Michelsen, K. A., Kralj-Iglič, V., and Iglič, A. (2006). Curvature Dependent Lateral Distribution of Raft Markers in the Human Erythrocyte Membrane. *Mol. Membr. Biol.*, 23, pp. 277–288.

Hagihara, Y., Goto, Y., Kato, H., and Yoshimura, T. (1995). Role of the N- and C-Terminal Domains of Bovine Beta 2-Glycoprotein I in its Interaction with Cardiolipin. *J. Biochem. (Tokyo)*, 118, pp. 129–136.

Haluska, C. K., Riske, K. A., Marchi-Artzner, V., Lehn, J. M., Lipowsky, R., and Dimova, R. (2006). Time Scales of Membrane Fusion Revealed by Direct Imaging of Vesicle Fusion with High Temporal Resolution. *Proc. Natl. Acad. Sci. USA*, 103, **43**, pp. 15841–15846. DOI: 10.173/pnas.0602766103.

Hamdan, R., Maiti, S. N., and Schroit, A. J. (2007). Interaction of [sup]2-Glycoprotein I with Phosphatidylserine Containing Membranes: Ligand Dependent Conformational Alterations Initiate Bivalent Binding. *Biochemistry*, 46, pp. 10612–10620.

Hamm, M., and Kozlov, M. M. (1998). Tilt Model of Inverted Amphiphilic Mesophases. *Eur. Phys. J. B*, 6, pp. 519–528.

Hammel, M., Kriechbaum, M., Gries, A., Kostner, G. M., Laggner, P., and Prassl, R. (2002). Solution Structure of Human and Bovine β_2-Glycoprotein I Revealed by Small-Angle X-ray Scattering. *J. Mol. Bio.*, 321, pp. 85–97.

Harder, T., and Simons, K. (1997). Caveolae, DIGs, and the Dynamics of Sphingolipid-Cholesterol Microdomains. *Curr. Opin. Cell. Biol.*, 9, pp. 534–542.

Harries, D., Ben-Shaul, A., and Szleifer, I. (2004). Enveloping of Charged Proteins by Lipid Bilayers. *J. Phys. Chem. B*, 108, pp. 1491–1496.

Hasselaar, P., Derksen, R. H., Oosting, J. D., Blokzijl, L., and de Groot, P. G. (1989). Synergistic Effect of Low Doses of Tumor Necrosis Factor and Sera from Patients with Systemic Lupus Erythematosus on the Expression of Procoagulant Activity by Cultured Endothelial Cells. *Thromb. Haemost.*, 62, pp. 654–660.

Hatlo, M. M., and Lue, L. (2009). A Field Theory for Ions near Charged Surfaces Valid from Weak to Strong Couplings. *Soft Matter.*, 5, pp. 125–133.

Heath, M. D., Henderson, B., and Perkin, S. (2010). Ion-Specific Effects on the Interaction between Fibronectin and Negatively Charged Mica Surfaces. *Langmuir*, 26, pp. 5304–5308.

Heerklotz, H., Binder, H., and Schmiedel, H. (1998). Excess Enthalpies of Mixing in Phospholipid-Additive Membranes. *J. Phys. Chem. B*, 102, pp. 5363–5368.

Heijnen, H. F. G., Schiel, A. E., Fijnheer, R., Geuze, H. J., and Sixma, J. J. (1999). Activated Platelets Release Two Types of Membrane Vesicles: Microvesicles by Surface Shedding and Exosomes Derived from Exocytosis of Multivesicular Bodies and Alpha-Granules. *Blood*, 94, pp. 3791–3799.

Heinrich, R., Gaestel, M., and Glaser, R. (1982). The Electric Potential Profile Across the Erythrocyte Membrane. *J. Theor. Biol.*, 96, pp. 2111–2231.

Heinrich, V., and Waugh, R. E. (1996). A Piconewton Force Transducer and its Application to Measurements of Bending Stiffness of Phospholipid Membrane. *Ann. Biomed. Eng.*, 24, pp. 595–605.

Helfrich, W. (1973). Elastic Properties of Lipid Bilayers: Theory and Possible Experiments. *Z. Naturforsch.*, 28, pp. 693–703.

Helfrich, W. (1974). Blocked Lipid Exchange in Bilayers and its Possible Influence on the Shape of Vesicles. *Z. Naturforsch.*, 29c, pp. 510–515.

Helfrich, W. (1995). Tension-Induced Mutual Adhesion and a Conjectured Superstructure of Lipid Membranes, in R. Lipowsky and E. Sackmann (eds.), *Structure and Dynamics of Membranes, Generic and Specific Interactions* (Elsevier), pp. 691–722.

Helfrich, W., and Prost, J. (1988). Intrinsic Bending Force in Anisotropic Membranes Made of Chiral Molecules. *Phys. Rev. A*, 38, pp. 3065–3068.

Helmholtz, H. (1879). Studienüber Elektrische Grenzschichten. *Ann. Phys.*, 7, pp. 337–382.

Heuser, J., and Reese, T. (1973). Evidence for Recycling of Synaptic Vesicle Membrane during Transmitter Release at the Frog Neuromuscular Junction. *J. Cell. Biol.*, 57, pp. 315–344.

Hill, T. L. (1986). *An Introduction to Statistical Thermodynamics* (General Publishing Company, Toronto, Canada).

Hirst, L. S., Ossowski, A., Fraser, M., Geng, J., Selinger, J. V., and Selinger, R. L. B. (2013). Morphology Transition in Lipid Vesicles Due to In-Plane Order and Topological Defects. *Proc. Natl. Acad. Sci. USA*, 110, 9, pp. 3242–3247. DOI: 10.1073/pnas.1213994110.

Holmes, C. E., Levis, J. E., and Ornstein, D. L. (2009). Activated Platelets Enhance Ovarian Cancer Cell Invasion in a Cellular Model of Metastasis. *Clin. Exp. Metab.*, 26, 7, pp. 653–661.

Holopainen, J. M., Angelova, M. I., T., and Kinnunen, P. K. J. (2000). Vectorial Budding of Vesicles by Asymmetrical Enzymatic Formation of Ceramide in Giant Liposomes. *Biophys. J.*, 78, pp. 830–838.

Holthius, J. C., van Meer, G., and Huitema, K. (2003). Lipid Microdomains, Lipid Translocation and the Organization of Intracellular Membrane Transport (review). *Mol. Membr. Biol.*, 20, pp. 231–241.

Horstman, L. L., Jy, W., Jimenez, J. J., Bidot, C., and Ahn, Y. S. (2004). New Horizons in the Analysis of Circulating Cell-Derived Microparticles. *Keio J. Med.*, 53, pp. 210–230.

Horstman. L. L., Jy, W., Schultz, D. R., Mao, W. W., and Ahn, Y. S. (1994). Complement-Mediated Fragmentation and Lysis of Opsonized Platelets: Ender Differences in Sensitivity. *J. Lab. Clin. Med.*, 123, pp. 515–525.

Hron, G., Kollars, M., Weber, H., Sagaster, V., Quehenberger, P., Eichinger, S., Kyrle, P. A., and Weltermann, A. (2007). Tissue Factor Positive Microparticles: Cellular Origin and Association with Coagulation Activation in Patients with Colorectal Cancer. *Thromb. Haemost.*, 97, pp. 119–123.

Huang, H. W. (2000). Action of Antimicrobial Peptides: Two-State Model. *Biochemistry*, 39, pp. 8347–8352.

Huber, V., Fais, S., Iero, M., Lugini, L., Canese, P., Squarcina, P., Zaccheddu, A., Colone, M., Arancia, G., Gentile, M., Seregni, E., Valenti, R., Ballabio, G., Belli, F., Leo, E., Parmiani, G., and Rivoltini, L. (2005). Human Colorectal Cancer Cells Induce T-cell Death through Release of Proapoptotic Microvesicles: Role in Immune Escape. *Gastroenterology*, 128, pp. 1796–1804.

Hugel, B., Martinez, M. C., Kunzelmann, C., and Freyssinet, J. M. (2005). Membrane Microparticles: Two Sides of the Coin. *Physiology (Bethesda)*, 20, pp. 22–27.

Hugel, B., Zobairi, F., and Freyssinet, J. M. (2004). Measuring Circulating Cell-Derived Microparticles. *J. Thromb. Haemost.*, 2, pp. 1846–1847.

Hughes, M., Hayward, C. P., Warkentin, T. E., Horsewood, P., Chorneyko, K. A., and Kelton, J. G. (2000). Morphological Analysis of Microparticle Generation in Heparin-Induced Thrombocytopenia. *Blood*, 96, pp. 188–194.

Hui, S. W., Stewart, T. P., and Boni, L. T. (1983). The Nature of Lipidic Particles and their Roles in Polymorphic Transitions. *Chem. Phys. Lipids*, 33, pp. 113–116.

Huica, R., Huica, S., and Moldoveanu, E. (2011). Flow Cytometric Assessment of Circulating Microparticles: Towards a More Objective Analysis. *Rom. Biotech. Lett.*, 16, 3, pp. 6271–6277.

Hurtig, J., Chiu, D. T., and Önfelt, B. (2010). Intercellular Nanotubes: Insights from Imaging Studies and Beyond. *WIREs Nanomed. Nanobiotechnol.*, 2, pp. 260–276.

Huttner, W. B., and Schmidt, A. A. (2002). Membrane Curvature: A Case of Endofilin. *Trends Cell Biol.*, 12, pp. 155–158.

Huttner, W. B., and Zimmerberg, J. (2001). Implications of Lipid Microdomains for Membrane Curvature, Budding and Fission. *Curr. Opin. Cell Biol.*, 13, pp. 478–484.

Hwang, W. C., and Waugh, R. A. (1997). Energy of Dissociation of Lipid Bilayer from the Membrane Skeleton of Red Blood Cells. *Biophys. J.*, 72, pp. 2669–2678.

Hyde, S., Anderson, S., Larsson, K., Blum, Z., Landth, T., Lidin, S., and Ninham, B. W. (1997). *The Language of Shape* (Elsevier, Amsterdam).

Ibarra-Armenta, J. G., Martin-Molina, A., and Quesada-Perez, M. (2009). Testing a Modified Model of the Poisson-Boltzmann Theory that Includes Ion Size Effects through Monte Carlo Simulations. *Phys. Chem. Chem. Phys.*, 11, pp. 309–316.

Iglič, A. (1997). A Possible Mechanism Determining the Stability of Spiculated Red Blood Cells. *J. Biomechanics*, 30, pp. 35–40.

Iglič, A., Hägerstrand, H., Veranič, P., Plemenitaš, A., and Kralj-Iglič, V. (2006). Curvature Induced Accumulation of Anisotropic Membrane Components and Raft Formation in Cylindrical Membrane Protrusions. *J. Theor. Biol.*, 240, pp. 368–373.

Iglič, A., Babnik, B., Fošnarič, M., Hägerstrand, H., and Kralj-Iglič, V. (2007a). On the Role of Anisotropy of Membrane Constituents in Formation of a Membrane Neck during Budding of Multicomponent Membrane. *J. Biomech.*, 40, pp. 579–585.

Iglič, A., Babnik, B., Gimsa, U., and Kralj-Iglič, V. (2005a). On the Role of Membrane Anisotropy in the Beading Transition of Undulated Tubular Membrane Structures. *J. Phys. A: Math. Gen.*, 38, pp. 8527–8536.

Iglič, A., Bohinc, K., Daniel, M., and Slivnik, T. (2004a). Effect of Circular Pore on Electric Potential of Charged Plate in Contact with Electrolyte Solution. *Electrotech. Rev. (Slovenia)*, 71, pp. 260.

Iglič, A., Brumen, M., and Svetina, S. (1997). Determination of the Inner Surface Potential of the Erythrocyte Membrane. *Bioelectrochem. Bioenerg.*, 43, pp. 97–103.

Iglič, A., Fošnarič, M., Hägerstrand, H., and Kralj-Iglič, V. (2004b). Coupling between Vesicle Shape and the Non-Homogeneous Lateral Distribution of Membrane Constituents in Golgi Bodies. *FEBS Lett.*, 574, pp. 9–12.

Iglič, A., Gongadze, E., and Bohinc, K. (2010). Excluded Volume Effect and Orientational Ordering near Charged Surface in Solution of Ions and Langevin Dipoles. *Bioelectrochemistry*, 79, 2, pp. 223–227.

Iglič, A., and Hägerstrand, H. (1999). Amphiphile Induced Spherical Microexovesicle Corresponds to an Extreme Local Area Difference between Two Monolayers of the Membrane Bilayer. *Med. Biol. Eng. Comput.*, 37, pp. 125–129.

Iglič, A., Hägerstrand, H., Bobrowska-Hägerstrand, M., Arrigler, V., and Kralj-Iglič, V. (2003). Possible Role of Phospholipid Nanotubes in Directed Transport of Membrane Vesicles. *Phys. Lett. A.*, 310, pp. 493–467.

Iglič, A., and Kralj-Iglič, V. (1994). Influence of Finite Size of Ions on Electrostatic Properties of Electric Double Layer. *Electrotech. Rev.*, 61, 3, pp. 127–133.

Iglič, A., and Kralj-Iglič, V. (2003). Effect of Anisotropic Properties of Membrane Constituents on Stable Shape of Membrane Bilayer Structure, in H. T. Tien, A. Ottova-Leitmannova (eds.), *Planar Lipid Bilayers (BLMs) and their Applications* (Elsevier SPC, Amsterdam, NL), pp. 143–172.

Iglič, A., Kralj-Iglič, V., and Hägerstrand, H. (1998). Amphiphile Induced Echinocyte-Spheroechinocyte Transformation of Red Blood Cell Shape. *Eur. Biophys. J.*, 27, pp. 335–339.

Iglič, A., Kralj-Iglič, V., and Majhenc, J. (1999). Cylindrical Shapes of Closed Bilayer Structures Correspond to an Extreme Area Difference between the Two Monolayers of the Bilayer. *J. Biomechanics*, 32, pp. 1343–1347.

Iglič, A., Kralj-Iglič, V., Božič, B., Bobrowska-Hägerstrand, M., and Hägerstrand, H. (2000). Torocyte Shapes of Red Blood Cell Daughter Vesicles. *Bioelectrochemistry*, 52, pp. 203–211.

Iglič, A., Lokar, M., Babnik, B., Slivnik, T., Veranič, P., Hägerstrand, H., and Kralj-Iglič, V. (2007b). Possible Role of Flexible Red Blood Cell Membrane Nanodomains in the Growth and Stability of Membrane Nanotubes. *Blood Cells Mol. Dis.*, 39, pp. 14–23.

Iglič, A., Slivnik, T., and Kralj-Iglič, V. (2007c). Elastic Properties of Biological Membranes Influenced by Attached Proteins. *J. Biomech.*, 40, pp. 2492–2500.

Iglič, A., Tzaphlidou, M., Remškar, M., Babnik, B., Daniel, M., and Kralj-Iglič, V. (2005b). Stable Shapes of Thin Anisotropic Nano-Strips. *Fuller. Nanotub. Car. N.*, 13, pp. 183–192.

Imani, R., Kabaso, D., Kreft, M. E., Gongadze, E., Penič, S., Elersič, K., Kos, A., Vŕranič, P., Zorec, R., and Iglič, A. (2012). Morphological alterations of T24 cells on flat end nanotubular TiO_2 surfaces. *Croat Med. J.*, 53, pp. 577–585.

Isambert, H. (1998). Understanding the Electroporation of Cells and Artificial Bilayer Membranes. *Phys. Rev. Lett.*, 80, pp. 3404–3407.

Israelachvili, J. (1997). *Intermolecular and Surface Forces* (Academic Press Limited, London, UK).

Israelachvili, J. N., and Wennerström, H. (1996). Role of Hydration and Water Structure in Biological and Colloidal Interactions. *Nature*, 379, pp. 219–225.

Iversen, T. G., Skotland, T., and Sandvig, K. (2011). Endocytosis and Intracellular Transport of Nanoparticles: Present Knowledge and Need for Future Studies. *Nano Today*, 6, 2, pp. 176–185. DOI: 10.1016/j.nanotod.2011.02.003.

Jackson, J. (1999). *Classical Electrodynamics* (J. Wiley and Sons. Inc., New York).

Jackson, M., and Chapman, E. (2008). The Fusion Necks of Ca(2+)-Triggered Exocytosis. *Nat. Struct. Mol. Biol.*, 15, pp. 684–689.

Jahn, R., Lang, T., and Südhof, T. (2003). Membrane Fusion. *Cell*, 112, pp. 519–533.

Jahn, R., and Scheller, R. (2006). SNAREs–Engines for Membrane Fusion. *Nat. Rev. Mol. Cell. Biol.*, 7, pp. 631–643.

Janša, R., Šuštar, V., Frank M., Susanj, P., Bester, J., Mancek-Keber, M., Krzan, M., Iglic, A. (2008). Number of Microvesicles in Peripheral Blood and Ability of Plasma to Induce Adhesion between Phospholipid Membranes in 19 Patients with Gastrointestinal Diseases. *Blood Cells Mol. Dis.*, 41, pp. 124–132.

Janich, P., and Corbeil, D. (2007). GM1 and GM3 Gangliosides Highlight Distinct Lipid Microdomains with the Apical Domain of Epithelial Cells. *FEBS Lett.*, 581, pp. 1783–1787.

Janowska-Wieczorek, A., Marquez-Curtis, L. A., Wysoczynski, M., and Ratajczak, M. Z. (2006). Enhancing Effect of Platelet-Derived Microvesicles on the Invasive Potential of Breast Cancer Cells. *Transfusion*, 46, 7, pp. 1199–1209.

Janowska-Wieczorek, A., Wysoczynski, M., Kijowski, J., Marques-Curtis, J. L., Machaliniski, B., Ratajczak, J., and Ratajczak, M. Z. (2005). Microvesicles Derived from Activated Platelets Induce Metastasis and Angiogenesis in Lung Cancer. *Int. J. Cancer*, 113, pp. 752–760.

Jesenek, D., Perutková, Š, Kralj-Iglič, V., Kralj, S., and Iglič, A. (2012). Exocytotic Fusion Pore Stability and Topological Defects in the Membrane with Orientational Degree of Ordering. *Cell Calcium*, 52, pp. 277–282.

Jesenek, D., Perutková, Š, Gozdzd, W., Kralj-Iglič, V., Iglič, A. and Kralj, S. (2013). Vesiculation of Biological Membrane Driven by Curvature

Induced Frustrations in Membrane Orientational Ordering, *Int. J. Nanomed.*, 8, pp. 677–687.

Johs, A., Hammel, M., Waldner, I., May, R. P., Laggner, P., and Prassl, R. (2006). Modular Structure of Solubilized Human Apolipoprotein B-100. *J. Biol. Chem.*, 28, pp. 19732–19739.

Jorgačevski, J., M. Fošnarič, N. V., Stenovec, M., Potokar, M., Kreft, M., Kralj-Iglič, V., Iglič, A., and Zorec, R. (2010). Fusion Pore Stability of Peptidergic Vesicles. *Mol. Membr. Biol.*, 27, pp. 65–80.

Junkar, I., Šuštar, V., Frank, M., Janša, V., Bedina-Zavec, A., Rozman, B., Mozetič, M., Hägerstrand, H., and Kralj-Iglič, V. (2009). Blood and Synovial Microparticles as Revealed by Atomic Force and Scanning Electron Microscope. *Op. Autoimmun. J.*, 1, pp. 50–58.

Jy, W., Horstman, L. L., Arce, M., and Ahn, Y. S. (1992). Clinical Significance of Platelet Microparticles in Autoimmune Thrombocytopenias. *J. Lab. Clin. Med.*, 119, pp. 334–345.

Jy, W., Tiede, M., Bidot, C. J., Horstman, L. L., Jimenez, J. J., Chirinos, J. and Ann, Y. S. (2007). Platelet Activation rather than Endothelial Injury Identifies Risk of Thrombosis in Subjects Positive for Antiphospholipid Antibodies. *Thromb. Res.*, 121, pp. 319–325.

Käs, J., and Sackmann, E. (1991). Shape Transitions and Shape Stability of Giant Phospholipid Vesicles in Pure Water Induced by Area-to-Volume Change. *Biophys. J.*, 60, pp. 825–844.

Kabaso, D., Gongadze, E., Elter, P. van Rienen, U., Gimsa, J., Kralj-Iglič, V., and Iglič, A. (2011a). Attachment of Rod-Like (BAR) Proteins and Membrane Shape. *Mini Rev. Med. Chem.*, 11, 4, pp. 272–282.

Kabaso, D., Gongadze, E., Perutková, Š., Kralj-Iglič, V., Matschegewski, C., Beck, U., van Rienen, U., and Iglič, A. (2011b). Mechanics and Electrostatics of the Interactions between Osteoblasts and Titanium Surface. *Comput. Meth. Biomech. Biomed. Eng.*, 14, 5, pp. 469–482.

Kabaso, D., Lokar, M., Kralj-Iglič, V., Veranič, P., and Iglič, A. (2011c). Temperature and Cholera Toxin B are Factors that Influence Formation of Membrane Nanotubes in RT4 and T24 Urothelial Cancer Cell Lines. *Int. J. Nanomed.*, 6, pp. 495–509.

Kabaso, D., Bobrovska, N., Góźdź, W., Gongadze, E., Kralj-Iglič, V., Zorec, R., and Iglič, A. (2012a). The Transport along Membrane Nanotubes Driven by the Spontaneous Curvature of Membrane Components. *Bioelectrochemistry*, 87, pp. 204–210.

Kabaso, D., Bobrovska, N., Gov, N. S., Kralj-Iglič, V., Veranic, P., and Iglič, A. (2012b). On the Role of Membrane Anisotropy and BAR Proteins in the Stability of Tubular Membrane Structures. *J. Biomech.*, 45, pp. 231–238.

Kachar, B., and Reese, T. S. (1982). Evidence for the Lipidic Nature of Tight Junction Strands. *Nature*, 296, pp. 464–466.

Kanduser, M., Fosnaric, M., Sentjurc, M., Kralj-Iglic, V., Hägerstrand, H., Iglic, A., and Miklavcic, D. (2003). Effect of Surfactant Polyoxyethylene Glycol (C12E8) on Electroporation of Cell Line DC3F. *Colloids Surf. A*, 214, pp. 205–217.

Kaneko, J., and Kamio, Y. (2004). Bacterial Two-Component and Hetero-Heptameric Pore-Forming Cytolytic Toxins: Structures, Pore-Forming Mechanism, and Organization of the Genes. *Biosci. Biotechnol. Biochem.*, 68, 5, pp. 981–1003. DOI: 10.1271/bbb.68.981.

Karagkiozaki, V., Logothetidis, S., and Vavoulidis, E. (2012). Nanomedicine Pillars and Monitoring Nano-Biointeractions, in S. Logothetidis (ed.), *Nanomedicine and Nanobiotechnology, NanoScience and Technology* (Springer Berlin Heidelberg), pp. 27–56. DOI 10.1007/978-3-642-24181-9.

Karatekin, E., Sandre, O., Guitouni, H., Borghi, N., Puech, P. H., and Brochard-Wyart, F. (2003). Cascades of Transient Pores in Giant Vesicles: Line Tension and Transport. *Biophys. J.*, 84, pp. 1734–1749.

Karlsson, A., Karlsson, R., Karlsson, M., Stromberg, A., Ryttsen, F., and Orwar, O. (2001). Molecular Engineering: Networks of Nanotubes and Containers. *Nature*, 409, pp. 150–152.

Kelf, T. A., Sreenivasan, V. K. A., Sun, J., Kim, E. J., Goldys, E. M., and Zvyagin, A. V. (2010). Non-Specific Cellular Uptake of Surface-Functionalized Quantum Dots. *Nanotechnology*, 21, 28, article number: 285105. DOI: 10.1088/0957-4484/21/28/285105.

Kertesz, Z., Yu, B. B., Steinkasserer, A., Haupt, H., Benham, A., and Sim, R. B. (1995). Characterization of Binding of Human β_2-Glycoprotein I to Cardiolipin. *Biochem. J.*, 310, pp. 315–321.

Khamashta, M. A., Harris, E. N., Gharavi, A. E., Derue, G., Gil, A., Vazquez, J. J., and Hughes, G. R. (1988). Immune Mediated Mechanism for Thrombosis: Antiphospholipid Antibody Binding to Platelet Membranes. *Ann. Rheum. Dis.*, 47, pp. 849–854.

Kim, H. K., Song, K. S., Park, Y. S., Kang, Y. H., Lee, Y. J., Lee, K. R., Kim, H. K., Ryu, K. W., Bae, J. M., and Kim, S. (2003). Elevated Levels of Circulating Platelet Microparticles, VEGF, I. L.–6 and RANTES in Patients with Gastric Cancer: Possible Role of a Metastatic Predictor. *Eur. J. Cancer*, 39, pp. 184–191.

Kim, Y., Yi, J., and Pincus, P. (2008). Attractions between Like-Charged Surfaces with Dumbbell-Shaped Counterions. *Phys. Rev. Lett.*, 101, p. 208305.

Kirk, G., Gruner, S. M., and Stein, D. L. (1984). A Thermodynamic Model of the Lamellar to Inverse Hexagonal Phase Transition of Lipid Membrane-Water Systems. *Biochemistry*, 23, pp. 1093–1102.

Kirkpatrick, S., Gelatt, C. D., and Vecchi, M. P. (1983). Optimization by Simulated Annealing. *Science, New Series*, 220, pp. 671–680.

Kirkwood, J. K. (1939). The Dielectric Polarization of Polar Liquids. *J. Chem. Phys.*, 7, 10, pp. 911–919.

Kirkwood, J. K., and Shumaker, J. B. (1952). The Influence of Dipole Moment Fluctuations on the Dielectric Increment of Proteins in Solution. *Proc. Natl. Acad. Sci. USA*, 38, pp. 855–862.

Kjellander, R. (1996). Ion-Ion Correlations and Effective Charges in Electrolyte and Macro-Ion Systems. *Ber. Bunsenger Phys. Chem.*, 100, pp. 894–904.

Kjellander, R., and Marčelja, S. (1988). Surface Interactions in Simple Electrolytes. *J. Phys. France*, 49, 6, pp. 1009–1015.

Knowles, D. W. L., Tilley, N., Mohandas, N., and Chasis, J. A. (1997). Erythrocyte Membrane Vesiculation: Model for the Molecular Mechanism of Protein Sorting. *Proc. Natl. Acad. Sci. USA*, 94, pp. 12969–12974.

Kobayashi, K., Kishi, M., Atsumi, T., Bertolaccini, M. L., Makino, H., Sakairi, N., Yamamoto, I., Yasuda, T., Khamashta, M. A., Hughes, G. R., Koike, T., Voelker, D. R., and Matsuura, E. (2003). Circulating Oxidized LDL Forms Complexes with β_2-Glycoprotein I: Implication as an Atherogenic Autoantigen. *J. Lipid Res.*, 44, pp. 716–726.

Koga, K., Matsumoto, K., Akiyoshi, T., Kubo, M., Yamanaka, N., Tasaki, A., Inakashima, H., Nakamura, M., Kuroki, S., Tanakam, M., and Katano, M. (2005). Purification, Characterization and Biological Significance of Tumor-Derived Exosomes. *Anticancer Res.*, 25, pp. 3703–3707.

Kohyama, T., Kroll, D. M., and Gompper, G. (2003). Budding of Crystalline Domains in Fluid Membranes. *Phys. Rev. E*, 68, p. 061905.

Kooijman, E., Chupin, V., Fuller, N., Kozlov, M., de Kruijff, B., Burger, K., and Rand, P. (2005). Spontaneous Curvature of Phosphatidic Acid and Lysophosphatidic Acid. *Biochemistry*, 44, pp. 2097–2102.

Korn, G. A., and Korn, T. M. (1968). *Mathematical Handbook for Scientists and Engineers* 2nd edn. (McGraw-Hill Book Comp., New York).

Kornyshev, A. A. (2007). Double-Layer in Ionic Liquids: Paradigm Change? *Chem. Phys. Lett.*, 111, pp. 5545–5557.

Kox, A. J., Michels, J. P. J., and Wiegel, F. W. (1980). Simulation of a Lipid Monolayer Using Molecular Dynamics. *Nature*, 287, 5780, pp. 317–319. DOI: 10.1038/287317a0.

Koyanagi, M., Brandes, R. P., Haendeler, J., Zeiher, A. M., and Dimmeler, S. (2005). Cell-to-Cell Connection of Endothelial Progenitor Cells with Cardiac Myocytes by Nanotubes: A Novel Mechanism for Cell Fate Changes? *Circ. Res.*, 96, pp. 1039–1041.

Kozlov, M. M., Leikin, S., and Rand, R. P. (1994). Bending, Hydration and Interstitial Energies Quantitatively Account for the Hexagonal-Lamellar-Hexagonal Reentrant Phase Transition in Dioleoylphosphatidylethanolamine. *Biophys. J.*, 67, pp. 1603–1611.

Kozlov, M., and Markin, V. (1983). Possible Mechanism of Membrane Fusion. *Biofizika*, 28, pp. 242–247.

Kralj-Iglič, V. (2012). Stability of Membranous Nanostructures as Key Mechanism in Cancer Progression. *Int. J. Nanomed.*, 7, pp. 3579–3596.

Kralj-Iglič, V., Iglič, A., Hägerstrand, H., and Peterlin, P. (2000). Stable Tubular Microexovesicles of the Erythrocyte Membrane Induced by Dimeric Amphiphiles. *Phys. Rev. E*, 61, pp. 4230–4234.

Kralj-Iglič, V., Svetina, S., and Zekš, B. (1996). Shapes of Bilayer Vesicles with Membrane Embedded Molecules. *Eur. Biophys. J.*, 24, pp. 311–321.

Kralj-Iglič, V., Heinrich, V., Svetina, S., and Žekš, B., (1999). Free Energy of Closed Membrane with Anisotropic Inclusions. *Eur. Phys. J. B*, 10, pp. 5–8.

Kralj-Iglič, V., Gomišček, G., Majhenc, J., Arrigler, V., and Svetina, S. (2001a). Myelin-Like Protrusions of Giant Phospholipid Vesicles Prepared by Electroformation. *Colloids. Surf. A*, 181, pp. 315–318.

Kralj-Iglič, V., Iglič, A., Gomišček, G., Sevšek, F., Arrigler, V., and Hägerstrand, H. (2002). Microtubes and Nanotubes of a Phospholipid Bilayer Membrane. *J. Phys. A: Math. Gen.*, 35, pp. 1533–1549.

Kralj-Iglič, V., Babnik, B., Gauger, D. R., May, S., and Iglič, A. (2006). Quadrupolar Ordering of Phospholipid Molecules in Narrow Necks of Phospholipid Vesicles, *J. Stat. Phys.*, 125, pp. 727–752.

Kralj-Iglič, V., Batista, U., Hägerstrand, H., Iglič, A., Majhenc, J. and Sok, M. (1998). On Mechanisms of Cell Plasma Membrane Vesiculation. *Radiol. Oncol.*, 32, pp. 119–123.

Kralj-Iglič, V., Hägerstrand, H., Veranič, P., Jezernik, K., and Iglič, A. (2005). Amphiphile-Induced Tubular Budding of the Bilayer Membrane. *Eur. Biophys. J.*, 34, pp. 1066–1070.

Kralj-Iglič, V., and Iglič, A. (1996). A Simple Statistical Mechanical Approach to the Free Energy of the Electric Double Layer Including the Excluded Volume Effect. *J. Phys II France*, 6, pp. 477–491.

Kralj-Iglič, V., Iglič, A., Bobrowska-Hägerstrand, M., and Hägerstrand, H. (2001b). Tethers Connecting Daughter Vesicles and Parent Red Blood Cell May Be Formed Due to Ordering of Anisotropic Membrane Constituents. *Colloid. Surf. A*, 180, pp. 57–64.

Kralj-Iglič, V., Remškar, M., and Iglič, A. (2004). Deviatoric Elasticity as a Mechanism Describing Stable Shapes of Nanotubes, in A. Riemer (ed.), *Horizons in World Physics* (Nova Science Publishers, Hauppauge, NY), 244, pp. 111–156.

Kralj-Iglič, V., and Veranič, P. (2007). Curvature-Induced Sorting of Bilayer Membrane Constituents and Formation of Membrane Rafts. *Advances in Planar Lipid Bilayer and Liposomes*, 5, pp. 129–149.

Krause, I., Blank, M., Fraser, A., Lorber, M., Stojanovich, L., Rovensky, J., and Shoenfeld, Y. (2005). The Association of Thrombocytopenia with Systemic Manifestations in the Antiphospholipid Syndrome. *Immunobiology*, 210, pp. 749–754.

Kravitz, M. S., and Shoenfeld, Y. (2005). Thrombocytopenic Conditions-Autoimmunity and Hypercoagulability: Commonalities and Differences in ITP, TTP, HIT, and APS. *Am. J. Hematol.*, 80, pp. 232–242.

Kroll, D. M., and Gompper, G. (1992). The Conformation of Fluid Membranes: Monte Carlo Simulations. *Science*, 255, pp. 968–971.

Kumar, P. B. S., and Rao, M. (1998). Shape Instabilities in the Dynamics of a Two-Component Fluid Membrane. *Phys. Rev. Lett.*, 80, pp. 2489–2492.

Kumar, P. B. S., Gompper, G., and Lipowsky, R. (2001). Budding Dynamics of Multicomponent Membranes. *Phys. Rev. Lett.*, 86, pp. 3911–3914.

Kuypers, F. A., Roelofsen, B., Berendsen, W., Op den Kamp, J. A. F., and van Deenen, L. L. M. (1984). Shape Changes in Human Erythrocytes Induced by Replacement of the Native Phosphatidiylcholine with Species Containing Various Fatty Acids. *J. Cell. Biol.*, 99, pp. 2260–2267.

Laggner, P., Kriechbaum, M., and Rapp, G. (1991). Structural Intermediates in Phospholipid Phase Transitions. *J. Appl. Crystal.*, 24, pp. 836–842.

Laidler, P., Gil, D., Pituch-Noworolska, A., Ciołczyk, D., Ksiazek, D., Przybyło, M., and Lityñska, A. (2000). Expression of Beta1-Integrins and N-Cadherin in Bladder Cancer and Melanoma Cell Lines. *Acta Biochim. Pol.*, 47, pp. 1159–1170.

Laiterä, T., and Lehto, K. (2009). Protein-Mediated Selective Enclosure of Early Replicators Inside of Membranous Vesicles: First Step towards

Cell Membranes. *Orig. Life Evol. Biosph.*, 39, 6, pp. 545–558. DOI: 10.1007/s11084-009-9171-8.

Lamers, E., Walboomers, X. F., Domanski, M., de Riet, J., van Delft, F. C., Luttge, R., Winnubst, L. A., Gardeniers, H. J., and Jansen, J. A. (2010). The Influence of Nanoscale Grooved Substrates on Osteoblast Behavior and Extracellular Matrix Deposition. *Biomaterials*, 31, pp. 3307–3316.

Lamperski, S., and Outhwaite, C. W. (2002). Exclusion Volume Term in the Inhomogeneous Poisson-Boltzmann Theory for High Surface Charge. *Langmuir*, 18, pp. 3423–3424.

Landau, L. D., and Lifshitz, E. M. (1997). *Theory of Elasticity*, 3rd edn, (Butterworth-Heinemann, Oxford).

Lange, J., Schlieps, K., Lange, K., and Knoll-Köhler, E. (1997). Activation of Calcium Signaling in Isolated Rat Hepatocytes is Accompanied by Shape Changes of Microvilli. *Exp. Cell Res.*, 234, 2, pp. 486–497. DOI: 10.1006/excr.1997.3652.

Lange, K. (2000). Regulation of Cell Volume via Microvillar Ion Channels. *J. Cell. Physiol.*, 185, 1, pp. 21–35. DOI: 10.1002/1097-4652(200010)185:1<21::AID-JCP2>3.0.CO;2-D.

Laradji, M., and Kumar, P. B. S. (2004). Dynamics of Domain Growth in Self-Assembled Fluid Vesicles. *Phys. Rev. Lett.*, 93, pp. 198105.

Larsson, K., and Tiberg, F. (2005). Periodic Minimal Surface Structures in Bicontinuous Lipid-Water Phases and Nanoparticles. *Curr. Opin. Coll. Interf. Sci.*, 9, pp. 365–369.

Lasic, D. D. (1998). Novel Applications of Liposomes. *Trends Biotechnol.*, 16, 7, pp. 307–321. DOI: 10.1016/S0167-7799(98)01220-7.

Lasic, D. D., and Barenholz, Y. (eds.) (1996). *Handbook of Nonmedical Applications of Liposomes* (CRC Press, Boca Raton).

Leckner, J. (1991). Summation of Coulomb Fields in Computer-Simulated Disordered Systems. *Physica. A.*, 176, pp. 485–498.

Lee, R. C., and Kolodney, M. S. (1987). Electrical Injury Mechanisms: Dynamics of the Thermal Response. *Plast. Reconstr. Surg.*, 80, pp. 663–671.

Leibler, S. (1986). Curvature Instability in Membranes. *J. Phys. (France)*, 47, pp. 507–516.

Leikin, S., Kozlov, M. M., Fuller, N. L., and Rand, R. P. (1996). Measured Effects of Diacylglycerol on Structural and Elastic Properties of Phospholipid Membranes. *Biophys. J.*, 71, pp. 2623–2632.

Leirer, C., Wunderlich, B., Myles, V. M., and Schneider, M. F. (2009). Phase Transition Induced Fission in Lipid Vesicles. *Biophys. Chem.*, 143, 1-2, pp. 106–109. DOI: 10.1016/j.bpc.2009.04.002.

Lekner, J. (1991). Summation of Coulomb Fields in Computer-Simulated Disordered Systems. *Physica. A.*, 176, pp. 485–498.

Leroueil, P. R., Hong, S. Y., Mecke, A., Baker, J. R., Orr, B. G., and Holl, M. M. B. (2007). Nanoparticle Interaction with Biological Membranes: Does Nanotechnology Present a Janus Face? *Accounts Chem. Res.*, 40, 5, pp. 335–342. DOI: 10.1021/ar600012y.

Levine, J. S., Branch, D. W., and Rauch, J. (2002). The Antiphospholipid Syndrome. *N. Engl. J. Med.*, 346, pp. 752–763.

Lew, V. L., Muallem, S., and Seymour, C. A. (1982). Properties of the Ca^{2+}-Activated k+ Channel in One-Step Inside-Out Vesicles from Human Red-Cell Membranes. *Nature*, 296, pp. 742–744.

Lewis, B. E., Wallis, D. E., Hursting, M. J., Levine, R. L., and Leya, F. (2006). Effects of Argatroban Therapy, Demographic Variables, and Platelet Count on Thrombotic Risks in Heparin-Induced Thrombocytopenia. *Chest*, 129, pp. 1407–1416.

Li, S., and Malmstadt, N. (2013). Deformation and Poration of Lipid Bilayer Membranes by Cationic Nanoparticles. *Soft Matter.*, 9, 20, pp. 4969–4976. DOI: 10.1039/c3sm27578g.

Li, X. (2013). Shape Transformations of Bilayer Vesicles from Amphiphilic Block Copolymers: A Dissipative Particle Dynamics Simulation Study. *Soft Matter.*, 9, pp. 11663–11670. DOI: 10.1039/c3sm52234b.

Lieber, M. R., and Steck, T. L. (1982a). A Description of the Holes in Human-Erythrocyte Membrane Ghosts, *J. Biol. Chem.*, 257, pp. 1651–1659.

Lieber, M. R., and Steck, T. L. (1982b). Dynamics of the Holes in Human-Erythrocyte Membrane Ghosts. *J. Biol Chem.*, 257, pp. 1660–1666.

Lin, A. J., Slack, N. L., Ahmad, A., George, C. X., Samuel, C. E., and Safinya, C. R. (2003). Three-Dimensional Imaging of Lipid Gene-Carriers: Membrane Charge Density Controls Universal Transfection Behavior in Lamellar Cationic Liposome-DNA Complexes. *Biophys. J.*, 84, pp. 3307–3316.

Lin, J. H., and Baumgaertner, A. (2000). Stability of a Melittin Pore in a Lipid Bilayer: A Molecular Dynamics Study. *Biophys. J.*, 78, pp. 1714–1724.

Lingwood, D., and Simons, K. (2010). Lipid Rafts as a Membrane-Organizing Principle. *Science*, 327, 5961, pp. 46–50. DOI: 10.1126/science.1174621.

Linhardt, R. J. (2004). Heparin-Induced Cancer Cell Death. *Chem. Biol.*, 11, pp. 420–422.

Lipowsky, R. (1991). The Conformation of Membranes. *Nature*, 349, 6309, pp. 475–481. DOI: 10.1038/349475a0.

Lipowsky, R., and Dimova, R. (2003). Domains in Membranes and Vesicles. *J. Phys. Condens. Matter.*, 15, pp. 531–545.

Litster, J. D. (1975). Stability of Lipid Bilayers and Red Blood Cell Membranes. *Phys. Lett.*, 53, pp. 193–194.

Lockett, V., Horne, M., Sedev, R., Rodopoulosb, T., and Ralstona, J. (2010). Differential Capacitance of the Double Layer at the Electrode/Ionic Liquids Interface. *Phys. Chem. Chem. Phys.*, 12, pp. 12499–12512.

Lockett, V., Sedev, R., Ralston, J., Horne, M., and Rodopoulos, T. (2008). Differential Capacitance of the Electrical Double Layer in Imidazolium Based Ionic Liquids: Influence of Potential, Cation Size, and Temperature. *J. Phys. Chem. C*, 1124, pp. 7486–7495.

Lokar, M., Urbanija, J., Frank, M., Hägerstrand, H., Rozman, B., Bobrowska-Hägerstrand, M., Iglič, A., and Kralj-Iglič, V. (2008). Agglutination of Like-Charged Red Blood Cells Induced by Binding of β_2-Glycoprotein I to Outer Cell Surface. *Bioelectrochemistry*, 73, pp. 110–116.

Lozado-Cassou, M., and Henderson, D. (1983). Application of the Hypernetted Chain Approximation to the Electrical Double Layer. Comparison with Monte Carlo Results for 2:1 and 1:2 Salts. *J. Phys. Chem.*, 87, pp. 2821–2824.

Lu, J., Getz, G., Miska, E. A. Alvarez-Saavedra, E., Lamb, J., Peck, D., Sweet-Cordero, A., Ebert, B. L., Mak, R. H., Ferrando, A. A., Downing, J. R., Jacks, T., Horvitz, H. R., and Golub, T. R. (2005). MicroRNA Expression Profiles Classify Human Cancers. *Nature*, 435, pp. 834–838.

Lubensky, T. C., and MacKintosh, F. C. (1993). Theory of "Ripple" Phases of Lipid Bilayers. *Phys. Rev. Lett.*, 71, pp. 1565–1568.

Lue, L., Zoeller, N., and Blankschtein, D. (1999). Incorporation of Nonelectrostatic Interactions in the Poisson-Boltzmann Equation. *Langmuir*, 15, pp. 3726–3730.

Luisi, P. L., Walde, P., and Oberholzer, T. (1999). Lipid Vesicles as Possible Intermediates in the Origin of Life. *Curr. Opin. Colloid. In.*, 4, 1, pp. 33–39. DOI: 10.1016/S1359-0294(99)00012-6.

Luzzati, V. (1997). Biological Significance of Lipid Polymorphism: The Cubic Phases. *Curr. Opin. Struct. Biol.*, 7, pp. 661–668.

Luzzati, V., Tardieu, A., Gulik-Krzywicki, T., Rivas, E., and Reiss-Husson, F. (1968). Structure of the Cubic Phases of Lipid-Water Systems. *Nature*, 220, pp. 485–488.

Maček-Lebar, A., Serša, G., Kranjc, S., Grošelj, A., and Miklavčič, D. (2002a). Optimisation of Pulse Parameters In Vitro for In Vivo Electrochemotherapy. *Anticancer Res.*, 22, pp. 1731–1736.

Maček-Lebar, A., Troiano, G. C., Tung, L., and Miklavčič, D. (2002b). Inter-Pulse Interval between Rectangular Voltage Pulses Affects Electroporation Threshold of Artificial Lipid Bilayers, in *IEEE Trans. Nanobiosci.*, 1, pp. 116–120.

Malev, V. V., Schagina, L. V., Gurnev, P. A., Takemoto, J. Y., Nestorovich, E. M., and Bezrukov, S. M. (2002). Syringomycin E channel: A Lipidic Pore Stabilized by Lipopeptide. *Biophys. J.*, 82, pp. 1985–1994.

Malinin, V. S., and Lentz, B. R. (2004). On the Analysis of Elastic Deformation in Hexagonal Phases. *Biophys. J.*, 86, pp. 3324–3328.

Mallat, Z., Hugel, B., Ohan, J., Lesche, G., Freyssinet, J. M., and Tedgui, A. (1999). Shed Membrane Microparticles with Procoagulant Potential in Human Atherosclerotic Plaques: A Role for Apoptosis in Plaque Thrombogenicity. *Circulation*, 99, pp. 348–353.

Manciu, M., and Ruckenstein, E. (2002). Lattice Site Exclusion Effect on the Double Layer Interaction. *Langmuir*, 18, pp. 5178–5185.

Manciu, M., and Ruckenstein, E. (2004). The Polarization Model for Hydration/Double Layer Interactions: The Role of the Electrolyte Ions. *Adv. Coll. Int. Sci.*, 112, pp. 109–128.

Marčelja, S. (1974). Chain Ordering in Liquid Crystal II. Structure of Bilayer Membranes. *Biochim. Biophys. Acta*, 367, pp. 165–176.

Marčelja, S. (1976). Lipid-Mediated Protein Interaction in Membranes. *Biochim. Biophys. Acta*, 455, pp. 1–7.

Mareš, T., Daniel, M., Perutková, Š., Perne, A., Dolinar, G., Iglič, A., Rappolt, M., and Kralj-Iglič, V. (2008). Role of Phospholipid Asymmetry in the Stability of Inverted Hexagonal Mesoscopic Phases. *J. Phys. Chem. B.*, 112, 51, pp. 16575–16584. doi: 10.1021/jp805715r.

Markin, V. S. (1981). Lateral Organization of Membranes and Cell Shapes. *Biophys. J.*, 36, pp. 1–19.

Markvoort, A. J., van Santen, R. A., and Hilbers, P. A. J. (2006). Vesicle Shapes From Molecular Dynamics Simulations. *J. Phys. Chem. B*, 110, 45, pp. 22780–22785. DOI: 10.1021/jp064888a.

Marrink, S. J., and Mark, A. E. (2004). Molecular View of Hexagonal Phase Formation in Phospholipid Membranes. *Biophys. J.*, 87, pp. 3894–3900.

Martens, S., Kozlov, M., and McMahon, H. (2007). How Synaptotagmin Promotes Membrane Fusion. *Science*, 316, pp. 1205–1208.

Martinez, M. C., Tesse, A., Zobairi, F., and Andriantsitohaina, R. (2005). Shed Membrane Microparticles from Circulating and Vascular Cells in

Regulating Vascular Function. *Am. J. Physiol. Heart Circ. Physiol.*, 288, pp. H1004–H1009.

Martinho, N., Damge, C., and Reis, C. P. (2011). Recent Advances in Drug Delivery Systems. *J. Biomater. Nanotechnol.*, 2, pp. 510–526. DOI: 10.4236/jbnb.2011.225062.

Marzesco, A., Wilsch-Bräuninger, M., Dubreuil, V., Janich, P., Langenfeld, K., Thiele, C., Huttner, W. B., and Corbeil, D. (2009). Release of Extracellular Membrane Vesicles from Microvilli of Epithelial Cells is Enhanced by Depleting Membrane Cholesterol. *FEBS Lett.*, 583, pp. 897–902.

Masedunskas, A., Porat-Shliom, N., and Weigert, R. (2012). Regulated Exocytosis: Novel Insights from Intravital Microscopy. *Traffic*, 13, pp. 1600-0854.

Masuda, M., Takeda, S., Sone, M., Ohki, T., Mori, H., Kamioka, Y., and Mochizuki, N. (2006). Endophilin BAR Domain Drives Membrane Curvature by Two Newly Identified Structure-Based Mechanism. *EMBO J.*, 25, pp. 2889–2897.

Mathivet, L., Cribier, S., and Devaux, P. F. (1996). Shape Change and Physical Properties of Giant Phospholipid Vesicles Prepared in the Presence of an A. C. Electric Field. *Biophys. J.*, 70, pp. 1112–1121.

Matsuura, E., Igarashi, Y., Fujimoto, M., Ichikawa, K., and Koike, T. (1990). Anticardiolipin Cofactor(s) and Differential Diagnosis of Autoimmune Disease. *Lancet*, 336, pp. 177–178.

Maurer-Spurej, E., Pfeiler, G., Maurer, N., Lindner, H., Glatter, O., and Devine, D. V. (2001). Room Temperature Activates Human Blood Platelets. *Lab Invest.*, 81, pp. 581–592.

Mavcic, B., Babnik, B., Iglic, A., Kanduser, M., Slivnik, T., and Kralj-Iglic, V. (2004). Shape Transformations of Giant Phospholipid Vesicles at High Concentrations of C12E8. *Bioelectrochemistry*, 63, pp. 183–187.

May, S. (2000). A Molecular Model for the Line Tension of Lipid Membranes. *Eur. Phys. J. E*, 3, pp. 37–44.

May, S. (2002). Membrane Perturbations Induced by Integral Proteins: Role of Conformational Restrictions of the Lipid Chains. *Langmuir*, 18, pp. 6356–6364.

May, S., and Ben-Shaul, A. (1999). Molecular Theory of Lipid-Protein Interaction and the L_α–H_{II} Transition. *Biophys. J.*, 76, pp. 751–767.

May, S., Iglič, A., Reščič, J., Maset, S., and Bohinc, K. (2008). Bridging Like-Charged Macroions through Long Divalent Rod-Like Ions. *J. Phys. Chem. B*, 112, pp. 1685–1692.

May, S., Kozlovsky, Y., Ben-Shaul, A., and Kozlov, M. M. (2004). Tilt Modulus of Lipid Monolayer. *Eur. Phys. J. E*, 14, pp. 299–308.

McLaughlin, S. (1989). The Electrostatic Properties of Membranes. *Ann. Rev. Biophys. Chem.*, 18, pp. 113–136.

McMahon, H. T., and Gallop, J. L. (2005). Membrane Curvature and Mechanisms of Dynamic Cell Membrane Remodelling. *Nature*, 438, pp. 590–596.

McNeil, H. P., Simpson, R. J., Chesterman, C. N., and Krilis, S. A. (1990). Anti-Phospholipid Antibodies are Directed against a Complex Antigen that Includes a Lipid-Binding Inhibitor of Coagulation: Beta2-Glycoprotein I (Apolipoprotein H). *Proc. Natl. Acad. Sci. USA*, 87, pp. 4120–4124.

McNiven, M. A., Kim, L., Krueger, E. W., Orth, J. D., Cao, H., and Wong, T. W. (2000). Regulated Interactions between Dynamin and the Actin-Binding Protein Cortactin Modulate Cell Shape. *J. Cell Bio.*, 151, 1, pp. 187–198. DOI: 10.1083/jcb.151.1.187.

Meleard, P., Gerbeaud, C., Pott, T., Fernandez-Puente, L., Bivas, I., Mitov, M. D., Dufourcq, J., and Bothorel, P. (1997). Bending Elasticities of Model Membranes: Influences of Temperature and Sterol Content. *Biophys. J.*, 72, pp. 2616–2629.

Memming, R. (2007). *Applications in Semiconductor Electrochemistry* (Wiley-VCH Verlag GmbH, Weinheim, Germany).

Metias, S. M., Lianidou, E., and Yousef, G. M. (2009). MicroRNAs in Clinical Oncology: At the Crossroads between Promises and Problems. *J. Clin. Pathol.*, 62, pp. 771–776.

Metropolis, N., Rosenbluth, A. W., Rosenbluth, M. N., Teller, A. H., and Teller, E. J. (1953). Equations of State Calculations by Fast Computing Machines. *Chem. Phys.*, 21, pp. 1087–1092.

Miao, L., Fourcade, B., Rao, M., Wortis, M., and Zia, R. K. P. (1991). Equilibrium Budding and Vesiculation in the Curvature Model of Fluid Lipid Vesicles. *Phys. Rev. E*, 43, pp. 6843–6856.

Miao, L., Seifert, U., Wortis, M., and Döbereiner, H. G. (1994). Budding Transitions of Fluid-Bilayer Vesicles: Effect of Area Difference Elasticity. *Phys. Rev. E*, 49, pp. 5389–5407.

Michelsen, A. E., Noto, A. T., Brodin, E., Mathiesen, E. B., Brosstad, F., and Hansen, J. B. (2009). Elevated Levels of Platelet Microparticles in Carotid Atherosclerosis and during the Postprandial State. *Thromb. Res.*, 123, pp. 881–886.

Mills, P., Anderson, C. F., and Record, M. T. (1985). Monte Carlo Studies of Counterion-DNA Interactions. Comparison of the Radial Distribution of

Counterions with Predictions of other Polyelectrolytes Theories. *J. Phys. Chem.*, 89, pp. 3984–3994.

Milner, S. T., and Safran, S. A. (1987). Dynamical Fluctuations of Droplet Emulsions and Vesicles. *Phys. Rev. A.*, 36, pp. 4371–4379.

Miyakis, S., Giannakopoulos, B., and Krilis, S. A. (2004). Beta 2 Glycoprotein I-Function in Health and Disease. *Thromb. Res.*, 114, pp. 335–346.

Miyamoto, V. K., and Stoecken, W. (1971). Preparation and Characteristics of Lipid Vesicles. *J. Membr. Biol.*, 4, 3, pp. 252. DOI: 10.1007/BF02431974.

Moestrup, S. K., Schousboe, I., Jacobsen, C., Leheste, J. R., Christensen, E. I., and Willnow, T. E. (1998). 2-Glycoprotein-I (Apolipoprotein H) and β_2-Glycoprotein-I-Phospholipid Complex Harbor a Recognition Site for the Endocytic Receptor Megalin. *J. Clin. Invest.*, 102, pp. 902–909.

Mohammadpour, R., Irajizad, A., Hagfeldt, A., and Boschloo, G. (2010). Comparison of Trap-State Distribution and Carrier Transport in Nanotubular and Nanoparticulate TiO_2 Electrodes for Dye-Sensitized Solar Cells. *Chem. Phys. Chem.*, 11, pp. 2140–2145.

Mohandas, N., and Evans, E. A. (1994). Mechanical Properties of the Red Cell Membrane in Relation to Molecular Structure and Genetic Defects. *Ann. Rev. Biophys. Biomel. Struct.*, 23, pp. 787–818.

Monsees, T. K., Barth, K., Tippelt, S., Heidel, K., Gorbunov, A., Pompe, W., Funk, R. H. W., Surface Patterning on Adhesion, Differentiation, and Orientation of Osteoblast-Like Cells. *Cell Tiss. Org.*, 180, pp. 81–95.

Monteith, D. K., Morgan, R. E., and Halstead, B. (2006). In Vitro Assays and Biomarkers for Drug-Induced Phospholipidosis. *Expert Opin. Drug Metab. Toxicol.*, 2, 5, pp. 687–696. DOI: 10.1517/17425255.2.5.687.

Moore, M. D., Di Scipio, R. G., Cooper, N. R., and Nemarrow, G. R. (1989). Hydrodynamic Electron Microscopic and Ligand Binding Analysis of the Epstein-Barr Virus/C3dg Receptor (CR2). *J. Biol. Chem.*, 264, pp. 20576–20582.

Moreira, A. G., and Netz, R. R. (2002). Simulations of Counterions at Charged Plates. *Eur. Phys. J. E*, 8, pp. 33–58.

Morel, O., Toti, F., Hugel, B., and Freyssinet, J. M. (2004). Cellular Microparticles: A Disseminated Storage Pool of Bioactive Vascular Effectors. *Curr. Opin. Hematol.*, 11, pp. 156–164.

Moroz, J. D., and Nelson, P. (1997). Dynamically Stabilized Pores in Bilayer Membranes. *Biophys. J.*, 72, pp. 2211–2216.

Mouritsen, O. G. (2005). *Life-As a Matter of Fat* (Springer Berlin Heidelberg).

Mrvar-Brečko, A., Šuštar, V., Janša, V., Štukelj R., Janša, R., Mujagic, E., Kruljc, P., Hägerstrand, H., Iglič, A., and Kralj-Iglič, V. (2010). Isolated

Microvesicles from Peripheral Blood and Body Fluids as Observed by Scanning Electron Microscope. *Blood Cell. Mol. Dis.*, 2010, 44, pp. 307–312.

Mukhopadhyay, R., Lim, G., and Wortis, M. (2002). Echinocyte Shapes: Bending, Stretching and Shear Determine Spicule Shape and Spacing. *Biophys. J.*, 82, pp. 1756–1772.

Müller, I., Klocke, A., Alex, M., Kotzsch, M., Luther, T., Morgenstern, E., Zieseniss, S., Zahler, S., Preissner, K., Engelmann, B. (2003). Intravascular Tissue Factor Initiates Coagulation via Circulating Microvesicles and Platelets. *FASEB J.*, Vol. 17, pp. 476–478.

Mullins, W. M. (1998). The Effect of Fermi Energy on Reaction of Water with Oxide Surfaces. *Surf. Sci.*, 217, pp. 459–467.

Murat, D., Byrne, M., and Komeili, A. (2010). Cell Biology of Prokaryotic Organelles. *Cold Spring Harb. Perspect. Bio.*, 2, 10, pp. a000422. DOI: 10.1101/cshperspect.a000422.

Murrow, L., and Debnath, J. (2013). Autophagy as a Stress-Response and Quality-Control Mechanism: Implications for Cell Injury and Human Disease. *Annu. Rev. Pathol.: Mech. Dis.*, 8, pp. 105–137. DOI: 10.1146/annurev-pathol-020712-163918.

Nagy, T., Henderson, D., and Boda, D. (2011). Simulation of an Electrical Double Layer Model with a Low Dielectric Layer between the Electrode and the Electrolyte. *J. Phys. Chem. B*, pp. 11409–11419.

Negoda, A., Kim, K. J., Crandall, E. D., and Worden, R. M. (2013). Polystyrene Nanoparticle Exposure Induces Ion-Selective Pores in Lipid Bilayers. *Biochim. Biophys. Acta*, 1828, 9, pp. 2215–2222. DOI: 10.1016/j.bbamem.2013.05.029.

Nelea, V., and Kaartinen, M. T. (2010). Periodic Beaded-Filament Assembly of Fibronectin on Negatively Charged Surface. *J. Struct. Biol.*, 170, pp. 50–59.

Netz, R. (2001). Electrostatistics of Counter-Ions at and between Planar Charged Walls: From Poisson-Boltzmann to the Strong-Coupling Theory. *Eur. Phys. J. E*, 5, pp. 557–574.

Neumann, E., Sowers, A. E., and Jordan, C. A. (eds.) (1989). *Electroporation and Electrofusion in Cell Biology* (Plenum Press, New York and London).

Nielsen, C., Goulian, M., and Andersen, O. S. (1998). Energetics of Inclusion-Induced Bilayer Deformations. *Biophys. J.*, 74, pp. 1966–1983.

Nielsen, B. S., Jorgensen, S., Fog, J. U. Søkilde, R., Christensen, I. J., Hansen, U., Brünner, N., Baker, A., Møller, S., and Nielsen, H. J. (2011). High Levels of MicroRNA-21 in the Stroma of Colorectal Cancers Predict

Short Disease-Free Survival in Stage II Colon Cancer Patients. *Clin. Exp. Metastasis.*, 28, pp. 27–38.

Nimpf, J., Bevers, E. M., Bomans, P. H., Till, U., Wurm, H., Kostner, G. M., and Zwaal, R. F. (1986). Prothrombinase Activity of Human Platelets is Inhibited by Beta 2-Glycoprotein-I. *Biochim. Biophys. Acta*, 884, pp. 142–149.

Nojima, J., Suehisa, E., Kuratsune, H., Machii, T., Koike, T., Kitani, T., Kanakura, Y., and Amino, N. (1999). Platelet Activation Induced by Combined Effects of Anticardiolipin and Lupus Anticoagulant IgG Antibodies in Patients with Systemic Lupus Erythematosus: Possible Association with Thrombotic and Thrombocytopenic Complications. *Thromb. Haemost.*, 81, pp. 436–441.

Nolde, N., Drobne, D., Valant, J., Padovan, I., and Horvat, M. (2006). Lysosomal Membrane Stability in Laboratory and Field-Exposed Terrestrial Isopods Porcellio Scaber (Isopoda, Crustacea). *Environ. Toxicol. Chem.*, 25, 8, pp. 2114–2122. DOI: 10.1897/05-593R1.1.

Nomura, S. (2004). Measuring Circulating Cell-Derived Microparticles. *J. Thromb. Haemost.*, 2, pp. 1847–1848.

Nossal, R. (2001). Energetics of Clathrin Basket Assembly. *Traffic*, 2, pp. 138–147.

Nowak, S. A., and Chou, T. (2008). Membrane Lipid Segregation in Endocytosis. *Phys. Rev. E*, 78, pp. 021908.

Oda, R., Huc, I., Schmutz, M., Candau, S. J., and MacKintosh, F. C. (1999). Tuning Bilayer Twist using Chiral Counterions. *Nature*, 399, pp. 566–569.

Oghaki, M., Kizuki, T., Katsura, M., and Yamashita, K. (2001). Manipulation of Selective Cell Adhesion and Growth by Surface Charges of Electrically Polarized Hydroxyapatite. *J. Biomed. Mater. Res.*, 57, 3, pp. 366–373.

Ogita, K., Ai, M., Tanaka, A., Ito, Y., Hirano, T., Yoshino, G., and Shimokado, K. (2007). Circadian Rhythm of Serum Concentration of Small Dense Low-Density Lipoprotein Cholesterol. *Clin. Chim. Acta*, 376, pp. 96–100.

Oldham, K. B. (2008). A Gouy-Chapman-Stern Model of the Double Layer at a (Metal)/(Ionic Liquid) Interface. *J. Electroanal. Chem.*, 613, pp. 131–138.

O'Meara, R. A. O., and Jackson, R. D. (1958). Cytological Observations on Carcinoma. *Irish J. Med. Sci.*, 391, pp. 327–328.

Önfelt, B., Nedvetzki, S., Yanagi, K., and Davis, D. M. (2004). Cutting Edge: Membrane Nanotubes Connect Immune Cells. *J. Immunol.*, 173, pp. 1511–1513.

Onsager, L. (1936). Electric Moments of Molecules in Liquids. *J. Am. Chem. Soc.*, 58, pp. 1486.

Oosawa, F. (1968). Interactions between Parallel Rod-Like Macro-Ions. *Biopolymers*, 6, pp. 1633–1647.

Oosawa, F. (1970). *Polyelectrolytes* (Marcel Dekker, New York).

Orozco, A. F., and Lewis, D. E. (2010). Flow Cytometric Analysis of Circulating Microparticles in Plasma. *Cytometry A.*, 77, 6, pp. 502–514 (PMC free article) (PubMed).

Osawa, M., Anderson, D. E., and Erickson, H. P. (2008). Reconstitution of Contractile FtsZ Rings in Liposomes. *Science*, 320, pp. 792–794.

Ott, M., Gogvadze, V., Orrenius, S., and Zhivotovsky, B. (2007). Mitochondria, Oxidative Stress and Cell Death. *Apoptosis*, 12, 5, pp. 913–922. DOI: 10.1007/s10495-007-0756-2.

Ottaviani, M., Ceresa, E., and Visca, M. (1985). Cation Adsorption at the TiO_2-Water Interface, *J. Colloid Inter. Sci.*, 108, pp. 114–122.

Outhwaite, C. W. (1976). A Treatment of Solvent Effect in the Potential Theory of Electrolyte Solution. *Mol. Phys.*, 31, 5, pp. 1345–1357.

Outhwaite, C. W. (1983). Towards a Mean Electrostatic Potential Treatment of an Ion-Dipole Mixture or a Dipolar System next to a Plane Wall. *Mol. Phys.*, 48, 3, pp. 599–614.

Outhwaite, C. W. (1986). A Modified Poisson-Boltzmann Equation for the Ionic Atmosphere around a Cylindrical Wall. *J. Chem. Soc. Faraday Trans. II*, 82, pp. 789–794.

Palm-Apergi, C., and Hallbrink, M. (2011). Calcium and Membrane Repair, in U. Langel (ed.), *Cell-Penetrating Peptides: Methods and Protocols*, Book Series: Methods in Molecular Biology, 683, pp. 157–164. DOI: 10.1007/978-1-60761-919-2_11.

Pap, E., Pállinger, E., Pásztói, M., and Falus, A. (2009). Highlights of a New Type of Intercellular Communication: Microvesicle-Based Information Transfer. *Inflamm. Res.*, 58, 1, pp. 1–8. (PubMed).

Park, J., Bauer, S., von der Mark, K., and Schmuki, P. (2007). Nanosize and Vitality: TiO_2 Nanotube Diameter Directs Cell Fate. *Nano Lett.*, 7, pp. 1686–1691.

Park, J., Bauer, S., Schlegel, K. A., Neukam, F. W., Mark, K. V., and Schmuki, P. (2009a). TiO_2 Nanotube Surfaces: 15 nm: An Optimal Length Scale of Surface Topography for Cell Adhesion and Differentiation. *Small*, 5, pp. 666–671.

Park, J., Bauer, S., Schmuki, P., and von der Mark, K. (2009b). Narrow Window in Nanoscale Dependent Activation of Endothelial Cell Growth and

Differentiation on TiO$_2$ Nanotube Surfaces. *Nano Lett.*, 9, pp. 3157–3164.

Pascual, M., Steiger, G., Sadallah, S., Paccaud, J. P., Carpentier, J. L., James, R., and Schifferli, J. A. (1994). Identification of Membrane Bound CR1 (CD35) in Human Urine: Evidence for its Release by Glomerular Podocytes. *J. Exp. Med.*, 179, pp. 889–899.

Patel, N., and Saute, R. (2011). Body Fluid Micro(mi)RNA as Biomarkers for Human Cancer. *J. Nucleic. Acids. Investig.*, 2, e1.

Pattanapanyasat, K., Noulsri, E., Fucharoen, S., Lerdwana, S., Lamchiagdhase, P., Siritanaratkul, N., and Webster, H. K. (2004). Flow Cytometric Quantitation of Red Blood Cell Vesicles in Thalassemia. *Cytometry B. Clin. Cytom.*, 57, pp. 23–31.

Pavelka, M., and Roth, J. (2010). *Functional Ultrastructure: Atlas of Tissue Biology and Pathology*, 2nd edn. (Springer, Wien Austria), pp. 365.

Pavlič, J. I., Genova, J., Zheliaskova, A., Iglič, A., and Mitov, M. D. (2010). Bending Elasticity of Lipid Membranes in Presence of β_2-Glycoprotein I in the Surrounding Solution. *J. Phys. Conf. Ser.*, 253, pp. 012064.

Pavlin, M., Kandušer, M., Reberšek, M., Pucihar, G., Hart, F. X., Magjarevic, R., and Miklavčič, D. (2005). Effect of Cell Electroporation on the Conductivity of a Cell Suspension. *Biophys. J.*, 88, pp. 4378–4390.

Pelchen-Matthews, A., Raposo, G., and Marsh, M. (2004). Endosomes, Exosomes and Trojan Viruses. *Trends Microbiol.*, 12, pp. 310–316.

Pencer, J., White, G. F., and Hallett, F. R. (2001). Osmotically Induced Shape Changes of Large Unilamellar Vesicles Measured by Dynamic Light Scattering. *Biophys. J.*, 81, 5, pp. 2716–2728.

Pereira, J., Alfaro, G., Goycoolea, M., Quiroga, T., Ocqueteau, M., Massardo, L., Pérez, C., Sáez, C., Panes, O., Matus, V., and Mezzano, D. (2006). Circulating Platelet-Derived Microparticles in Systemic Lupus Erythematosus: Association with Increased Thrombin Generation and Procoagulant State. *Thromb. Haemost.*, 95, pp. 94–99.

Perutková, Š., Daniel, M., Dolinar, G., Rappolt, M., Kralj-Iglič, V., and Iglič, A. (2009). Stability of the Inverted Hexagonal Phase, in A. Leitmannova Liu (ed.), *Advances in Planar Lipid Bilayers and Liposomes* (Elsevier, Amsterdam), 9, pp. 237–278.

Perutková, Š., Daniel, M., Rappolt, M., Pabst, G., Dolinar, G., Kralj-Iglič V., and Iglič, A. (2011). Elastic Deformations in Hexagonal Phases Studied by Small Angle X-Ray Diffraction and Simulations. *Phys. Chem. Chem. Phys.*, 13, pp. 3100–3107.

Perutková, Š., Frank, M., Bohinc, K., Bobojevič, K., Zelko, J., Rozman, B., Kralj-Iglič, V., and Iglič, A. (2010a). Interaction between Equally Charged Membrane Surfaces Mediated by Positively and Negatively Charged Nanoparticles. *J. Membr. Biol.*, 236, pp. 43–53.

Perutková, Š., Frank-Bertoncelj, M., Rozman, B., Fošnarič, M., Kralj-Iglič, V., and Iglič, A. (2013). Influence of Ionic Strength and Beta2-Glycoprotein in Concentration on Agglutination of Like-Charged Phospholipid Membranes. *Coll. Surf. B*, 111, pp. 699–706.

Perutková, Š., Kralj-Iglič, V., Frank, M., and Iglič, A. (2010b). Mechanical Stability of Membrane Nanotubular Protrusions Influenced by Attachment of Flexible Rod-Like Proteins. *J. Biomech.*, 43, pp. 1612–1617.

Peter, B. J., Kent, H. M., Mills, I. G., Vallis, Y., Butler, P. J. G., Evans, P. R., and McMahon, H. T. (2004). BAR Domains as Sensors of Membrane Curvature: The Amphiphysin BAR Structure. *Science*, 303, pp. 495–499.

Petrov, A. G., and Derzhanski, A. (1976). On Some Problems in the Theory of Elastic and Flexoelectric Effects of Bilayer Lipid Membranes and Biomembranes. *J. Phys.*, Supplement 37, pp. C3–155.

Piccin, A., Murphy, W. G., and Smith, O. P. (2007). Circulating Microparticles: Pathophysiology and Clinical Implications. *Blood Rev.*, 21, 3, pp. 157–171. (PubMed).

Pierangeli, S. S., Colden-Stanfield, M., Liu, X., Barker, J. H., Anderson, G. L., and Harris, E. N. (1999). Antiphospholipid Antibodies from Antiphospholipid Syndrome Patients Activate Endothelial Cells In Vitro and In Vivo. *Circulation*, 99, pp. 1997–2002.

Pike, L. J. (2006). Rafts Defined: A Report on the Keystone Symposium on Lipid Rafts and Cell Function. *J. Lipid Res.*, 47, pp. 1597–1598.

Pisetsky, D. S. (2009). Microparticles as Biomarkers in Autoimmunity: From Dust Bin to Center Stage. *Arth. Res. Therapy*, 11, 6, pp. 135.

Pollard, T. D., and Cooper, J. A. (2009). Actin, a Central Player in Cell Shape and Movement. *Science*, 326, 5957, pp. 1208–1212. DOI: 10.1126/science.1175862.

Polz, E., and Kostner, G. M. (1979). The Binding of Beta2-Glycoprotein-I to Human Serum Lipoproteins: Distribution among Density Fractions. *FEBS Lett.*, 102, pp. 183–186.

Popat, K. C., Chatvanichkul, K. I., Barnes, G. L., Latempa, T. J., Grimes, C. A., and Desai, T. A. (2007). Differentiation of Marrow Stromal Cells Cultured on Nanoporous Alumina Surfaces. *J. Biomed. Mater. Res. A.*, 80, pp. 955–964.

Popat, K. C., Daniels, R. H., Dubrow, R. S., Hardev, V., and Desai, T. A. (2006). Nanostructured Surfaces for Bone Biotemplating Applications. *J. Orthop. Res.*, 24, pp. 619–627.

Powel, K. (2009). Ahead of the Curve. *Nature*, 460, pp. 318–320.

Price, B. E., Rauch, J., Shia, M. A., Walsh, M. T., Lieberthal, W., Gilligan, H. M., O'Laughlin, T., Koh, J. S., and Levine, J. S. (1996). Anti-Phospholipid Autoantibodies Bind to Apoptotic, but Not Viable, Thymocytes in a Beta2-Glycoprotein I-Dependent Manner. *J. Immunol.*, 157, pp. 2201–2208.

Prokopi, M., Pula, G., Mayr, U. Devue, C., Gallagher, J., Xiao, Q, Boulanger, C. M., Westwood, N., Urbich, C., Willeit, J., Steiner, M., Breuss, J., Xu, Q., Kiechl, S., and Mayr, M. (2009). Proteomic Analysis Reveals Presence of Platelet Microparticles in Endothelial Progenitor Cell Cultures. *Blood*, 114, 3, pp. 723–732. (PubMed).

Puckett, S., Pareta, R., and Webster, T. J. (2008). Nano Rough Micron Patterned Titanium for Directing Osteoblast Morphology and Adhesion. *Int. J. Nanomed.*, 3, pp. 229–241.

Rabinovich, A. L., and Lyubartsev, A. P. (2013). Computer Simulation of Lipid Membranes: Methodology and Achievements. *Polym. Sci. Ser. C*, 55, 1, pp. 162–180. DOI: 10.1134/S1811238213070060.

Rajendran, L., Masilamani, M., Solomon, S., Tikkanen, R., Stuermer, C. A., Plattner, H., and Illges, H. (2003). Asymmetric Localization of Flotillins/Reggies in Preassembled Platforms Confers Inherent Polarity to Hematopoietic Cells. *Proc. Natl. Acad. Sci. USA*, 100, pp. 8241–8246.

Rand, R. P., Fuller, N. L., Gruner, S. M., and Parsegian, V. A. (1990). Membrane Curvature, Lipid Segregation and Structural Transitions for Phospholipids under Dual-Solvent Stress. *Biochemistry*, 29, pp. 76–87.

Raphael, R. M., and Waugh, R. E. (1996). Accelerated Interleaflet Transport of Phosphatidylcholine Molecules in Membranes under Deformation. *Biophys. J.*, 71, pp. 1374–1388.

Rappolt, M. (2006). The Biologically Relevant Lipid Mesophases as "Seen" by X-Rays. *Advances in Planar Lipid Bilayer and Liposomes*, 5, pp. 253–283.

Rappolt, M. (2012). Synchrotron Light for Characterizing the Formation of Curved Membranes and Membrane Fusion Processes. *Advances in Planar Lipid Bilayers and Liposomes*, 17 (Elsevier). (in print)

Rappolt, M., Hickel, A., Bringezu, F., and Lohner, K. (2003). Mechanism of the Lamellar/Inverse Hexagonal Phase Transition Examined by High Resolution X-Ray Diffraction. *Biophys. J.*, 84, pp. 3111–3122.

Rappolt, M., Hodzic, A., Sartori, B., Ollivon, M., and Laggner, P. (2008). Conformational and Hydrational Properties during the L_β- to L_α- and L_α- to H_{II}-Phase Transition in Phosphatidylethanolamine. *Chem. Phys. Lipids*, 154, pp. 46–55.

Rappolt, M., Laggner, P., and Pabst, G. (2004). Structure and Elasticity of Phospholipid Bilayers in the Lalpha Phase: A Comparison of Phosphatidylcholine and Phosphatidylethanolamine Membranes, in S. G. Pandalai (ed.), *Recent Research Developments in Biophysics*, (Transworld Research Network, Trivandrum), 3, Part II, pp. 363–392.

Rappolt, M., and Pabst, G. (2008). Flexibility and Structure of Fluid Bilayer Interfaces, in K. Nag (ed.), *Structure and Dynamics of Membranous Interfaces* (John Wiley & Sons, Inc., Hoboken, NJ), pp. 45–81.

Rapuano, B. E., and MacDonald, D. E. (2011). Surface Oxide Net Charge of a Titanium Alloy: Modulation of Fibronectin-Activated Attachment and Spreading of Osteogenic Cells. *Coll. Surf. B*, 82, pp. 95–103.

Raspaud, E., Olvera de la Cruz, M., Sikorav, J. L., and Livolant, F. (1998). Precipitation of DNA by Polyamines: A Polyelectrolyte Behavior. *Biophys. J.*, 74, pp. 381–393.

Ratajczak, M. Z. (2006). Microvesicles: From "Dust to Crown". *Blood*, 108, pp. 2885–2886.

Ratajczak, J., Miekus, K., Kucia, M. Zhang, J., Reca, R., Dvorak, P., and Ratajczak, M. Z. (2006a). Embryonic Stem Cell-Derived Microvesicles Reprogram Hematopoietic Progenitors: Evidence for Horizontal Transfer of mRNA and Protein Delivery. *Leukemia*, 20, pp. 847–856.

Ratajczak, J., Wysoczynski, M., Hayek, F., Janowska-Wieczorek, A., and Ratajczak, M. Z. (2006b). Membrane-Derived Microvesicles: Important and Underappreciated Mediators of Cell to Cell Communication. *Leukemia*, 20, pp. 1487–1495.

Rauch, U., and Antoniak, S. (2007). Tissue Factor-Positive Microparticles in Blood Associated with Coagulopathy in Cancer. *Thromb. Haemost.*, 97, pp. 9–18.

Reasor, M. J., and Kacew, S. (2001). Drug-Induced Phospholipidosis: Are There Functional Consequences? *Exp. Biol. Med.*, 226, 9, pp. 825–830.

Reviakine, I., and Brisson, A. (2000). Formation of Supported Phospholipid Bilayers from Unilamellar Vesicles Investigated by Atomic Force Microscopy. *Langmuir*, 16, pp. 1806–1815.

Reynwar, B. J., Illya, G., Harmandaris, V. A., Muller, M. M., Kremer, K., and Deserno, M. (2007). Aggregation and Vesiculation of Membrane Proteins by Curvature-Mediated Interactions. *Nature*, 447, pp. 461–464.

Robert, S., Poncelet, P., Lacroix, R. Arnaud, L., Giraudo, L., Hauchard, A., Sampol, J., and Dignat-George, F. (2009). Standardization of Platelet-Derived Microparticle Counting using Calibrated Beads and a Cytomics C500 Routine Flow Cytometer: A First Step towards Multicenter Studies? *J. Thromb. Haemost.*, 7, 1, pp. 190–197. (PubMed).

Roelofsen, B., Kuypers, F. A., Op den Kamp, J. A. F., and Deenen, L. L. M. (1989). Influence of Phosphatidylcholine Molecular Species Composition on Stability of the Erythrocyte Membrane. *Biochem. Soc. Trans.*, 17, pp. 284–286.

Röper, K., Corbeil, D., and Huttner, W. B. (2000). Retention of Prominin in Microvilli Reveals Distinct Cholesterol-Based Lipid Microdomains in the Apical Plasma Membrane. *Nat. Cell Biol.*, 2, pp. 582–592.

Roubey, R. A. (1996). Immunology of the Antiphospholipid Antibody Syndrome. *Arthritis Rheum.*, 39, pp. 1444–1454.

Roux, A., Cappello, G., Cartaud, J., Prost, J., Goud, B., and Bassereau, P. (2002). A Minimal System Allowing Tubulation with Molecular Motors Pulling on Giant Liposomes. *Proc. Natl. Acad. Sci. USA*, 99 (Roux), pp. 5394–5399.

Rumsby, M. G., Trotter, J., Allan, D., and Michell, R. H. (1966). Recovery of Membrane Micro-Vesicles from Human Erythrocytes Stored for Transfusion: A Mechanism for the Erythrocyte Discocyte-to-Spherocyte Shape Transformation. *Biochem. Soc. Trans.*, 5, pp. 126–128.

Rustom, A., Saffrich, R., Markovič, I., Walther, P., and Gerdes, H. H. (2004). Nanotubular Highways for Intercellular Organelle Transport. *Science*, 303, pp. 1007–1010.

Sáenz, J. P., Sezgin, E., Schwille, P., and Simons, K. (2012). Functional Convergence of Hopanoids and Sterols in Membrane Ordering. *Proc. Natl. Acad. Sci. USA*, 109, 35, pp. 14236–14240. DOI: 10.1073/pnas.1212141109.

Sabatier, F., Roux, V., Anfosso, F., Camoin, L., Sampol, J., and Dignat-George, F. (2002). Interaction of Endothelial Microparticles with Monocytic Cells in Vitro Induces Tissue Factor-Dependent Procoagulant Activity. *Blood*, 99, pp. 3962–3970.

Sackmann, E. (1994). Membrane Bending Energy Concept of Vesicle and Cell Shapes and Shape Transitions. *FEBS Lett.*, 346, pp. 3–16.

Sadar, J., and Chan, D. (2000). Long-Range Electrostatic Attractions between Identically Charged Particles in Confined Geometries and the Poisson-Boltzmann Theory. *Langmuir*, 16, pp. 324–331.

Safinya, C. R., Sirota, E. B., Roux, D., and Smith, G. S. (1989). Universality in Interacting Membranes: The Effect of Cosurfactants on the Interfacial Rigidity. *Phys. Rev. Lett.*, 62, pp. 1134–1137.

Safran, A. (1994). *Statistical Thermodynamics of Surfaces, Interfaces, and Membranes* (Addison-Wesley Publishing Company, Colorado, USA).

Saitoh, A., Takiguchi, K., Tanaka, Y., and Hotani, H. (1998). Opening-up of Liposomal Membranes by Talin. *Proc. Natl. Acad. Sci. USA*, 95, pp. 1026–1031.

Sakashita, A., Urakami, N., Ziherl, P., and Imai, M. (2012). Three-Dimensional Analysis of Lipid Vesicle Transformations. *Soft Matter*, 8, 33, pp. 8569–8581. DOI: 10.1039/c2sm25759a.

Salzer, U., and Prohaska, R. (2003). Segregation of Lipid Raft Proteins during Calcium-Induced Vesiculation of Erythrocytes. *Blood*, 101, pp. 3751–3753.

Schara, K., Janša, V., Šuštar, V., Dolinar, D., Lokar, M., Kralj-Iglič, V., Veranič, P., and Iglič, A. (2009). Mechanisms for the Formation of Membranous Nanostructures in Cell-to-Cell Communications. *Cell. Mol. Biol. Lett.*, 14, pp. 636–656.

Schmitz, G., and Müller, G. (1991). Structure and Function of Lamellar Bodies, Lipid-Protein Complexes Involved in Storage and Secretion of Cellular Lipids. *J. Lipid Res.*, 32, 10, pp. 1539–1570.

Schousboe, I. (1980). Binding of Beta2-Glycoprotein I to Platelets: Effect of Adenylate Cyclase Activity. *Thromb. Res.*, 19, pp. 225–237.

Schwarzenbacher, R., Zeth, K., Diederichs, K., Gries, A., Kostner, G. M., Laggner, P., and Prassl, R. (1999). Crystal Structure of Human β_2-Glycoprotein I: Implications for Phospholipid Binding and the Antiphospholipid Syndrome. *EMBO J.*, 18, pp. 6228–6239.

Seddon, J. M., Robins, J., Gulik-Krzywicki, T., and Delacroix, H. (2000). Inverse Micellar Phases of Phospholipids and Glycolipids. *Phys. Chem. Chem. Phys.*, 2, pp. 4485–4493.

Seddon, J. M., and Templer, R. H. (1995). Polymorphism of Lipid-Water Systems, in, A. J. Hoff, R. Lipowsky, and E. Sackmann (eds.), *Handbook of Biological Physics: Structure and Dynamics of Membranes—from Cells to Vesicles* (Elsevier SPC, Amsterdam, NL), 1A, pp. 97–160.

Segota, S., and Tezak, D. (2006). Spontaneous Formation of Vesicles. *Adv. Colloid Inter. Sci.*, 121, 1–3, pp. 51–75. DOI: 10.1016/j.cis.2006.01.002.

Seifert, U. (1993). Curvature-Induced Lateral Phase Segregation in Two-Component Vesicles. *Phys. Rev. Lett.*, 70, pp. 1335–1338.

Seifert, U. (1997). Configurations of Fluid Membranes and Vesicles. *Adv. Phys.*, 46, pp. 13–137.

Seifert, U., Shillcock, J., and Nelson, P. (1996). Role of Bilayer Tilt Difference in Equilibrium Membrane Shapes. *Phys. Rev. Lett.*, 77, pp. 5237–5240.

Selinger, J. V., MacKintosh, F. C., and Schnur, J. M. (1996). Theory of Cylindrical Tubules and Helical Ribbons of Chiral Lipid Membranes. *Phys. Rev. E*, 53, pp. 3804–3818.

Sellam, J., Proulle, V., Jüngel, A. Ittah, M., Miceli Richard, C., Gottenberg, J. E., Toti, F., Benessiano, J., Gay, S., Freyssinet, J. M., and Mariette, X. (2009). Increased Levels of Circulating Microparticles in Primary Jögren's Syndrome, Systemic Lupus Erythematosus and Rheumatoid Arthritis and Relation with Disease Activity. *Arthritis Res. Ther.*, 11, 5, pp. R156 (PMC free article) (PubMed).

Sens, P., and Gov, N. (2007). Force Balance and Membrane Shedding at the Red-Blood-Cell Surface. *Phys. Rev. Lett.*, 98, pp. 018102.

Sens, P., and Turner, M. S. (2004). Theoretical Model for the Formation of Caveolae and Similar Membrane Invaginations. *Biophys. J.*, 86, pp. 2049–2057.

Sens, P., and Turner, M. S. (2006). The Forces that Shape Caveolae, in C. J. Fielding (ed.), *Lipid Rafts and Caveolae* (Wiley-VCH Verlag, Weinheim), pp. 25–44.

Shah, M. D., Bergeron, A. L., Dong, J. F., and Lopez, J. A. (2008). Flow Cytometric Measurement of Microparticles: Pitfalls and Protocol Modifications. *Platelets*, 19, 5, pp. 365–372. (PubMed).

Shai, Y. (1999). Mechanism of the Binding, Insertion and Destabilization of Phospholipid Bilayer Membranes by Alpha-Helical Antimicrobial and Cell Non-selective Membrane-Lytic Peptides. *Biochim. Biophys. Acta*, 1462, pp. 55–70.

Shedden, K., Xie, X. T., Chandaroy, P., Chang, Y. T., and Rosania, G. R. (2003). Expulsion of Small Molecules in Vesicles Shed by Cancer Cells: Association with Gene Expression and Chemosensitivity Profiles. *Cancer Res.*, 63, pp. 4331–4337.

Sheetz, M. P., and Singer, S. J. (1974). Biological Membranes as Bilayer Couples. A Molecular Mechanism of Drug-Induced Interactions. *Proc. Natl. Acad. Sci. USA*, 72, pp. 4457.

Shet, A. S., Aras, O., Gupta, K., Hass, M. J., Rausch, D. J., Saba, N., Koopmeiners, L., Key, N. S., and Hebbelet, R. P. (2003). Sickle Blood Contains Tissue

Factor-Positive Microparticles Derived from Endothelial Cells and Monocytes. *Blood.*, 102, pp. 2678–2683.

Shet, A. S., Key, N. S., and Hebbel, R. P. (2004). Measuring Circulating Cell-Derived Microparticles. *J. Thromb. Haemost.*, 2, pp. 1848–1850.

Shlomovitz, R., and Gov, N. S. (2008). Physical Model of Contractile Ring Initiation in Dividing Cells. *Biophys. J.*, 94, pp. 1155–1168.

Shlomovitz, R., Gov, N. S., Roux, A. (2011). Membrane-Mediated Interactions and the Dynamics of Dynamin Oligomers on Membrane Tubes. *New J. Phys.*, 13, 065008.

Shukla, S. D., Billah, M. M., Coleman, R., Finean, J. B., and Michell, R. H. (1978). Modulation of the Organization of Erythrocyte Membrane Phospholipids by Cytoplasmic ATP. The Susceptibility of Isoionic Human Erythrocytes Ghosts to Attack by Detergents and Phospholipase C. *Biochim. Biophys. Acta.*, 509, 1, pp. 48–57.

Siegel, D. P. (1986). Inverted Micellar Intermediates and the Transitions between Lamellar, Cubic and Inverted Hexagonal Lipid Phases. II. Implications for Membrane-Membrane Interactions and Membrane Fusion. *Biophys. J.*, 49, pp. 1171–1183.

Siegel, D. P. (1988). Inverted Micellar Intermediates and the Transitions between Lamellar, Cubic and Inverted Hexagonal Lipid Phases. *Biophys. J.*, 49, pp. 1155–1170.

Siegel, D. P. (1993). Energetics of Intermediates in Membrane Fusion: Comparison of Stalk and Inverted Micellar Intermediate Mechanisms. *Biophys. J.*, 65, pp. 2124–2140.

Siegel, D. P. (1999). The Modified Stalk Mechanism of Lamellar/Inverted Phase Transitions and its Implications for Membrane Fusion. *Biophys. J.*, 76, pp. 291–313.

Simak, J., and Gelderman, M. P. (2006). Cell Membrane Microparticles in Blood and Blood Products: Potentially Pathogenic Agents and Diagnostic Markers. *Transfus. Med. Rev.*, 20, pp. 1–26.

Simantov, R., LaSala, J. M., Lo, S. K., Gharavi, A. E., Sammaritano, L. R., Salmon, J. E., and Silverstein, R. L. (1995). Activation of Cultured Vascular Endothelial Cells by Antiphospholipid Antibodies. *J. Clin. Invest.*, 96, pp. 2211–2219.

Simons, K., and Gerl, M. J. (2010). Revitalizing Membrane Rafts: New Tools and Insights. *Nat. Rev. Mol. Cell Biol.*, 11, pp. 688–699.

Simons, K., and Ikonen, E. (1997). Functional Rafts in Cell Membranes. *Nature*, 387, pp. 569–572.

Singer, S. J., and Nicolson, G. L. (1972). The Fluid Mosaic Model of the Structure of Cell Membranes. *Science*, 175, pp. 720–731.

Smeets, R., Kolk, A., Gerressen, M., Driemel, O., Maciejewski, O., Hermanns-Sachweh, B., Riediger, D., and Stein, J. M. (2009). A New Biphasic Osteoinductive Calcium Composite Material with a Negative Zeta Potential for Bone Augmentation. *Head Face Med.*, 5, 13. DOI: 10.1186/1746-160X-5-13.

Smith, I. O., Baumann, M. J., and McCabe, L. R. (2004). Electrostatic Interactions as a Predictor for Osteoblast Attachment to Biomaterials. *J. Biomed. Mater. Res. A*, 70, pp. 436–441.

Smith, K. A., Jasnow, D., and Balazs, A. C. (2007). Designing Synthetic Vesicles that Engulf Nanoscopic Particles. *J. Chem. Phys.*, 127, pp. 084703.

Sodin-Šemrl, S., Frank, M., Ambrožič, A., Pavlič, J., Šuštar, V., Čučnik, S., Božič, B., Kveder T., and Rozman, B. (2008). Interactions of Phospholipid Binding Proteins with Negatively Charged Membrane: Beta2-Glycoprotein I as a Model Mechanism. *Advances in Planar Lipid Bilayer and Liposomes*, 8, pp. 243–273.

Solum, N. O. (1999). Procoagulant Expression in Platelets and Defects Leading to Clinical Disorders. *Arterioscler Thromb. Vasc. Biol.*, 19, 12, pp. 2841–2846.

Sorice, M., Circella, A., Misasi, R., Pittoni, V., Garofalo, T., Cirelli, A., Pavan, A., Pontieri, G. M., and Valesini, G. (2000). Cardiolipin on the Surface of Apoptotic Cells as a Possible Trigger for Antiphospholipid Antibodies. *Clin. Exp. Immunol.*, 122, pp. 277–284.

Sorre, B., Callan-Jones, A., Manneville, J.-B., Nassoy, P., Joanny, J.-F., Prost, J., Goud, B., and Bassereau, P. (2009). Curvature-Driven Lipid Sorting Needs Proximity to a Demixing Point and is Aided by Proteins. *PNAS*, 106, pp. 5622–5626.

Sperb, R. (1998). Alternative to Ewald Summation. *Mol. Simul.*, 20, pp. 179–200.

Sperotto, M. M. (1997). A Theoretical Model for the Association of Amphiphilic Transmembrane Peptides in Lipid Bilayers. *Eur. Biophys. J.*, 26, pp. 405–416.

Staneva, G., Seigneuret, M., Koumanov, K., Trugnan, G., and Angelova, M. I. (2005). Detergents Induce Raft-Like Domains Budding and Fission from Giant Unilamellar Heterogeneous Vesicles. A Direct Microscopy Observation. *Chem. Phys. Lipids*, 136, pp. 55–66.

Stark, G. (2005). Functional Consequences of Oxidative Membrane Damage. *J. Membr. Biol.*, 205, 1, pp. 1–16. DOI: 10.1007/s00232-005-0753-8.

Steinhardt, R. A. (2005). The Mechanisms of Cell Membrane Repair: A Tutorial Guide to Key Experiments. *Cell Injury: Mechanisms, Responses and Repair* (Book Series: Annals of the New York Academy of Sciences), 1066, pp. 152–165. DOI: 10.1196/annals.1363.017.

Stenovec, M., Kreft, M., Poberaj, I., Betz, W., and Zorec, R. (2004). Slow Spontaneous Secretion from Single Large Dense-Core Vesicles Monitored in Neuroendocrine Cells. *FASEB J.*, 18, pp. 1270–1272.

Stern, O. (1924). Zur Theorie der Elektrolytischen Doppelschicht. *Z. Elektrochemie.*, 30, pp. 508–516.

Stevenson, J. L., Choi, S. H., Wahrenbrock, M., Varki, A., and Varki, N. M. (2005). Heparin Effects in Metastasis and Trousseau Syndrome: Anticoagulation is Not the Primary Mechanism. *Haem. Rep.*, 1, pp. 59–60.

Stokke, B. T., Mikkelsen, A., and Elgsaeter, A. (1986). The Human Erythrocyte Membrane Skeleton may be an Ionic Gel. *Eur. Biophys. J.*, 13, pp. 203–218.

Štukelj, R. et al. (2013). *Gen. Phys. Biophys. 2013*, In print.

Sun, M., Graham, J. S., Hegedüs, B., Marga, F., Zhang, Y., and Forgacs, G. (2005). Multiple Membrane Tethers Probed by Atomic Force Microscopy. *Biophys. J.*, 89, pp. 4320–4329.

Šuštar, V., Bedina-Zavec, A., Štukelj, R., Frank, M., Bobojevič, G., Janša, R., Ogorevc, E., Kruljc, P., Mam, K., Šimunič, B., Manček-Keber, M., Jerala, R., Rozman, B., Veranič, P., Hägerstrand, H., and Kralj-Iglič, V. (2011a). Nanoparticles Isolated from Blood: A Reflection of Vesiculability of Blood Cells during the Isolation Process. *Int. J. Nanomed.*, 6, pp. 2737–2748.

Šuštar, V., Bedina-Zavec, A., Štukelj, R., Frank, M., Ogorevc, E., Janša, R., Mam, K., Veranič, P., and Kralj-Iglič, V. (2011b). Post-Prandial Rise of Microvesicles in Peripheral Blood of Healthy Human Donors. *Lipids Health Dis.*, 10, pp. 47.

Šuštar, V., Janša, R., Frank, M., Hägerstrand, H., Kržan, M., Iglič, A., and Kralj-Iglič, V. (2009). Suppression of Membrane Microvesiculation: A Possible Anticoagulant and Anti-Tumor Progression Effect of Heparin. *Blood Cells Mol. Dis.*, 42, pp. 223–227.

Svendsen, C., Spurgeon, D. J., Hankard, P. K., and Weeks, J. M. (2004). A Review of Lysosomal Membrane Stability Measured by Neutral Red Retention: Is it a Workable Earthworm Biomarker? *Ecotoxicol. Environ. Safety*, 57, 1, pp. 20–29. DOI: 10.1016/j.ecoenv.2003.08.009.

Svetina, S., Ottova-Leitmannova, A., and Glaser, R. (1982). Membrane Bending Energy in Relation to Bilayer Couples Concept of Red Blood Cell Shape Transformations. *J. Theor. Biol.*, 94, pp. 13.

Szajnik, M., Czystowska, M., Szczepanski, M. J., Mandapathil, M., and Whiteside, T. L. (2010). Tumor-Derived Microvesicles Induce, Expand and Up-Regulate Biological Activities of Human Regulatory T Cells (TReg). *PLoS One.*, 5, 7, pp. e11469. (PMC free article) (PubMed).

Szleifer, I., Kramer, D., Ben-Shaul, A., Gelbart, W. M., and Safran, S. A. (1990). Molecular Theory of Curvature Elasticity in Surfactant Films. *J. Chem. Phys.*, 92, pp. 6800.

Tam, C., Idone, V., Devlin, C., Fernandes, M. C., Flannery, A., He, X. X., Schuchman, E., Tabas, I., and Andrews, N. W. (2010). Exocytosis of Acid Sphingomyelinase by Wounded Cells Promotes Endocytosis and Plasma Membrane Repair. *J. Cell Biol.*, 189, 6, pp. 1027–1038. DOI: 10.1083/jcb.201003053

Taupin, C., Dvolaitzky, M., and Sauterey, C. (1975). Osmotic-Pressure Induced Pores in Phospholipid Vesicles. *Biochemistry*, 14, pp. 4771–4775.

Taylor, D. D., and Black, P. H. (1987). Neoplastic and Developmental Importance of Plasma Membrane Vesicles. *Am. Zool.*, 26, pp. 411–415.

Taylor, D. D., Chou, I. N., and Black, P. H. (1983a). Isolation of Plasma-Membrane Fragments from Cultured Murine Melanoma-Cells. *Biochem. Bioph. Res. Com.*, 113, pp. 470–476.

Taylor, D. D., Homesley, H. D., and Doellgast, G. J. (1983b). Membrane-Associated Immunoglobulins in Cysts and Ascites Fluids of Ovarian Cancer Patients. *Am. J. Reprod. Immunol.*, 3, pp. 7–11.

Tenchov B. G., MacDonald R. C., and Siegel, D. P. (2006). Cubic Phases in Phosphatidylcholine-Cholesterol Mixtures: Cholesterol as Membrane "hFusogen". *Biophys. J.*, 91, pp. 2508–2516.

Teng, N. C., Nakamura, S., Takagi, Y., Yamashita, Y., Ohgaki, M., and Yamashita, K. (2000). A New Approach to Enhancement of Bone Formation by Electrically Polarized Hydroxyapatite. *J. Dent. Res.*, 80, pp. 1925–1929.

Thiagarajan, P., Le, A., and Benedict, C. R. (1999). β_2-Glycoprotein I Promotes the Binding of Anionic Phospholipid Vesicles by Macrophages. *Arterioscler. Thromb. Vasc. Biol.*, 19, pp. 2807–2811.

Thiele, C., Hannah, M. J., Fahrenholz, F., and Huttner, W. B. (1999). Cholesterol Binds to Synaptophysin and is Required for Biogenesis of Synaptic Vesicles. *Nat. Cell. Biol.*, 2, pp. 2–49.

Thurmond, R. L., Otten, D., Brown, M. F., and Beyer, K. (1994). Structure and Packing of Phosphatidylcholines in Lamellar and Hexagonal Liquid Crystalline Mixtures with a Nonionic Detergent: A Wide-Line

Deuterium and Phosphorus-31 NMR Study. *J. Phys. Chem.* 98, pp. 972–983.

Tian, A., and Baumgart, T. (2009). Sorting of Lipids and Proteins in Membrane Curvature Gradients. *Biophys. J.*, 96, pp. 2676–2688.

Tien, H. T., and Ottova, A. (2003). The Lipid Bilayer Concept: Experimental Realization and Current Application, in H. T. Tien and A. Ottova-Leitmannova (eds.), *Planar Lipid Bilayers (BLMs) and their Applications* (Elsevier, Amsterdam, London), pp. 1–74.

Tomita, T., Sugawara, T., and Wakamoto, Y. (2011). Multitude of Morphological Dynamics of Giant Multilamellar Vesicles in Regulated Nonequilibrium Environments. *Langmuir*, 27, 16, pp. 10106–10112. DOI: 10.1021/la2018456.

Torrie, G. M., and Valleau, J. P. (1982). Electrical Double-Layers. 4. Limitations of the Gouy-Chapman Theory. *J. Phys. Chem.*, 86, pp. 3251–3257.

Tresset, G. (2008). Generalized Poisson-Fermi Formalism for Investigating Size Correlation Effects with Multiple Ions. *Phys. Rev. E*, 78, pp. 061506.

Trizac, E., and Raimbault, J. L. (1999). Long-Range Electrostatic Interactions between Like-Charged Colloids: Steric and Confinement Effects. *Phys. Rev. E*, 60, 6, pp. 6530–6533.

Troiano, G. C., Tung, L., Sharma, V., and Stebe, K. J. (1998). The Reduction in Electroporation Voltages by the Addition of a Surfactant to Planar Lipid Bilayers. *Biophys. J.*, 75, pp. 880–888.

Troutier, A. L., and Ladaviere, C. (2007). An Overview of Lipid Membrane Supported by Colloidal Particles. *Adv. Colloid. Interf. Sci.*, 133, pp. 1–21.

Tsafrir, I., Caspi, Y., Guedeau, M. A., Arzi, T., and Stavans, J. (2003). Budding and Tubulation of Highly Oblate Vesicles by Anchored Amphiphilic Molecules. *Phys. Rev. Lett.*, 91, pp. 138102.

Turner, D. C., and Gruner, S. M. (1999). X-ray Diffraction Reconstruction of the Inverted Hexagonal (H_{II}) Phase in Lipid-Water Systems. *Biophys. J.*, 31, pp. 1340–1355.

Tushuizen, M. E., Nieuwland, R., Rustemeijer, C., Hensgens, B. E., Sturk, A., Heine, R. J., and Diamant, M. (2007). Elevated Endothelial Microparticles following Consecutive Meals are Associated with Vascular Endothelial Dysfunction in Type 2 Diabetes. *Diabetes Care*, 30, pp. 728–730.

Tushuizen, M. E., Nieuwland, R., Scheffer, P. G., Sturk, A., Heine, R. J., and Diamant, M. (2006). Two Consecutive High-Fat Meals Affect Endothelial-Dependent Vasodilation, Oxidative Stress and Cellular

Microparticles in Healthy Men. *J. Thromb. Haemostas.*, 4, pp. 1003–1010.

Umalkar, D. G., Rajesh, K. S., Bangale, G. S., Rathinaraj, B. S., Shinde, G. V., and Panicker, P. S. (2011). Applications of Liposomes in Medicine: A Review. *Pharma Sci. Monitor*, 2, 2, pp. 24–39.

UNEP (1997). *Report of the Meeting of Experts to Review the MED POL Biomonitoring Programme.* UNEP(OCA)/MED WG. 132/7 (Athens, Greece).

Urbanija, J., Tomšič, N., Lokar, M., Ambrožič, A., Čučnik, S., Rozman, B., Kandušer, M., Iglič, A., and Kralj-Iglič, V. (2007). Coalescence of Phospholipid Membranes as a Possible Origin of Anticoagulant Effect of Serum Proteins. *Chem. Phys. Lipids*, 150, pp. 49–57.

Urbanija, J., Babnik, B., Frank, M., Tomšič, N., Rozman, B., Kralj-Iglič, V., and Iglič, A. (2008a). Attachment of β_2-Glycoprotein I to Negatively Charged Liposomes may Prevent the Release of Daughter Vesicles from the Parent Membrane. *Eur. Biophys. J.*, 37, pp. 1085–1095.

Urbanija, J., Bohinc, K., Bellen, A., Maset, S., Iglič, A., Kralj-Iglič, V., and Sunil Kumar, P. B. (2008b). Attraction between Negatively Charged Surfaces Mediated by Spherical Counterions with Quadrupolar Charge Distribution. *J. Chem. Phys.*, 129, pp. 105101.

Usenik, P., Vrtovec, T., and Pernuš, F. (2011). Automated Tracking and Analysis of Phospholipid Vesicle Contours in Phase Contrast Microscopy Images. *Med. Biol. Eng. Comput.*, 49, pp. 957–966.

Vachon, V., Laprade, R., and Schwartz, J. L. (2012). Current Models of the Mode of Action of Bacillus thuringiensis Insecticidal Crystal Proteins: A Critical Review. *J. Invertebr. Pathol.*, 11, 1, pp. 1–12. DOI: 10.1016/j.jip.2012.05.001.

Valant, J., Drobne, D., and Novak, S. (2012). Effect of Ingested Titanium Dioxide Nanoparticles on the Digestive Gland Cell Membrane of Terrestrial Isopods. *Chemosphere*, 87, 1, pp. 19–25. DOI: 10.1016/j.chemosphere.2011.11.047.

Valant, J., Drobne, D., Sepcic, K., Jemec, A., Kogej, K., and Kostanjsek, R. (2009). Hazardous Potential of Manufactured Nanoparticles Identified by In Vivo Assay. *J. Hazard. Mater.*, 171, 1–3, pp. 160–165.

Valenti, R., Huber, V., Iero, M., Filipazzi, P., Parmiani, G., and Rivoltini, L. (2007). Tumor-Released Microvesicles as Vehicles of Immunosuppression. *Cancer Res.*, 67, pp. 2912–2915.

Vardjan, N., Stenovec, M., Jorgaéevski, J., Kreft, M., and Zorec, R. (2007). Subnanometer Fusion Necks in Spontaneous Exocytosis of Peptidergic Vesicles. *J. Neurosci.*, 27, pp. 4737–4746.

Velikonja, A., Santhosh, P. B., Gongadze, E., Kulkarni, M., Eleršič, K., Perutková, Š., Kralj-Iglič, V., Poklar Ulrih, N., and Iglič, A. (2013). Interaction between Dipolar Lipid Headgroups and Charged Nanoparticles Mediated by Water Dipoles and Ions. *Int. J. Mol. Sci.*, 14, pp. 15312–15329.

Vella, L. J., Greenwood, D. L. V., Cappai, R., Scheerlinck, J. P., and Hill, A. F. (2008). Enrichment of Prion Protein in Exosomes Derived from Ovine Cerebral Spinal Fluid. *Vet. Immunol. Immunop.*, 124, pp. 385–393.

Veranič, P., Lokar, M., Schütz, G. J., Weghuber, J., Wieser, S., Hägerstrand, H., Kralj-Iglič, V., and Iglič, A. (2008). Different Types of Cell-to-Cell Connections Mediated by Nanotubular Structures, *Biophys. J.*, 95, pp. 4416–4425.

Verma, A., and Stellacci, F. (2010). Effect of Surface Properties on Nanoparticle-Cell Interactions. *Small*, 6, 1, pp. 12–21. DOI: 10.1002/smll.200901158.

Verwey, E. J., and Overbeek, J. T. G. (1948). *Theory of Stability of Lyophobic Colloids* (Elsevier Publishing Company, New York).

Vesel, A., Junkar, I., Cvelbar, U., Kovac, J., and Mozetic, M. (2008). Surface Modification of Polyester by Oxygen-and Nitrogen-Plasma Treatment. *Surf. Interf. Anal.*, 40, pp. 1444–1453.

Vidulescu, C., Clejan, S., and O'Connor, K. C. (2004). Vesicle Traffic through Intercellular Bridges in D. U. 145 Human Prostate Cancer Cells. *J. Cell Mol. Med.*, 8, pp. 388–396.

von Wilmowsky, C., Bauer, S., Lutz, R., Meisel, M., Neukam, F. W., Toyoshima, T., Schmuki, P., Nkenke, E., and Schlegel, K. A. (2009). In Vivo Evaluation of Anodic TiO_2 Nanotubes: An Experimental Study in the Pig. *J. Biomed. Mater. Res. B Appl. Biomater.*, 89, pp. 165–171.

Wagenknecht, D. R., and McIntyre, J. A. (1992). Interaction of Heparin with Beta2-Glycoprotein I and Antiphospholipid Antibodies in Vitro. *Thromb. Res.*, 68, pp. 495–500.

Wagner, G. M., Chiu, D. T. Y., Yee, M. C., and Lubin, B. H. (1986). Red Cell Vesiculation: A Common Membrane Physiological Event. *J. Lab. Clin. Med.*, 108, pp. 315–324.

Walboomers, F. F., and Jansen, J. A. (2001). Cell and Tissue Behaviour on Micro-Grooved Surface. *Odontology*, 89, pp. 2–11.

Walde, P., Cosentino, K., Engel, H., and Stano, P. (2010). Giant Vesicles: Preparations and Applications. *Chembiochem.*, 11, 7, pp. 848–865. DOI: 10.1002/cbic.201000010.

Wang, F., Xia, X. F., and Sui, S. F. (2002). Human Apolipoprotein H may have Various Orientations when Attached to Lipid Layer. *Biophys. J.*, 83, pp. 985–993.

Wang, M. J., and Petersen, N. O. (2013). Lipid-Coated Gold Nanoparticles Promote Lamellar Body Formation in A549 Cells. *Biochim. Biophys. Acta,* 1831, 6, pp. 1089–1097. DOI: 10.1016/j.bbalip.2013.01.018.

Wang, S. X., Cai, G. P., and Sui, S. F. (1998). The Insertion of Human Apolipoprotein H into Phospholipid Membranes: A Monolayer Study. *Biochem. J.,* 335, pp. 225–232.

Wang, W., Yang, L., and Huang, H. (2007). Evidence of Cholesterol Accumulated in High Curvature Regions: Implication to the Curvature Elastic Energy for Lipid Mixtures. *Biophys. J.,* 92, pp. 2819–2830.

Warkentin, T. E., Hayward, C. P., Boshkov, L. K., Santos, A. V., Sheppard, J. A. I., Bode, A. P., and Kelton, J. G. (1994). Sera from Patients with Neparin-Induced Thrombocytopenia Generate Platelet-Derived Microparticles with Procoagulant Activity: An Explanation for the Thrombotic Complications of Heparin-Induced Thrombocytopenia. *Blood,* 84, pp. 3691–3699.

Watkins, S. C., and Salter, R. D. (2005). Functional Connectivity between Immune Cells Mediated by Tunneling Nanotubules. *Immunity,* 23, pp. 309–318.

Waugh, R. E. (1996). Elastic Energy of Curvature-Driven Bump Formation on Red Blood Cell Membrane. *Biophys. J.,* 70, pp. 1027–1035.

Wesołowska, O., Michalak, K., Maniewska, J., and Hendrich, A. B. (2009). Giant Unilamellar Vesicles: A Perfect Tool to Visualize Phase Separation and Lipid Rafts in Model Systems. *Acta Biochim. Pol.,* 56, 1, pp. 33–39.

White, N. M., and Yousef, G. M. (2010). MicroRNAs: Exploring a New Dimension in the Pathogenesis of Kidney Cancer. *BMC Med.,* 8, pp. 65.

Whiteside, T. L. (2005). Tumour-Derived Exosomes or Microvesicles: Another Mechanism of Tumour Escape from the Host Immune System? *British J. Cancer,* 92, pp. 209–211.

Widder, D. V. (1947). *Advanced Calculus* (Prentice-Hall, Inc., New York).

Wiegel, F. W., and Strating, P. (1993). Distribution of Electrolytes with Excluded Volume around a Charged DNA Molecule. *Mod. Phys. Lett. B.,* 7, 7, pp. 483–490.

Willems, G. M., Janssen, M. P., Pelsers, M. M. A. I., Comfurius, P., Galli, M., Zwaal, R. F. A., and Bevers, E. M. (1996). Role of Divalency in the High Affinity Binding of Anticardiolipin Antibody-β_2-Glycoprotein I Complexes to Lipid Membranes. *Biochemistry,* 35, pp. 13833–13842.

Williams, P. L., James, R. C., and Roberts, S. M. (eds.) (2000). *Principles of Toxicology: Environmental and Industrial Applications,* 2nd edn. (John Wiley & Sons, Inc., New York, USA).

Wilson, D. L., Kump, K. S., Eppell, S. J., and Marchant, R. E. (1995). Morphological Restoration of Atomic Force Microscopy Images. *Langmuir*, 11, pp. 265–272.

Wolf, H., Rols, M. P., Boldt, E., Neumann, E., and Teissie, J. (1994). Control by Pulse Parameters of Electric Field-Mediated Gene-Transfer in Mammalian Cells. *Biophys. J.*, 66, pp. 524–531.

Wolf, P. (1967). The Nature and Significance of Platelet Products in Human Plasma. *Br. J. Haematol.*, 13, pp. 269–288.

Yaghmur, A., Laggner, P., Zhang, S., and Rappolt, M. (2007). Tuning Curvature and Stability of Monoolein Bilayers by Short Surfactant-Like Designer Peptides. *PLoS One*, 2, pp. e479.

Yaghmur, A., Paasonen, L., Yliperttula, M., Urtti, A., and Rappolt, M. (2010). Structural Elucidation of Light Activated Vesicles. *J. Phys. Chem. Lett.*, 1, pp. 962–996.

Yaghmur, A., and Rappolt, M. (2012). Structural Characterization of Lipidic Systems under Nonequilibrium Conditions. *Eur. Biophys. J.*, 41, 10, pp. 831–840.

Yamaguchi, T., Kajikawa, T., and Kimoto, E. (1991). Vesiculation Induced by Hydrostatic-Pressure in Human Erythrocytes. *J. Biochem.*, 3, pp. 355–359.

Yamashita, Y., Masum, S. M., Tanaka, T., Tamba, Y., and Yamazaki, M. (2002). Shape Changes of Giant Unilamellar Vesicles of Phosphatidylcholine Induced by a de novo Designed Peptide Interacting with their Membrane Interface. *Langmuir*, 18, pp. 9638–9641.

Young, E. (2008). The Anti-Inflammatory Effects of Heparin and Related Compounds. *Thromb. Res.*, 122, pp. 743–752.

Yuan, H. Y., Huang, C. J., and Zhang, S. L. (2010). Dynamic Shape Transformations of Fluid Vesicles. *Soft Matter*, 6, 18, pp. 4571–4579. DOI: 10.1039/c0sm00244e.

Zelko, J., Iglič, A., Kralj-Iglič, V., and Kumar, P. B. S. (2010). Effects of Counterion Size on the Attraction between Similarly Charged Surfaces. *J. Chem. Phys.*, 133, 20, pp. 204901.

Zemel, A., Fattal, D. R., and Ben-Shaul, A. (2003). Energetics and Self-Assembly of Amphipathic Peptide Pores in Lipid Membranes. *Biophys. J.*, 84, pp. 2242–2255.

Zhang, R., and Nguyen, T. T. (2008). Model of Human Immunodeficiency Virus Budding and Self-Assembly: Role of the Cell Membrane. *Phys. Rev. E*, 78, pp. 051903.

Zimmerberg, J., and Kozlov, M. M. (2006). How Proteins Produce Cellular Curvature. *Nat. Rev. Mol. Cell Biol.*, 7, pp. 9–19.

Zuckermann, M. J., and Heimburg, T. (2001). Insertion and Pore Formation Driven by Adsorption of Proteins onto Lipid Bilayer Membrane-Water Interfaces. *Biophys. J.*, 81, pp. 2458–2472.

Zupanc, J., Drobne, D., Drašler, B., Valant, J., Iglič, A., Kralj-Iglič, V., Makovec, D., Rappolt, M., Sartori, B., and Kogej, K. (2012). Experimental Evidence for the Interaction of C-60 Fullerene with Lipid Vesicle Membranes. *Carbon* 50, 3, pp. 1170–1178. DOI: 10.1016/j.carbon.2011.10.030.

Zwaal, R. F. (1978). Membrane and Lipid Involvement in Blood Coagulation. *Biochim. Biophys. Acta*, 515, pp. 163–205.

Zwaal, R. F., Comfurius, P., and van Deenen, L. L. (1997). Membrane Asymmetry and Blood Coagulation. *Nature*, 268, pp. 358–360.

Index

ADE model *see* area-difference-elasticity model
adhesion 68, 238, 249, 290, 320, 325, 331, 335–337, 376, 397, 423, 424, 426, 427, 430–432, 435, 436
  cation-mediated 331
  cation-mediated fibronectin 335
  cellular 45, 47, 327, 330, 332
  electrostatic 324
  osteoblast 327, 328, 330, 336, 337
  protein-mediated 335
adhesion mediators 430
AFM *see* atomic force microscopy
agglutination 313, 316, 321, 325
anisotropic inclusions 167, 170, 351, 356, 357, 359–363, 370, 444
anisotropic membrane constituents 210–213, 224–228, 348, 349
anisotropic nanodomains 187–189, 191, 193, 200, 204, 205, 207, 210, 212, 217
anisotropic phospholipids 99, 129
antibodies 237, 411, 421, 422, 424–426
anti-phospholipid syndrome (APS) 421, 426, 435, 436
APS *see* anti-phospholipid syndrome
APS patients 426, 445

area-difference-elasticity model (ADE model) 145, 148, 152–154, 213
atomic force microscopy (AFM) 71, 74, 236, 320, 391, 397, 404
average orientation 100, 103, 171, 222, 224, 225, 229, 269, 306, 316, 318

Bikerman equation 257, 261, 264, 285, 287
Bikerman model 265, 266, 285
bilayer membrane 138, 146, 163, 182–185, 187, 193, 199, 231, 362, 370
  charged 242, 322, 348, 357–359, 370
  closed 149
  flat 164
  isotropic lipid 190
  planar 351, 353, 356
  two-component 223
bilayers 41, 42, 62, 63, 84, 88, 89, 99, 113, 115, 116, 120, 135, 144, 145, 164, 172, 173, 200
biological membranes 41, 42, 44–48, 50, 52, 54, 56, 58–60, 65, 155, 181–184, 186, 188, 209–218, 233, 245, 246
biological systems
  non-lamellar phases 88, 89
  charged 245
biopolymers 155, 168, 245

Bjerrum length 268, 270, 296, 311, 313
blood 386, 390–393, 396, 397, 401, 404–413, 415–417, 419, 421, 434, 448
  human 406, 410
  mare 392, 406, 410
blood cells 400, 405, 406, 412, 416, 417, 429
blood cholesterol 417, 418, 421
blood plasma 74, 316, 404
blood sampling 408, 409, 412, 416, 417
body fluids 385, 386, 390, 397, 421
Boltzmann constant 20, 251
Boltzmann distribution function 247, 261, 266
Boltzmann factor 21, 278, 279, 281
Boltzmann, Ludwig 20
Booth generalization 276
Booth model 276
Born, Max 9
boundary conditions 129, 250, 261, 264, 267, 272, 280, 291, 302, 313, 333, 352, 355
Bragg–Williams approximation 184, 223
bridging nanotubes 374–379, 381

cancer 386, 387, 391, 411, 434, 446, 447
  colon 402
  colorectal 386, 447
  gastric 447
  pancreatic 393, 396
cancer cells 390, 411, 416, 435
carbohydrates 42, 45–47, 83, 418
cell death 55, 365–367
cell fragments 407, 417
cell membranes 44–47, 50, 51, 53, 62, 65, 66, 191, 234, 236, 330, 335, 339, 347, 366, 367, 369, 387, 388
  apical 53
  eukaryotic 47, 53
  osteoblast 328
  parent 215
  vesiculating 444
cells 45–53, 56, 57, 66–68, 193, 194, 234–236, 250–254, 325–327, 335–337, 366, 367, 371, 372, 374–377, 379–381, 385, 415–417, 430–432
  apoptotic 236, 289, 422
  deformed 406, 407
  endothelial 326, 390, 391, 411, 417, 422
  epithelial 45, 52, 417
  eukaryotic 45, 53, 54, 66, 219, 374
  mast 434
  mesenchymal 217
  metastatic cancer 434
  mobile 416
  neoplastic 411
  non-transfected 377
  osteoblast 337
  prokaryotic 53
  residual 392
  sedimented 398, 400, 401
  smooth muscle 326
  tumour 391, 416
  vesiculating 445
cell swelling 52
charge density 306, 328, 342, 359, 364
charged lipids 148, 238, 342–345, 351
charged membranes 237, 290, 309, 317, 318, 320, 342, 348, 349, 359, 362, 425, 435
charged membrane surfaces 236, 238, 268, 289, 294, 303, 317, 320, 322, 324, 325

charged nanoparticles 249, 289, 292–297, 302, 304, 307–312, 314–320, 341–345
charged proteins 239, 242, 320, 322, 328–331, 342
charged surfaces 246–250, 257–259, 261, 264, 266–268, 271–274, 278, 281, 283–285, 291–295, 302–307, 309, 310, 312–320, 328–330
cholesterol 46, 47, 147, 188, 191, 388, 418, 419, 447
coions 246–248, 253, 254, 256, 258, 261–263, 269, 270, 278, 309, 315, 318, 320
complexes 10, 146, 155, 321, 350
   anisotropic lipid 228
   anisotropic prominin–lipid 187
   anisotropic protein–lipid 193
   immune 417
   macroion–membrane 342
   nanoparticle–membrane 343
configurational entropy 30, 165, 223, 232, 235, 247, 251, 254, 256, 292, 296, 323, 335
correlation 275, 319, 412, 418, 420, 444, 446–448
   charge–charge 319
   direct ion–ion 249
   inter-ionic 292
   intra-ionic 292
   intra-particle 319
   negative 420
   particle–particle 292
   structural 275, 276
counterions 246–248, 250–254, 257–259, 261–264, 266, 269, 270, 272, 278, 280–282, 284, 291–293, 295, 309, 310, 318, 320
   Fermi–Dirac 260, 264, 266
curvature deviator 100, 141, 158, 166, 233, 356

average 203
   intrinsic 87, 124, 189, 212, 227
   spontaneous 171
curvatures 78–82, 84–87, 89, 107–111, 128, 135–137, 141, 142, 150, 152, 153, 156–158, 164–166, 197, 222–225, 233, 332–336
   deviatoric 166
   edge 335
   finite 328, 332
   inverse 77
   isotropic 209
   local 99, 100, 135, 157, 165
   mesoscopic spherical 163
   spherical 163, 174
   unfavourable 186
curvature tensors 100, 136, 157, 201, 203, 204
cylindrical protrusion 139, 141, 204, 206
cytochalasin B 191, 194
cytochalasin D 374, 376

deformation 42, 85, 116, 135, 167–169, 173, 174, 177, 233, 235, 342, 343
   elastic 135, 343
   lipid 177
   saddle 173
   tilt 171
   twist 173
detergent molecules 195, 197
detergents 65, 101, 195–197, 200, 349, 350, 365, 369, 388
   dimeric 200
   echinocytogenic 198, 199
   gemini 350
   single-chained 369
digestive gland cells 46, 53, 57, 60, 67, 75

dipole 270, 274–277, 280, 282, 283
disease 386, 387, 408, 417, 418, 447
  autoimmune 391
  gastrointestinal 446, 448
  intestinal 447
disorders 21, 63, 445, 448
  cellular phospholipid storage 56
  pathological 444
  thromboembolic 421
distribution 18, 19, 21, 22, 38, 149, 246, 264, 266, 269, 294, 328, 339, 344
  internal 425
  orientational 223
  spatial 246, 320, 325
domains 94, 183, 191, 238, 245, 320, 322–324, 330, 424

EDL *see* electric double layer
eigenenergy 21, 25
eigenfunction 10, 25
elastic energy 116, 157, 158, 162, 197, 198, 235, 241, 243, 351, 383
electric double layer (EDL) 246, 247, 249, 257, 267, 268, 281, 285, 290, 293, 307, 334, 424, 425
electric field 6, 7, 64, 92, 261, 264, 274, 275, 280, 307, 310, 333–335, 364, 366
electrostatic energy 249, 250, 258, 280, 292, 298, 349, 351, 352, 355, 360, 425
energy 7–13, 18, 19, 104–112, 116–120, 122, 123, 125, 126, 128, 130–136, 144, 145, 159–163, 165, 183–186, 204–206, 232–235, 238–240
  chemical 31
  deviatoric 140, 141
  discrete 4, 10
  electrical 31
  free 33–35, 116–120, 122–124, 132, 133, 135–138, 154, 155, 184–186, 221–225, 227–229, 234, 235, 258, 259, 261–263, 292, 293, 348–351, 355–359
  hydration 119
  internal 11–13, 23
  intrinsic 168
  kinetic 5, 9, 12, 13
  mechanical 13, 31
  osmotic 117
  potential 5, 9, 267
  shear 198
  single-inclusion 358
  single-nanodomain 155, 168
  thermal 267, 270, 280, 311
  Van der Waals 119
  void-filling 110, 123
ensemble
  canonical 17–21
  microcanonical 17
entropy 11, 14, 24, 28, 190, 205, 232, 246, 249–253, 255
  isolated system 14
  orientational 304, 311, 312
  translational 311
equilibrium 14, 32, 39, 40, 108, 109, 111, 135, 161, 168, 297, 302, 313, 339, 383
  global 259, 262
  thermal 271, 312
erythrocytes 60, 61, 181, 195, 196, 372, 390, 395, 400, 401, 411, 417, 429, 430, 432
  deformed 395
  manipulated 372
Euler-Lagrange equations 128, 138, 174, 203, 260, 263

FEM *see* finite element method

FIB *see* focused ion beam
finite element method (FEM) 274
flexible rod-like proteins (FRPs) 231–235, 239
fluctuations 92, 123, 221, 248, 344, 394, 425, 437, 438, 443
  critical 444
  long wavelength 92, 97
  thermal 43, 141, 154, 344, 436, 438
fluid 46
  chylous 398, 400
  human cerebrospinal 402
  synovial 397, 402–404, 417
focused ion beam (FIB) 49, 54, 60
Fourier coefficients 439–442
Fröhlich model 275
FRPs *see* flexible rod-like proteins
functional density theory 249, 256, 266, 269, 309, 317, 319, 320
fusion neck 213, 219–229

Gauss–Bonnet theorem 149, 197
Gaussian curvature 80–82, 85, 128
Gaussian saddle-splay constant 176, 241
GC model *see* Gouy–Chapman model
giant phospholipid vesicles (GPVs) 92, 95, 96, 143, 289, 290, 414, 422, 425–427, 430, 431–435, 437, 438, 439, 443, 444, 446, 447
giant unilamellar vesicles (GUVs) 61, 62, 64, 66, 73, 147, 154, 235–237
Gibbs, John Willard 16
GI equation *see* Gongadze–Iglič equation
GI model *see* Gongadze–Iglič model
Gongadze–Iglič equation (GI equation) 279, 280, 286

Gongadze–Iglič model (GI model) 276–287
Gouy–Chapman model 247–249, 256, 257, 264–268, 273, 307, 342, 348, 352
GPVs *see* giant phospholipid vesicles
GUVs *see* giant unilamellar vesicles

Hamaker constant 107, 116
Hamilton function 9
Hamilton operator 25
Hamilton, William Rowan 9
Heisenberg uncertainty principle 8
Heisenberg, Werner 8
Helfrich–Evans bending energy 107, 122, 136, 145, 195
Helfrich–Evans membrane 196
Helfrich Hamiltonian form 103, 137
Helmholz free energy 185
Helmholtz plane 257
hemifusion stalk 219, 221, 229
HNC approximation *see* hypernetted chain approximation
Hook's law 120
human urothelial line (RT4) cell 212
hydrocarbon chains 41, 42, 46, 88, 89, 113, 121, 122, 125, 133, 135, 143, 351
hypernetted chain approximation, 248, 249

images 10, 60, 71, 210, 394–396, 407, 413, 438, 442
  binary 438
  electron microscope 338
  fluorescence microscope 93, 212

mirror 287
phase contrast 375
vesicle 439
IMIs *see* micellar intermediates, inverted
insertion
  cone-angle 242
  cone-like 242
  inverted cone-like 242
integrin molecules 330, 335–339
interaction constants 105, 108, 122, 167, 171, 177, 178, 190, 193, 242, 356, 357
interaction energy 185, 204, 351
internal charge distribution 293, 303, 309, 328–331
interstitial energy 112, 116–120, 122, 132–134
inverted hexagonal phase 76, 87–90, 112–115, 117–123, 125, 126, 132–134
  stability 112
ionic strength 325, 347, 349, 352, 362–364, 370
ions 245–249, 253, 256–258, 266, 267, 269, 271, 273, 274, 276, 278, 281, 284, 287, 303, 307, 313
  dimensionless 265–267, 281, 290
  divalent 249
  finite-sized 265, 284, 303
  monovalent 267, 269, 274
irreversible process 14
isotropic continuum 144
isotropic inclusions 167, 228, 362
isotropic molecules 109, 110
isotropic nanodomains 215, 217

Jordan, Pascual 9

Kirkwood model 275

Kirkwood–Onsager–Fröhlich theory 275

lamellar bodies 48, 49, 57
lamellar phase 88, 116, 117, 123, 130, 131, 133
Lagrange–Euler differential equation 151, 186
Lagrange multiplier 20, 80, 201, 203, 204, 260
  α 20
  β 20
  global 151, 186, 260, 263, 297
  local 129, 151, 260, 263, 270
Langevin–Bikerman equation 284
Langevin–Bikerman model 275, 281, 284, 328, 332, 334
Langevin Poisson-Boltzmann equation (LPB equation) 271, 273
Langevin Poisson-Boltzmann model (LPB model) 268, 269, 272, 275, 276, 280, 283, 284
lattice 28–30, 36, 122, 184, 185, 205, 222
lattice constant 256, 264–267, 281
lattice sites 31, 36, 251, 254, 256, 261, 264, 265, 278
  concentration 35
laws of Newton 5, 6, 11
laws of thermodynamics
  first 12, 13, 33
  second 14, 33
  third 14
layers 41, 48, 135, 136, 138, 144, 196, 197, 204, 222, 226, 228, 246, 304, 432, 443
  diffuse 267, 281
  phospholipid 425
  saturated 267, 281
LDs *see* line defects
leukocytes 400, 401, 416, 417, 430, 432, 434

line defects (LDs) 13, 134
light scattering (LS) 71, 411
lipid bilayers 41–43, 48, 54, 59,
    61, 62, 144, 146, 149,
    161–163, 168–170, 173, 174,
    176, 347–349, 351, 352, 356
  one-component 148
  planar 350, 353
  relaxed 164
  symmetric 162
  unilammellar 83
lipid cylinders 122, 124, 126
lipid layer 170, 231, 241, 242, 322,
    351, 358
lipid molecules 41, 46, 83, 85–87,
    99, 100, 103, 104, 106–108,
    110, 111, 114–117, 119, 120,
    122–124, 130, 131, 135–137,
    161–163, 350
lipid monolayer 63, 84, 85, 99,
    106–108, 116, 117, 122, 123,
    134, 137, 144, 170, 351
lipids 42–47, 53, 60–63, 114, 115,
    117, 124–126, 153, 161–165,
    167–169, 182–184, 227–229,
    232, 350–352, 358, 438
  cationic 341
  disturbed 242
  neutral 61
  oriented 148, 153
  perturbed 358
  saturated 53
  single-chained 83
  uncharged 358
lipid tails 89, 112, 121, 132
lipid tilt 162–164, 169, 177
lipid tubes 112, 121, 134
lipid vesicles 41–43, 59–64, 66,
    68, 71–76, 343, 344, 349
  charged 343, 344
  giant 228
  multilammellar 72
  spherical 42, 44
  unilamellar 72, 235

lipoproteins 220, 233, 350, 417
liposomes 148, 181, 233, 371,
    373
LPB equation *see* Langevin
    Poisson-Boltzmann equation
LPB model *see* Langevin
    Poisson-Boltzmann model
LS *see* light scattering

Macro-ions 311, 316, 318,
    341–345
  lipid-coated 342
  negative 311
  rod-like 318, 319
Maxwell–Boltzmann distribution
    function 31
Maxwell equations 6, 7
Maxwell, James Clerk 6
MC simulations *see* Monte Carlo
    simulations
mechanics
  classical 3–5, 8, 9, 11, 12
  quantum 3, 4, 7–10, 12, 28
membrane 45–47, 50, 51,
    141–144, 154, 156–159,
    161–166, 183–186, 190–193,
    209–212, 226–229, 231–233,
    239–243, 380, 381, 387–389,
    429–439
  artificial 181
  binary 342
  boundary 59
  curved 350
  cytoplasmic 53
  damaged 58
  flat 204, 343, 380
  gondola 379, 381
  heterogeneous 211
  leukocyte 431
  liposome 154, 181
  macrophage 447
  mother 214, 421, 427,
    429–432, 436

multicomponent 221, 222
nuclear 48
permeable 49
phospholipid 94, 369
platelet 444, 445, 447
pore-free 353, 355
saddle-like 241
tube 373
two-component 383
membrane bilayer 155, 156, 163, 176, 185, 197, 199, 233, 238, 356, 358, 367, 393
membrane components 47, 73, 146, 211, 213, 221, 307, 343, 381–383
membrane constituents 47, 87, 209–211, 213, 215, 218, 221–224, 228, 229, 307, 349, 367, 368, 385, 387, 388, 390, 391, 437
membrane curvatures 81, 85, 160, 162, 174, 184, 239, 307, 341, 385, 388, 412
membrane domains 182, 190, 207, 215
membrane elasticity 81, 168, 369
membrane inclusions 63, 156, 350, 351, 358–360, 362, 363, 367–370
membrane layers 91, 143, 144, 146, 195, 196, 222–225, 241, 289, 389, 437, 438, 444
membrane lipids 52, 148, 183
membrane nanodomains 146, 155–157, 160–162, 164, 166–170, 172, 174, 176, 183–186, 211, 222, 228
membrane nanotubes 209, 215, 377, 381
membrane neck 165, 213, 214, 220, 221, 436
membrane pores 50, 347–350, 352, 357, 358, 367, 369

circular 351
hydrophilic 348, 365, 367
membrane proteins 47, 162, 164, 169, 183, 212, 215
flexible 168
globular 155
integral 447
membrane protrusions 191, 194, 206, 232, 235
membrane rafts 47, 193, 388, 389, 418
membrane regions 162, 164, 185, 186, 239
curved 147, 212, 358, 387, 389, 418
curved tubular 182, 189
flat 188, 205, 206
neck-shaped 210
spheroidal 383
tubular-shaped 193
membrane rim 348, 352, 357, 359
membrane skeleton 196, 198, 199
membrane surface 47, 156, 157, 161, 163, 166, 214, 222, 233, 234, 236, 238, 239, 241, 245, 246, 312, 320, 322
curved 241
flat 293
tubular 239
membrane vesiculation 341, 413, 420, 421, 427, 435–437, 439, 441, 443
micellar intermediates
inverted (IMIs) 112
rod-like (RMIs) 113
micelles 62, 85, 107, 245
microvesicles 392, 400, 401
charged 422
isolated 401
platelet-derived 422
model
area difference elasticity 228
constitutive 195
fluid mosaic 387–389

Helfric–Evans membrane elasticity 191
hydration 268
lattice 28, 30, 31, 35, 38, 250, 252, 253
lattice statistics 257
mean-field 287
membrane raft 389
microscopic interaction 241
molecular 114
nucleation 132
primitive electrolyte 249
two-energy state 102, 104
two-orientation 104
model parameters 129. 139, 140, 154, 169, 207, 228, 265, 267, 305, 315, 319, 345, 248
estimation 169–179
molecules
 amphiphilic 195, 245
 anisotropic 109–111, 124, 132
 charged 245
 choleratoxin 341
 cholesterol 46
 fibronectin 331
 monolayers 61, 63, 84–87, 106–108, 113, 114, 120, 128–130, 134, 145, 164, 171–173, 242
 curved 132
 homogeneous 99
 lamellar 126
 perturbation decay 243
 phospholipid 119, 121
 planar 87
 surfactant 245
Monte Carlo simulations (MC simulations) 248, 257, 293, 303–306, 309, 313–315, 317, 319, 320, 328, 343–345
Monte Carlo technique 248

nanodomains 155–157, 159–161, 165, 182–193, 195, 200, 204–206, 209–213, 215, 222, 348–350, 356, 366–368, 370, 388, 389
 membrane-embedded 184
 mobile 188
 monomeric 205, 206
 prominin 187–189, 193, 206
 prominin–lipid 188
 protein-induced 369
nanoparticles 50, 51, 58, 64, 65, 67, 240, 293–296, 299, 302–305, 307, 309–312, 316, 319, 408, 410
 biological 220
 divalent 249, 305
 hydrophilic gold 76
 organic 245
 rod-like 306
 spherical-charged 307
nanorough regions 336, 340
nanotubes 181, 190, 214–217, 232, 326, 327, 335, 338, 371, 372, 374–380, 382, 437
nanovesicles 385, 390, 397, 399, 401–403, 411, 417, 419, 446, 447
N-ethylmaleimide-sensitive factor attachment protein (SNARE) 220
Newton, Issac 5
non-equilibrium state 21, 32

Onsager model 275
organelles 45, 47, 56, 374, 378, 379
 lipid-bounded 54
 primitive 54
organisms 32, 50, 52, 57, 448
 biological 88
 living 31

orientations 100, 102, 158, 160, 166, 172, 236, 240, 295, 305, 307, 311, 315, 316, 318, 328, 329
   horizontal-like 236, 320
   in-plane 157, 162, 443
   orthogonal 307
   random 316

PB equation *see* Poisson–Boltzmann equation
PBS *see* phosphate buffer saline
phosphate buffer saline (PBS) 393, 423, 428, 429
Planck constant 8
Planck, Max 8
platelets 289, 390, 391, 405, 409, 411–413, 415–417, 422, 430, 432, 434, 444, 446–448
Poisson–Boltzmann equation (PB equation) 247, 248, 257, 261, 265–267, 269, 274, 287, 292, 352, 353
Poisson–Boltzmann model *see also* Gouy–Chapman model 342
pores 213, 219, 221, 347–349, 351, 352, 355, 357–364, 366, 367, 370
   circular 349, 355
   hydrophilic 348, 358–360, 362, 370
   stable 363, 364
   transient 369
pore size 75, 347, 359–361, 364, 370
probability density 9, 10, 302, 311
properties
   dynamic 63
   elastic 168, 231, 233, 241, 367
   intrinsic 68, 148, 349
   macroscopic 11, 12
   mechanical 46
   metabolic 54
   physiochemical 56
   structural 75
   topographical 327
proteins 42, 45–47, 53, 55, 155, 156, 161–171, 174–178, 183, 220, 227–229, 233–236, 238–241, 243, 320, 328, 329, 387
   bound-charged 320
   carrier 47
   cell recognition 47
   channel 47
   enzymatic 47
   globular 293
   intercalated 168
   long-lived 56
   membrane-embedded 156, 170, 171
   plasma 289
   prion 385
   receptor 47
   rod-like 240
   spheroidal 328
   surface-bound 330
protrusions 92–97, 138–144, 146, 188, 189, 191, 193, 198, 204, 207, 374, 375, 380, 429, 431, 436–441, 443
   cell-surface 52
   flattened 191
   hydrophobic 231, 241–243, 322
   myelin 439, 441
   platelet 431
   rod-like 193
   vesicular 215

RBCs *see* red blood cells
receptors 220, 385, 412
   growth factor 215
   membrane-bound 432
   osteogenic cell 332

putative cell surface 424
red blood cell ghosts 347, 363
red blood cells (RBCs) 61, 218, 289, 321, 325, 372, 445
relative dielectric permittivity 250, 268, 269, 272–277, 279, 280, 283–285, 328
RMIs *see* micellar intermediates, rod-like

samples 74, 91, 391, 393, 397–402, 404, 405, 408, 415, 417, 423, 428, 431
  biological 397
  donor plasma 290
  dried 199
scanning electron microscopy (SEM) 46, 49, 57, 72–75, 381, 391, 393–397, 401, 402, 404–407, 413
Schrödinger equation 9, 10, 25, 26
Schrödinger, Erwin 9
SEM *see* scanning electron microscopy
simulations 63, 134, 293, 343
  computer 62, 63, 248
  molecular dynamic 287
  numerical 63
SNARE N-ethylmaleimide-sensitive factor attachment protein
Stirling approximation 19, 29, 37, 185
stress 52, 53, 55, 57, 123, 167
  mechanical 52, 417
  osmotic 65, 114, 117
  thermal 417
stretching moduli 121, 123, 125, 130–132
surfactants 63, 83, 364, 365, 367

tails 26, 27, 83, 104, 106, 113, 136
  hydrocarbon 42, 120, 121, 348
  hydrophobic 42, 46, 62, 63
  tension 58, 239, 348, 349, 351, 352, 358, 360, 367, 377, 378
  interfacial 343
  lateral membrane 154
thermodynamic variables 11, 12, 16, 21, 32
TNTs *see* tunnelling nanotubes
transport 12, 49, 50, 52, 59, 91, 371, 373, 381, 388, 416
  cellular 50
  extracellular 341
  free vesicle 381
  gene 108
  intercellular 182
  intra-tubular particle 371
  nanotubule-directed 382
tunnelling nanotubes (TNTs) 182, 372, 374, 377, 381

vesicles 41, 42, 49, 58–65, 67, 68, 91–97, 143, 144, 148, 192, 214–216, 218–227, 344, 345, 372, 373, 393, 394, 396, 397, 422, 423, 438
  bilayer 136, 168
  cardiolipin 423
  carrier 382
  charged 423
  endosomal 56
  free 427
  fused 213
  giant phospholipid 422
  globular 97
  lysosomal 56
  multilamellar 42, 44, 76
  neutral 423
  pear-shaped 153
  phospholipid 289
  prolate 201

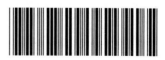